Essence of
CLINICAL ENDOCRINOLOGY

Essence of
CLINICAL ENDOCRINOLOGY

Authors

Tofail Ahmed
MBBS DEM PhD
Chief Executive Officer
Distance Learning Program (DLP) of Diabetic Association of Bangladesh
BIRDEM General Hospital
Dhaka, Bangladesh

Tania Tofail
MBBS MRCP (UK) SCE (UK) MD (Endocrinology)
PhD Student
Department of Endocrinology
Bangabandhu Sheikh Mujib Medical University (BSMMU)
Dhaka, Bangladesh

Foreword

Hajera Mahtab

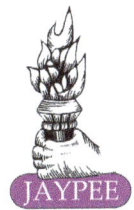

JAYPEE BROTHERS MEDICAL PUBLISHERS
The Health Sciences Publisher
New Delhi | London

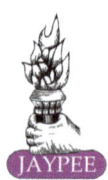 **Jaypee Brothers Medical Publishers (P) Ltd**

Headquarters
EMCA House
23/23-B, Ansari Road, Daryaganj
New Delhi 110 002, India
Landline: +91-11-23272143, +91-11-23272703
+91-11-23282021, +91-11-23245672
E-mail: jaypee@jaypeebrothers.com

Overseas Office
JP Medical Ltd.
83, Victoria Street, London
SW1H 0HW (UK)
Phone: +44-20 3170 8910
Fax: +44(0)20 3008 6180
E-mail: info@jpmedpub.com

Corporate Office
Jaypee Brothers Medical Publishers (P) Ltd.
4838/24, Ansari Road, Daryaganj
New Delhi 110 002, India
Phone: +91-11-43574357
Fax: +91-11-43574314
E-mail: jaypee@jaypeebrothers.com

EU GPSR Authorised Representative
LOGOS EUROPE, 9 rue Nicolas Poussin
17000, LA ROCHELLE, France
Phone: +33 (0) 6 67 93 73 78
Email: Contact@logos europe.eu

Website: www.jaypeebrothers.com
Website: www.jaypeedigital.com

© 2024, Jaypee Brothers Medical Publishers

The views and opinions expressed in this book are solely those of the original contributor(s)/author(s) and do not necessarily represent those of editor(s) or publisher of the book.

All rights reserved. No part of this publication may be reproduced, stored or transmitted in any form or by any means, electronic, mechanical, photocopying, recording or otherwise, without the prior permission in writing of the publishers.

All brand names and product names used in this book are trade names, service marks, trademarks or registered trademarks of their respective owners. The publisher is not associated with any product or vendor mentioned in this book.

Medical knowledge and practice change constantly. This book is designed to provide accurate, authoritative information about the subject matter in question. However, readers are advised to check the most current information available on procedures included and check information from the manufacturer of each product to be administered, to verify the recommended dose, formula, method and duration of administration, adverse effects and contraindications. It is the responsibility of the practitioner to take all appropriate safety precautions. Neither the publisher nor the author(s)/editor(s) assume any liability for any injury and/or damage to persons or property arising from or related to use of material in this book.

This book is sold on the understanding that the publisher is not engaged in providing professional medical services. If such advice or services are required, the services of a competent medical professional should be sought.

Every effort has been made where necessary to contact holders of copyright to obtain permission to reproduce copyright material. If any have been inadvertently overlooked, the publisher will be pleased to make the necessary arrangements at the first opportunity.

Inquiries for bulk sales may be solicited at: jaypee@jaypeebrothers.com

*Essence of Clinical Endocrinology / **Tofail Ahmed, Tania Tofail***

First Edition: **2024**

ISBN: 978-93-5696-439-6

DEDICATION

The book is dedicated to two National Professors

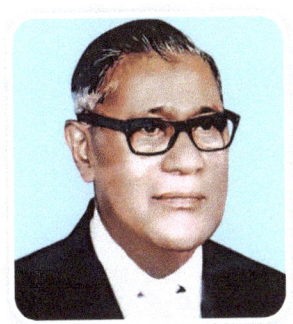

M Ibrahim
(3-12-1911 to 6-9-1989)
For being my mentor who paved my path to become an endocrinologist

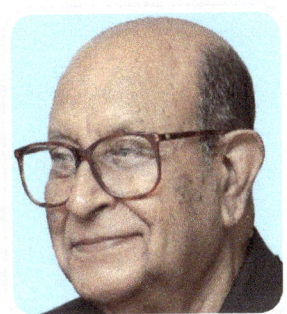

MR Khan
(1-8-1928 to 5-11-2016)
Who inspired me to be an author

Foreword

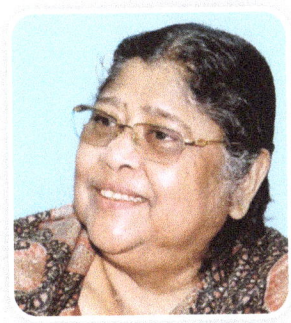

Hajera Mahtab MBChB (Liverpool) DTM&H (Liverpool)
FCPS (Pakistan) and FRCP (Edinburgh)
Emeritus Professor of Medicine and Endocrinology
Bangladesh Institute of Health Science (BIHS)
Dhaka, Bangladesh

It is my pleasure and privilege to write an introduction for the book titled *"Essence of Clinical Endocrinology"* written by Professor Tofail Ahmed and Dr Tania Tofail.

I know Professor Tofail Ahmed since he joined BIRDEM as a student of Diploma Course of Endocrinology in 1986. Subsequently, he completed his PhD in Endocrinology successfully.

He is a sincere and dedicated academic with several publications, books, book chapters, and papers including quite a few in peer-reviewed journals. Currently, he is heading very successfully the Distance Learning Program of Diabetic Association of Bangladesh, which has gained recognition at home and abroad.

This book is well written. Each chapter begins with relevant anatomy and physiology. In the case of common and difficult scenario it is supplemented with simple decision-making steps. Adequate tables, figures, flowcharts, and boxes have been used to make the subject clear and easier to understand. It will be of use to clinical endocrinologists, medical specialists, general practitioners, and related health professionals. Medical students will also be benefitted.

I wish them success in the publication of this book!

Preface

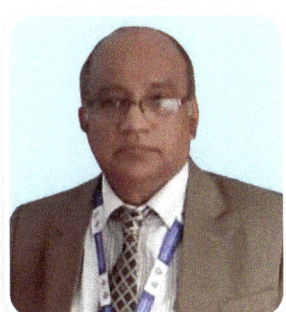

Tofail Ahmed

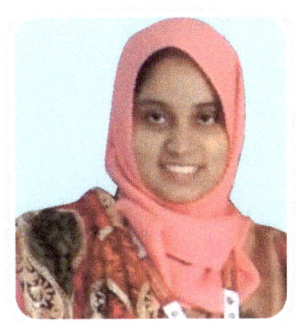

Tania Tofail

The inspiration of writing this book comes from the hands-on training I got from Late National Professor MR Khan (legendry pediatrician of the country) during drafting of our book *"Essence of Endocrinology"* back in 1997. My workplace also plays an important role for it. Since 1988, I started working in the endocrinology outpatient department of BIRDEM with Professor Emeritus Hajera Mahtab (the pioneer endocrinologist of the country) after completing Diploma in Endocrinology from BIRDEM. At that time, this was the only referral institute of Endocrinology in the country. I had ample opportunities of dealing with common, uncommon, and also rare endocrine cases. Initially, clinical challenges were more because of limited diagnostic and therapeutic facilities for most of the diseases but with time remarkable improvements happened.

I was fortunate to do few fundamental works in endocrinology, such as (1) clinical and biochemical research on Lean Young Diabetic (Malnutrition-related Diabetes Mellitus) of Bangladesh as a PhD student, (2) a monography publication on thyroid diseases with data of our laboratory, and (3) receiving hands-on training on assisted reproductive techniques (ART) in Singapore National University. As a teaching faculty, I have experience in teaching as well as examination activities of BIRDEM, University of Dhaka, Bangladesh, and Bangabandhu Sheik Mujib Medical University (BSMMU). I retired as a Professor of Endocrinology in 2017. I am a founder member of Bangladesh Endocrine Society, served as President of American Association of Clinical Endocrinology (AACE), Bangladesh Chapter (2017 to 2019) and General Secretary of South Asian Federation of Endocrine Societies (SAFES) from 2015 to 2017.

There were two different aims during writing this book. One is to make physicians and medical students more accustomed with clinical endocrinology for which each chapter begins with relevant anatomy and physiology and common but tricky scenarios are supplemented with decision-making investigation steps (DMIS) and the other aim is to improve skill-sharing opportunities between endocrinologist and allied specialist (imaging specialist, laboratory scientist, physiologist, endocrine surgeons, oncologists, etc.) by appropriately highlighting current multidisciplinary workups for disorders including incidentalomas, assisted reproductive techniques, etc.

I would like to mention that the coauthor of the book is my daughter. She has an excellent academic track having five gold medals during her MBBS course and one chancellor's gold medal for MD in Endocrinology. She has completed MRCP (UK) and SEC in Endocrinology and Diabetology from UK and currently a PhD fellow in BSMMU.

I am fortunate to have so many brilliant students, friendly teachers, colleagues, and friends who supported me unconditionally for my work, and I express my sincere gratitude to them.

Acknowledgments

We remember with gratitude all of those who inspired us to write the book. To mention, mostly they are my beloved students, friends, teachers, and senior colleagues, including my mentor Professor Hajera Mahtab.

I am fortunate to have very supportive family. The physician members—wife Dr Tahmina Kabir (Consultant Obstetrics and Gynecology), eldest son Dr Towhid (Consultant Prosthodontist), and son-in-law Dr Rayhan (Consultant Orthopedic)—provided constant support and inspiration in every job of a long draft preparation phase. The rest of the members—youngest son Towfiq (Automobile Engineer) and two daughters-in-law Omee (Lawyer) and Sorba (Engineer)—were always deeply concerned for our project. Our four grandchildren—Daneen, Tahsin, Mohsin, and Mihu—are the precious gifts of God for the family. We acknowledge their contribution.

I acknowledge my nephew Professor Massod Paveez, Professor of Histopathology, for providing histopathological pictures of thyroid malignancies for the book.

Our gratitude to Shri Jitendar P Vij (Group Chairman), Mr Ankit Vij (Managing Director), Mr MS Mani (Group President), Ms Chetna Malhotra (Senior Director—Professional Publishing, Marketing and Business Development), and Mr Anirban Mukherjee (Development Editor) of M/s Jaypee Brothers Medical Publishers (P) Ltd, New Delhi, India.

Contents

CHAPTER 1: Endocrinology 1

CHAPTER 2: Disorders of Pituitary Gland 11

CHAPTER 3: Disorders of Thyroid Gland 28

CHAPTER 4: Disorders of Parathyroid Gland 52

CHAPTER 5: Disorders of Adrenal Gland 68

CHAPTER 6: Diabetes Mellitus and Insulinoma 92

CHAPTER 7: Disorders of Growth and Development 125

CHAPTER 8: Reproductive Medicine 153

Index 187

Abbreviations

A	Alpha cell	CMZ	Carbimazole
ACD	Atherosclerotic cardiovascular diseases	CNS	Central nervous system
ACT	Anaplastic carcinoma thyroid	COCs	Combined oral contraceptives
ACTH	Adrenocorticotropic hormone	CPA	Cyproterone acetate
ADH	Antidiuretic hormone	CPP	Constitutional precocious puberty
ADP	Adenosine diphosphate	CRF	Corticotropin-releasing factor
ADT	Androgen deprivation therapy	CRH	Corticotropin-releasing hormone
AITD	Autoimmune thyroid disease	CS	Cushing's syndrome
ALT	Alanine transaminase	CSS	Constitutional short stature
AMA	Antimicrosomal antibody	CT	Computed tomography
ANF	Atrial natriuretic factor	CTS	Constitutional tall stature
AR	Autosomal recessive	CVA	Cerebrovascular accident
ART	Assisted reproductive technique	D	Delta cell
AST	Aspartate aminotransferase	DA	Dopamine
ATA	Antithyroglobulin antibody	DCI	Daily calorie intake
ATP	Adenosine triphosphate	DCT	Distal convoluted tubule
B	Beta cell	dDAVP	Desmopressin
BIPSS	Bilateral simultaneous inferior petrosal sinus sampling	DHEA	Dehydroepiandrosterone
		DHEAS	Dehydroepiandrosterone sulfate
BMD	Bone mass density	DI	Diabetes insipidus
BMI	Body mass index	DIC	Disseminated intravascular coagulation
BS	Bartter syndrome	DKA	Diabetic ketoacidosis
BWS	Beckwith–Wiedemann syndrome	DM	Diabetes mellitus
CAD	Coronary artery disease	DMIS	Decision-making investigation steps
CAH	Congenital adrenal hyperplasia	DXA	Dual-energy X-ray absorptiometry
CD	Cushing's disease	E_2	Estradiol
CDC	Clinical growth chart	EMG	Electromyography
CDI	Cranial diabetes insipidus	ERT	Estrogen replacement therapy
CEA	Carcinoembryonic antigen	ET	Embryo transfer
CF	Calorie factor	FBG	Fasting blood glucose
CGM	Continuous glucose monitoring	FCPD	Fibrocalculous pancreatic diabetes
cGMP	Cyclic guanosine monophosphate	FFA	Free fatty acid
CHF	Congestive heart failure	FHH	Familial hypocalciuric hypercalcemia
CL	Corpus luteum		

FNAB-PTH	Fine-needle aspiration biopsy-parathyroid hormone	IGT	Impaired glucose tolerance
		IQ	Intelligence quotient
FNAC	Fine-needle aspiration cytology	IR	Insulin resistance
FRAX	Fracture Risk Assessment Tool	ISD	Inhibited sexual desire
FSH	Follicle-stimulating hormone	IUGR	Intrauterine growth retardation
FT_4	Free thyroxine	IUI	Intrauterine insemination
FTC	Follicular thyroid carcinoma	IVF	In vitro fertilization
GD	Grave's disease	LARC	Long-acting reversible contraceptives
GDM	Gestational diabetes mellitus	LDL	Low-density lipoprotein
GH	Growth hormone	LH	Luteinizing hormone
GHIF	Growth hormone inhibitory factor	LMB	Laurence–Moon–Biedl
GHIS	Growth hormone insensitivity syndrome	LODST	Low-dose overnight dexamethasone suppression test
GHR	Growth hormone receptor	MAO-I	Monoamine oxidase inhibitors
GHRD	Growth hormone receptor deficiency	MAS	McCune–Albright syndrome
GHRF	Growth hormone-releasing factor	MCT	Medullary carcinoma of thyroid
GLP1	Glucagon-like peptide-1	MEDAC	Multiple endocrine deficiency-Addison disease-candidiasis
GLUT2	Glucose transporter 2		
GnRH	Gonadotropin-releasing hormone	MEN	Multiple endocrine neoplasia
GS	Gitelman syndrome	MEN1	Multiple endocrine neoplasia type 1
GSS	Genetic short stature	MEN4	Multiple endocrine neoplasia type 4
GTS	Genetic tall stature	MHR	Maximum heart rate
HbA1c	Hemoglobin A1c	MMI	Methimazole
HBS	Hungry bone syndrome	MNG	Multinodular goiter
HC	Hip circumference	MNT	Medical nutrition therapy
hCG	Human chorionic gonadotropin	MRI	Magnetic resonance imaging
HDL	High-density lipoprotein	MRKH	Mayer–Rokitansky–Küster–Hauser
HFI	Hyperostosis frontalis interna	MS	Metabolic syndrome
HGU	Hepatic glucose output	MTHFR	Methylenetetrahydrofolate reductase
HLA	Human leukocyte antigen	NCDs	Noncommunicable diseases
HONK	Hyperglycemic hyperosmolar nonketotic coma	NDI	Nephrogenic diabetes insipidus
		NE	Norepinephrine
HPLC	High-pressure liquid chromatography	NPE	Nocturnal penile erection
HR complex	Hormone-receptor complex	NPO	Nothing per oral
HRE	Hormone response element	OGTT	Oral glucose tolerance test
HRT	Hormone replacement therapy	PCOS	Polycystic ovary syndrome
IBW	Ideal body weight	PE	Premature ejaculation
ICSI	Intracytoplasmic sperm injection	PET	Positron emission tomography
IDF	International Diabetes Federation	PGE1	Prostaglandin E1
IFG	Impaired fasting glucose	PGS	Pubertal growth spurt
IGF-1	Insulin-like growth factor-1		

PH	Pubic hair	SPL	Stretched penile length
PHP	Pseudohypoparathyroidism	SRC	Sexual response cycle
PLID	Prolapse lumbar intervertebral disc	SSRI	Selective serotonin reuptake inhibitor
POF	Premature ovarian failure	STD	Sexually transmitted disease
POMC	Precursor hormone pro-opiomelanocortin	STIs	Sexually transmitted infections
POPs	Progestin-only pills	SU	Sulfonylurea
Posm	Plasma osmolality	T1DM	Type 1 diabetes mellitus
PP	Primary polydipsia	T2DM	Type 2 diabetes mellitus
PPHP	Pseudopseudohypoparathyroidism	T_3	Triiodothyronine
PRA	Plasma renin activity	T_4	Thyroxine
PRL	Prolactin	TAL	Thick ascending limb
PRLIF	Prolactin inhibitory factor	TBG	Thyroxine-binding globulin
PSS	Psychosocial short stature	TESA	Testicular sperm aspiration
PTC	Papillary thyroid carcinoma	TFT	Thyroid function test
PTH	Parathyroid hormone	TG	Triglyceride
PTHrP	Parathyroid hormone-related protein	TPN	Total parenteral nutrition
PTU	Propylthiouracil	TPO	Thyroid peroxidase
PWLS	Prader–Willi–Lambert	TRH	Thyrotropin-releasing hormone
Rads	Radiation absorption dose	TSH	Thyroid-stimulating hormone
RAIU	Radioactive iodine uptake	TSI	Thyroid-stimulating immunoglobulin
RBS	Random blood sugar	UFC	Urinary free cortisol
RTA	Renal tubular acidosis	Uosm	Urine osmolality
SD	Standard deviation	USG	Ultrasonography
SERMs	Selective estrogen receptor modulators	VLDL	Very low-density lipoprotein
SGA	Small for gestational age	VMA	Vanillylmandelic acid
SIAD	Syndrome of inappropriate ADH secretion	WBS	Williams–Beuren syndrome
SMBG	Self-monitoring of blood glucose	WC	Waist circumference
SPACE	Single potential analysis of cavernous electrical activity	WFS	Waterhouse–Friderichsen syndrome
		WHR	Waist-hip ratio

CHAPTER 1

Endocrinology

- Features of hormones
  - Chemical features of hormones
- Hormone structure
- Sources and sites of actions of some hormones
- Metabolic areas of hormonal regulation
- Mechanism of hormone action
  - Class I: Hormones that bind with intracellular mobile receptors
  - Class II: Hormones that bind with fixed cell surface receptors
- Endocrine function tests
  - Single sample assay
  - Serial sample assay
  - Paired sample assay
  - Dynamic test

This chapter is an introduction to general and clinical endocrinology. It covers general features and chemical structures of important hormones. Practical use of blood levels of hormones to ascertain their health/disorders states. Beginners may face difficulties in understanding a few endocrine function tests, but they will definitely solve in relevant chapter study. This chapter contains 12 Figures, 4 Tables, and 5 Flowcharts to illustrate its text.

INTRODUCTION

The study of biomedical science concerning biomolecule termed "Hormone" (hormone—a Greek word that means "I excite") is called "Endocrinology." It is a branch of medicine that is not only concerned with therapeutics of individual's diseases related to hormone(s) but also has involvement in preventive and community/social medicine. Hormones are signaling biomolecules with a capacity of regulating subcellular metabolic events in specific cells called as their target cells. The endocrine system consists of several hormone-producing glands situated in different parts of the body. Hormones exert different regulatory functions. The diseases of the endocrine system are usually related to deficient or excess secretion of a hormone and relatively rare from resistance or oversensitivity of a hormone. **Figure 1** summarizes these facts of endocrine disorders with examples.

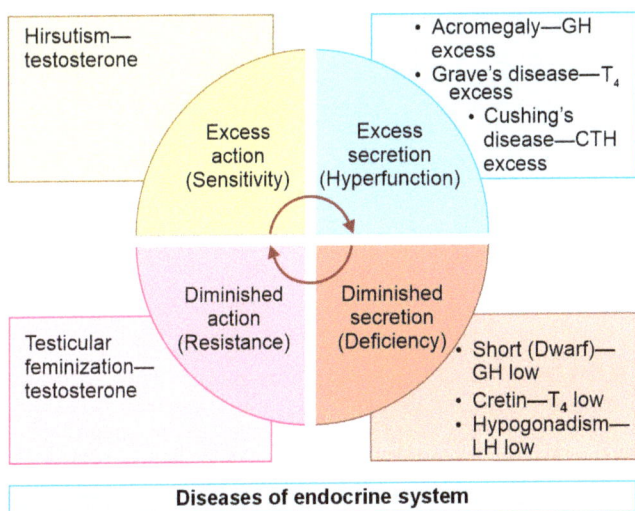

FIG. 1: Hormonal disorders arise from excess/diminished amount or excess/diminished action of a hormone.
(CTH: corticotropic hormone; GH: growth hormone; LH: luteinizing hormone; T_4: thyroxine)

FEATURES OF HORMONES

There are many features that can describe the similarities between different hormones. Some of them are given here:
- Hormones are synthesized in and secreted from specialized cells (usually organized as glands).
- They travel to their target cell via blood.
- Blood concentrations of individual hormones are strikingly low (usually in the range of pmol/L or nmol/L).
- Hormone regulates cell function/metabolism and thereby of tissues, organs, and ultimately the individual. The regulatory property is not an autonomy of a hormone rather they work in cooperation with nervous system and endocrine system; for example, cortico-hypothalamic-pituitary controls.
- There is also feedback regulation between endocrine glands (TSH and T_4; ACTH, cortisol, etc.) and hormones with electrolytes [parathormone (PTH) and serum Ca^{++}; aldosterone serum Na^+, etc.].

■ Chemical Features of Hormones

Chemical structure of hormones provides a fundamental basis to classifying them into groups or classes. There are three groups/classes of hormones shown here.
Chemically hormones belong to three different groups:
1. *Group I*: Proteins and peptide hormones: (A) Glycoproteins—thyroid-stimulating hormone (TSH), follicle-stimulating hormone (FSH), luteinizing hormone (LH), and human chorionic gonadotropin (hCG). (B) Polypeptide—adrenocorticotropic hormone (ACTH), growth hormone (GH), and insulin
2. *Group II*: Steroids—cortisol and testosterone
3. *Group III*: Amines—thyroxine (T_4), tri-iodthyronine (T_3), and epinephrine

Flowchart 1 describes the chemical structure-based classification of hormones.

HORMONE STRUCTURE

The primary structure of some important hormones of human body along with molecular weights of different groups of hormones is shown in **Figures 2 to 5**.

Group IA: Protein and peptide (polypeptide) hormones produced by anterior pituitary and beta cells of pancreases from amino acids in a single chain (**Figs. 2A to C**).

Group IB: Protein and peptide (polypeptide) hormones produced by ectodermal gland from amino acids with two subunits of which one (alpha) is common for all (**Figs. 3A to D**).

Group II: Steroid hormones, produced by mesodermal gland from cholesterol molecule (**Figs. 4A and B**).

Group III: Amine hormones produced by thyroid and adrenal medullary cells from amino acids (**Figs. 5A to C**).

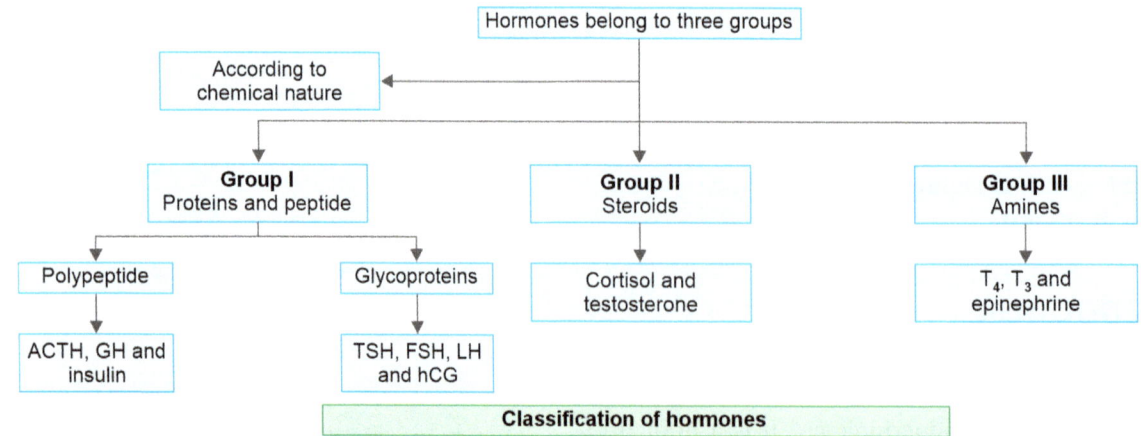

FLOWCHART 1: Classification/grouping of hormones on the basis of chemical structure.
(ACTH: adrenocorticotropic hormone; FSH: follicle-stimulating hormone; GH: growth hormone; LH: luteinizing hormone; TSH: thyroid-stimulating hormone; hCG: human chorionic gonadotropin; T_3: tri-iodthyronine; T_4: thyroxine)

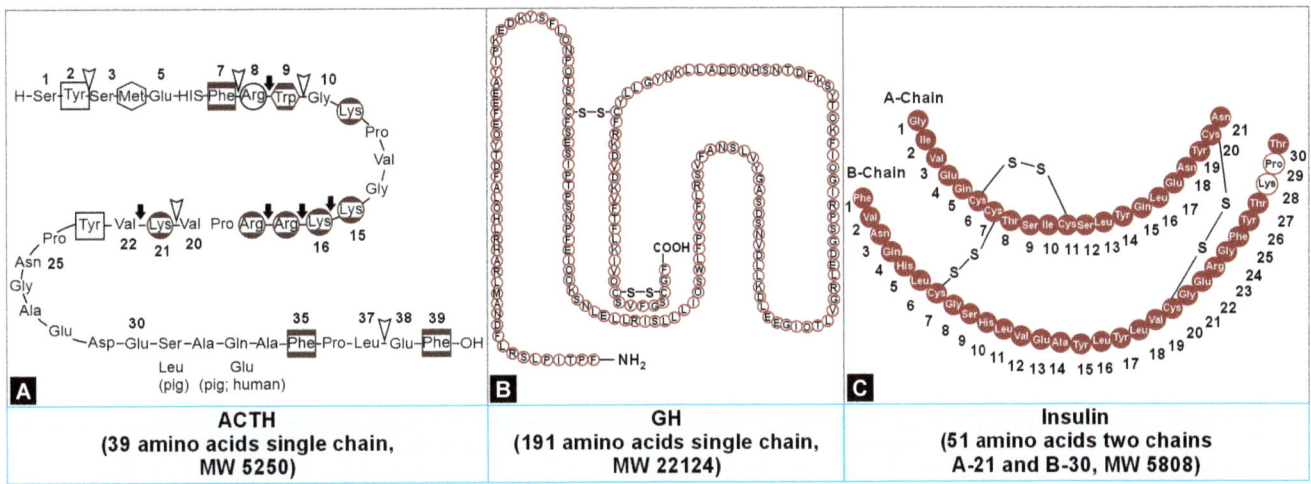

FIGS. 2A TO C: Primary structure and molecular weight (MW) of group IA hormones: Adrenocorticotropic hormone (ACTH), growth hormone (GH), and insulin.

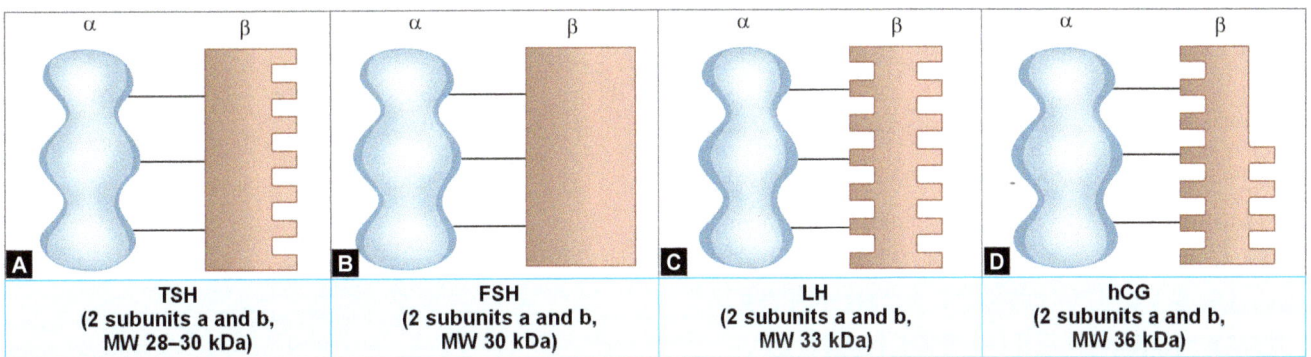

FIGS. 3A TO D: Primary structure and molecular weight (MW) of group IB hormones: Thyroid-stimulating hormone (TSH), follicle-stimulating hormone (FSH), luteinizing hormone (LH), and human chorionic gonadotropin (hCG).

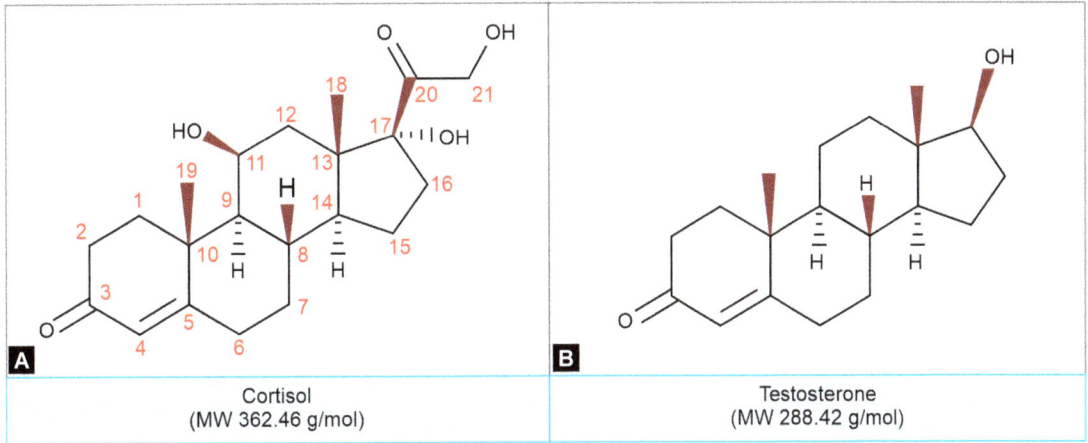

FIGS. 4A AND B: Primary structure and molecular weight (MW) of group II hormones: Cortisol and testosterone.

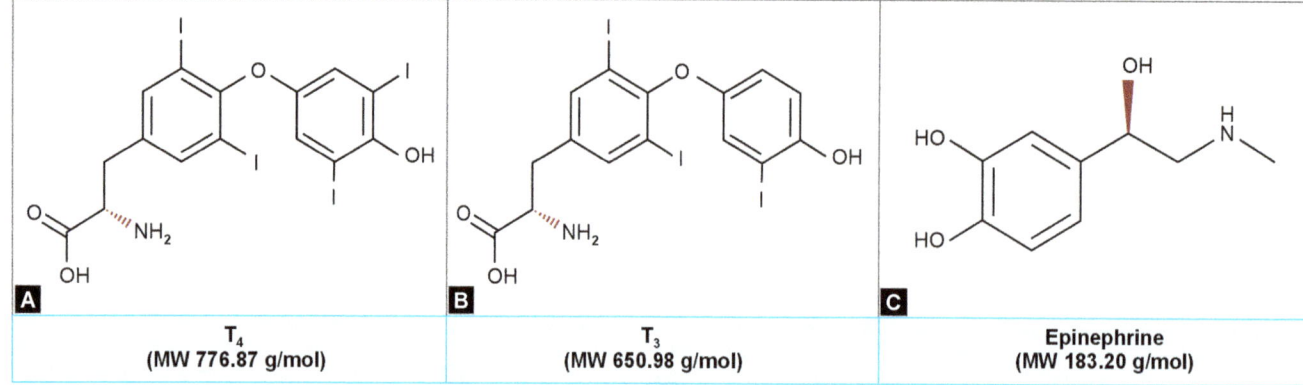

FIGS. 5A TO C: Primary structure and molecular weight (MW) of group III hormones: T_4, T_3, and epinephrine.

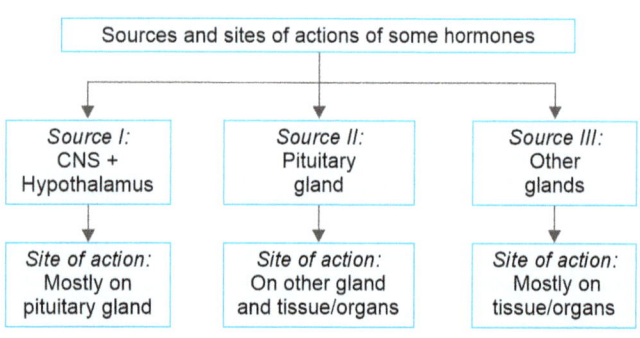

FLOWCHART 2: Sources and sites of actions of some hormones.

SOURCES AND SITES OF ACTIONS OF SOME HORMONES (FLOWCHART 2)

- *Source I:*
  o CNS + hypothalamus
  o Site of action: Mostly on pituitary gland
- *Source II:*
  o Pituitary gland (anterior + posterior hormones)
  o Site of action: On other gland and tissue/organs
- *Source III:*
  o Other glands (thyroid, parathyroid, pancreases, adrenal cortex, and gonads)
  o Site of action: Mostly on tissue/organs

METABOLIC AREAS OF HORMONAL REGULATION

Hormones regulate four metabolic areas **(Fig. 6)**:
1. *Metabolic area I*: Reproduction
2. *Metabolic area II*: Growth and development
3. *Metabolic area III*: Energy production, utilization, and storage
4. *Metabolic area IV*: Internal environment maintenance

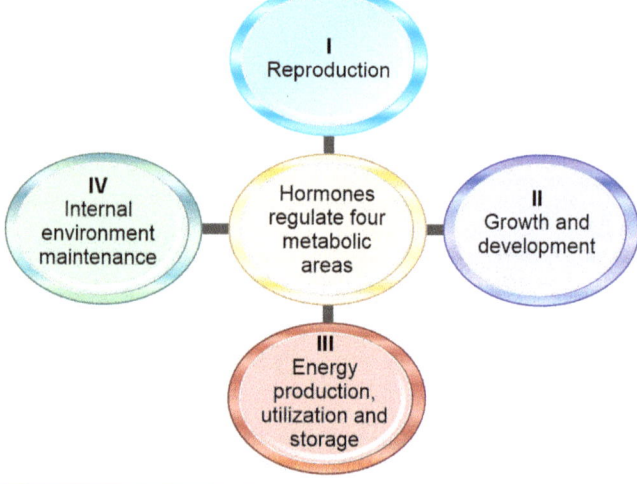

FIG. 6: There are four metabolic areas of hormonal regulation. (1) Reproductive; (2) Growth and development; (3) Energy production, utilization, and storage; (4) Internal environment maintenance.

MECHANISM OF HORMONE ACTION

Hormones are signaling molecules. The phenomenon of hormonal action starts by binding of a hormone with its specific receptors those are located in its target cells. There are two different sites of a hormone receptor. One is fixed on the cell surface and the other one is mobile, which lies inside the cell (in cytoplasm or within nucleus) **(Fig. 7)**. To describe the mechanism of action of hormone, hormones are grouped into two classes:
1. *Class I*: Hormones that bind with intracellular mobile receptors.
2. *Class II*: Hormones that bind with cell-surface fixed receptors.

Class I: Hormones that Bind with Intracellular Mobile Receptors

- These hormones are lipophilic molecules. Therefore, they can easily diffuse through the plasma membrane and the receptor molecules have high affinity for the hormone.
  - *Step 1*: Initially, hormone and its receptor form the hormone-receptor complex (HR complex).
  - *Step 2*: The HR complex undergoes to "activation reaction". This is a temperature and salt-dependent phenomenon that changes in size, conformation, and surface charge so that the complex gets the ability to bind to chromosome.
  - *Step 3*: The activated HR complex binds with the specific DNA [called hormone response element (HRE)] and activates the specific genes.
  - *Step 4*: The activated gene then synthesizes specific protein in the cytoplasm and thereby brings metabolic response of the hormone **(Fig. 8)**.
- Steroid hormones and fatty acids hormones are lipid soluble; therefore, they can easily pass through the plasma membrane.
- Their receptor lies inside the cell and can freely float in the cytoplasm. The enzymatic activity of the cell for biochemical changes occurs after the binding of hormone to the specific receptor.
- Receptors of testosterone, progesterone, estrogen, cortisol, and thyroxine are located inside the nucleus.

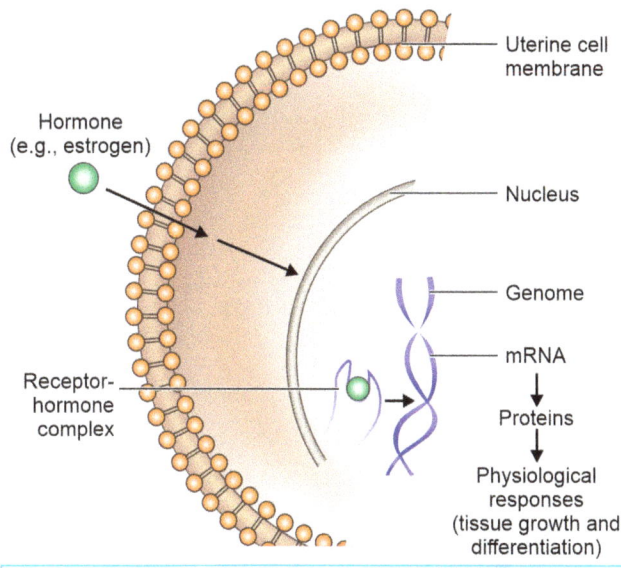

Mobile receptor mechanism of hormone action

FIG. 8: Four steps: (1) Hormone enters in the cell; (2) Receptor-hormone form; (3) Activation of gene; (4) Protein (enzyme) forms to regulate cell function.

- The HR complex within the nucleus initiates transcription of the DNA to form specific mRNA.
- The mRNAs then initiate protein synthesis in the cytoplasm, causing enzymatic changes in the cell.

Class II: Hormones that Bind with Fixed Cell Surface Receptors

These hormone molecules are larger in size and hydrophilic. Therefore, they cannot diffuse through the plasma membrane. Their receptor molecules are fixed in the cell membrane.

- *Step 1*: Initially, hormone and its receptor form the HR complex.
- *Step 2*: HR complex releases some intracellular substances (called second messengers).
  The HR complex undergoes to "activation reaction." This is a temperature and salt- dependent phenomenon that changes in size, conformation, and surface charge so that the complex gets ability to bind to chromosome.
- *Step 3*: The second messengers activate the specific genes and bring other effects (e.g., ion and channel activity, activity of intracellular proteins, or interfere metabolic regulation) for metabolic regulation.

There are several second messenger molecules, e.g., cyclic adenosine monophosphate (cAMP), cytidine cyclic monophosphate (cCMP), calcium, phosphatidylinositides, and unknown messengers. Multiple hormones can utilize a common second messenger.

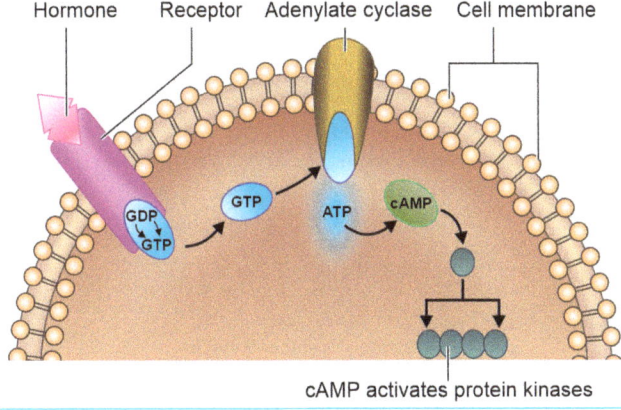

Mechanism of hormone action

FIG. 7: Hormones are target specific and bind to the specific receptor. On the basis of binding of hormone on their specific receptor, the mechanism of hormonal action is categorized into two groups—(1) Fixed membrane receptor mechanism and (2) Mobile receptor mechanism.
(ATP: adenosine triphosphate; cAMP: cyclic adenosine monophosphate; GTP: guanosine triphosphate)

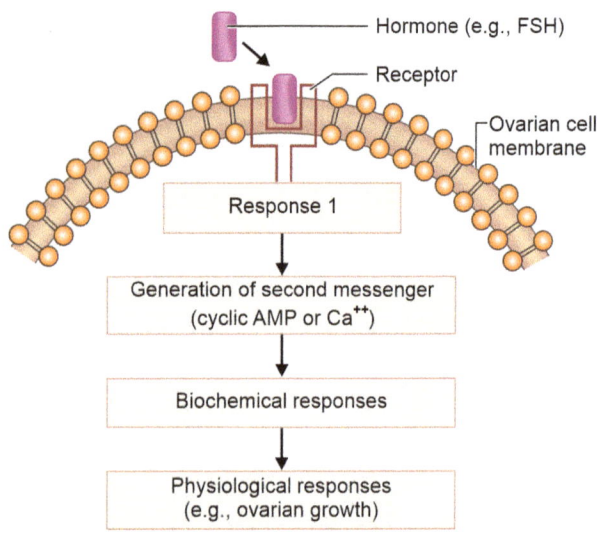

FLOWCHART 3: Three steps: (1) Receptor-hormone form at cell membrane; (2) Generate a second messenger within cell; (3) Second messenger regulate cell function.
(AMP: adenosine monophosphate; FSH: follicle-stimulating hormone)

Class II hormones are again subclassified on the basis of their second messenger molecule.

Examples of these hormones are given according to their subclass:
- *cAMP is the second messenger*: Acetylcholine, glucagon, ACTH, antidiuretic hormone (ADH), PTH, calcitonin, TSH, FSH, LH, hCG, corticotropin-releasing hormone (CRH), etc.
- *Cyclic guanosine monophosphate (cGMP) is the second messenger*: Arial natriuretic factor (ANF).
- *Calcium or phosphatidylinositides (or both) is the second messenger*: Gonadotropin-releasing hormone (GnRH), thyrotropin-releasing hormone (TRH); α-1 adrenergic catecholamines, oxytocin, and gastrin.
- *The second messenger is unknown*: Insulin, GH, and prolactin (PRL) **(Flowchart 3)**.

ENDOCRINE FUNCTION TESTS

For diagnosis as well as during monitoring of treatment, a precise measurement of hormone(s) level in blood/other body fluid plays a vital role. It directly provides information whether the hormone is within normal range or abnormal (hyper/hypofunction). Normal range of a particular hormone is ascertained by measuring of a hormone value in a healthy population and is usually expressed as a range, but it may be expressed as 95% confidence interval also.

However, for diagnosis, a hormone level of an individual is not always able to separate normal from abnormal states. This is because many endocrine disorders pass through subtle degrees of glandular dysfunction, and compensatory mechanism(s) may be active. So other types of sample assay are advocated. There are four different types of hormone sample assay **(Flowchart 4)**.
1. Single sample assay
2. Serial hormone assay
3. Paired sample assay
4. Dynamic tests

Nowadays, for diagnosis, endocrine function tests are mostly performed by paired test of a hormone with its tropic hormone. Dynamic tests either by stimulation or suppression of glands show greater accuracy even in preclinical state or stage of dysfunctions.

Single Sample Assay

A single value is informative of whether it is within normal range or abnormal (high/low), indicating normal or abnormal (hyper/hypo) function status of the gland **(Flowchart 5)**. Examples include:
- As in case thyroid function level of free T_4 within normal range (euthyroximia), above (hyperthyroximia), or below (hypothyroximia) are equivalent to euthyroidism, hyperthyroidism, and hypothyroidism, respectively. Such a simple interpretation does not fit always.

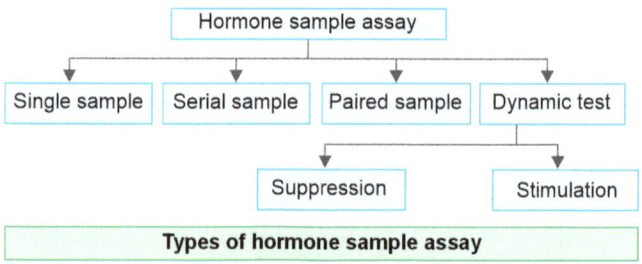

FLOWCHART 4: There are four different types hormone sample assay: (1) Single sample assay; (2) Serial hormone assay; (3) Paired sample assay; (4) Dynamic tests.

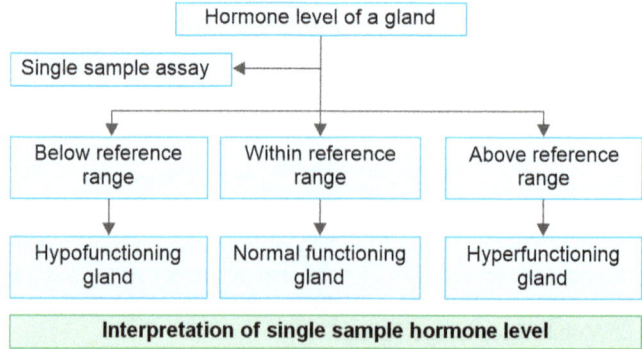

FLOWCHART 5: Normal range-based interpretation are simple interpretation but does not fit always. There are many pit falls in such tests.

- If there is glandular dysfunction and compensatory mechanism could maintain the hormonal level within normal range as in compensated hypo- or hyperthyroidism. Or in case where fluctuation of secretion is a feature of the gland as in diurnal rhythms of cortisol, monthly cyclical partum of estrogen, and progesterone secretion.

Serial Sample Assay

Serial sample assay can provide a better understanding of endocrine function particularly where there is fluctuation in secretion. And a single measurement of a hormone has the risks of both false positivity as well as false negativity. Serial samples taken can improve the scenario in many occasions; for example: (1) samples in different times of a day—diurnal rhythm of cortisol, (2) samples in different days of the menstrual cycle—day 22 progesterone of a regular cycle women to understand ovulation, and (3) samples in different ages—LH at during puberty onset **(Figs. 9 to 11)**.

Examples:
- Two-sample cortisol assay (morning and evening): Normally the evening value is around 50% of morning value. This diurnal variation may be lost in early stage of Cushing's disease.
- Measurement of progesterone on day 22 of a regular cycle woman. A value > 30 units is considered a conceptual cycle, which means ovulation plus luteal sufficiency of the cycle.
- Measurement of LH during day and during sleep at night in boys and girls may document nocturnal LH surges. It can be the first clue for ensuring puberty.

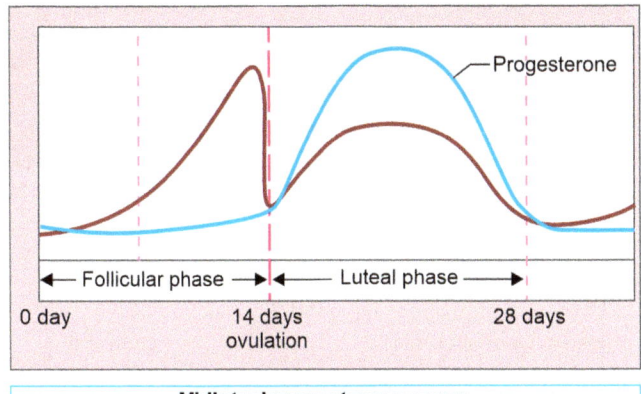

Midluteal progesterone assay

FIG. 10: Measurement of progesterone on day 22 of a regular cycle woman. A value > 30 units considered conceptual cycle, which means ovulation plus luteal sufficiency of the cycle.

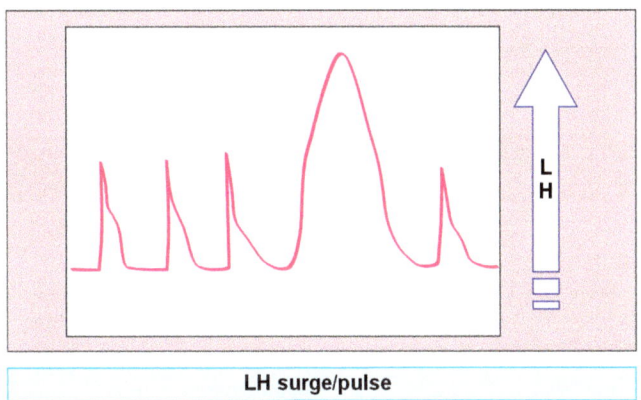

LH surge/pulse

FIG. 11: Measurement of luteinizing hormone (LH) in blood during day and during sleep at night in boys and girls can document nocturnal LH surges. It can be the first clue of ensuring puberty.

Paired Sample Assay

Paired tests such as hormone plus its tropic hormone or a hormone plus a molecule that keeps a strong correlation with the hormone are assayed from one sample. These approaches have improved endocrine function test for identifying cases at preclinical stage and also for classifying the disorder as primary or not **(Tables 1 and 2)**.

Example: FT_4 assay paired with TSH can produce nine different combination states or classes.
Measurement of PTH plus calcium assay:
- Normal PTH and normal Ca^{++} means functional status of parathyroid normal
- High PTH and high Ca^{++} means primary hyperparathyroidism
- High PTH and low Ca^{++} means primary hypoparathyroidism

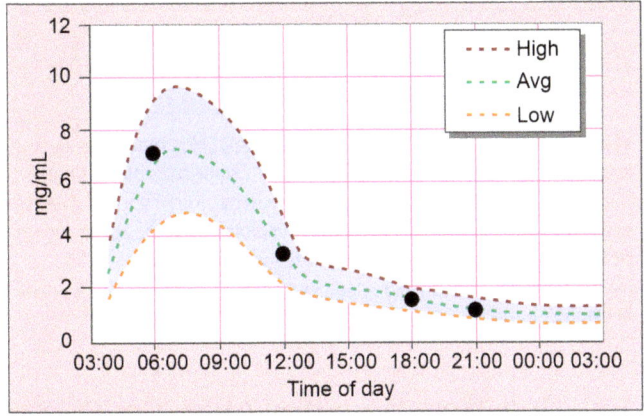

Diurnal variation of cortisol secretion allow two-sample assay test

FIG. 9: Two-sample cortisol assay: (1) Morning (8–9 AM) and (2) Evening (5 PM) is done. Normally the evening value is around 50% of morning value. This diurnal variation may be lost in early stage of Cushing's disease.

CHAPTER 1: Endocrinology

TABLE 1: Thyroxine (FT$_4$) assay paired with thyroid-stimulating hormone (TSH) can produce nine different combination states or class.

Paired test can classify functional status of thyroid into nine classes

Class 2 Primary hypothyroid FT$_4$ low TSH high FT$_4$ L	TSH H	Class 4 Compensated hypothyroid FT$_4$ normal TSH high FT$_4$ N	TSH H	Class 7 Secondary hyperthyroid FT$_4$ high TSH high FT$_4$ H
Class 8 Isolated hypothyroximia FT$_4$ low TSH normal FT$_4$ L	TSH N	Class 1 Euthyroid FT$_4$ normal TSH normal FT$_4$ N	TSH N	Class 9 Isolated hyperthyroximia FH$_4$ high TSH normal FT$_4$ H
Class 6 Secondary hypothyroid FT$_4$ low TSH low	TSH L	Class 5 Compensated hyperthyroid FT$_4$ normal TSH low	TSH L	Class 3 Primary hyperthyroid FT$_4$ high TSH low

Inference: There are nine classes in this classification system.

TABLE 2: Parathormone (PTH) paired with calcium can determine parathyroid gland function.

	Serum PTH low	Serum PTH normal	Serum PTH high
Serum Ca^{++} high			Primary hyperparathyroidism
Serum Ca^{++} normal		Normal parathyroid	
Serum Ca^{++} low	Primary hypoparathyroidism		

■ Dynamic Test

These tests involve the use of an exogenous agent to manipulate body's hormonal milieu for the diagnosis. Dynamic endocrine tests are done when information(s) provided by single or paired hormone assay is insufficient particularly to deal with subtle cases. These are of two different subtypes as described here.

1. *Stimulation test*: Summation tests are utilized in a situation where hypofunction is suspected. They perturb the endogenous control mechanism to access the reserve capacity to synthesize and secrete hormones. This is done in two general ways.
   i. Tropic hormone is administered to test the reserve of the target gland's hormone production capacity.
      Examples:
      a. TRH is used to see TSH secreting capacity of thyrotrophic cells of anterior pituitary gland **(Fig. 12)**.

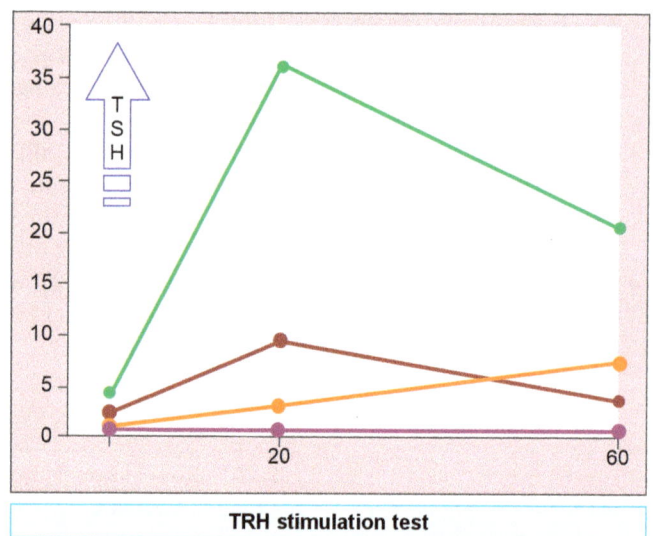

TRH stimulation test

FIG. 12: TRH (200 µg) is given as IV bolus; TSH is measures at 0, 20, and 60 minutes. TSH is flat (<2 mU/L) in hyperthyroidism (Line 1); Exaxateted response (>25 mU/L) in hypothyroidism (Line 4); Delayed response in hypothalamic Hypothyroidism (Line 2); in normal person 20 minutes value >60 minutes value (Line 3).
(IV: intravenous; TRH: thyroid-releasing hormone; TSH: thyroid-stimulating hormone)

   b. hCG or LH is used to testosterone secreting capacity of Leydig cells of testis.
   c. GnRH is used to see FSH and LH of gonadotropic cells of anterior pituitary gland.
   ii. A stimulatory agent or factor is administered to test the tropic production capacity.

Examples:
  a. Clomiphene citrate administered orally—acts on hypothalamus to increase gonadotropin hormone secretion (by decreasing the negative feedback) and increase the gonadal steroid secretion by gonads.
  b. Hypoglycemia is induced by insulin administration and causes cerebral cortical stress resulting in increased GnRH and corticotropin-releasing factor (CRF) of hypothalamus, which stimulate GH and ACTH secretion from the anterior pituitary and then ACTH stimulates adrenal cortex to secret cortisol. **Table 3** summarizes some commonly used stimulation tests.
2. *Suppression test*: Suppression tests are utilized in a situation where hyperfunction is suspected. They determine whether a negative feedback control is intact or not.

Examples:
  i. *Dexamethasone suppression tests*: Dexamethasone is given in a suspected Cushing's syndrome to assess its capacity to inhibit ACTH secretion by anterior pituitary, and thus cortisol is produced by the adrenal glands.
  ii. *TSH suppression test*: Thyroid hormones (T_3/T_4) are given to assess their ability to suppress TSH secretion by thyrocytes of anterior pituitary and thereby inhibit radioiodine uptake by thyroid gland.

Failure to suppression by such test indicates either there is autonomy in secretion from gland or there is ectopic source of hormone production. **Table 4** summarizes some commonly used suppression tests.

TABLE 3: Commonly used stimulation test.

	Organ/system	Stimulus	Response measured
1	Adrenal	ACTH	Cortisol
		Upright posture	Renin and aldosterone
2	Gonad	hCG	Testosterone and its precursors
3	Hypothalamus and pituitary	Hypoglycemia (insulin)	GH and ACTH
		L-dopa	GH
		Exercise	GH
		Clonidine	GH
		Water deprivation	ADH action (urine osmolality)
4	Pituitary	TRH	TSH and prolactin
		GnRH	FSH and LH
		CRF	ACTH
5	Thyroid	TSH	T_4, T_3, and radioiodine uptake
6	Pancreas	Glucose	OGTT and insulin

(ACTH: adrenocorticotropic hormone; ADH: antidiuretic hormone; CRF: corticotropin-releasing factor; FSH: follicle-stimulating hormone; GH: growth hormone; GnRH: gonadotropin-releasing hormone; hCG: human chorionic gonadotropin; LH: luteinizing hormone; OGTT: oral glucose tolerance test; TRH: thyroid-releasing hormone; TSH: thyroid-stimulating hormone; T_3: triiodothyronine; T_4: thyroxine)

TABLE 4: Commonly used suppression tests.

	Organ/system	Suppressor	Response measured
1	Adrenal	Dexamethasone	Cortisol
		Saline	Renin and aldosterone
2	Hypothalamus and pituitary	Glucose	GH and ACTH
3	Thyroid	T_3 and T_4	TSH, radioiodine uptake
4	Pancreas	Fasting	Glucose and insulin

(ACTH: adrenocorticotropic hormone; GH: growth hormone; TSH: thyroid-stimulating hormone; T_3: triiodothyronine; T_4: thyroxine)

FURTHER READINGS

1. Anatomy & Physiology by ©2017 Rice University. Textbook content produced by OpenStax. [online] Available from https://openstax.org/ [Last accessed August, 2023].
2. Standring S (Ed). Gray's Anatomy: The Anatomical Basis of Clinical Practice, 41st edition. [online] Available from https://www.amazon.com/Garys-Anatomy-Henry-Gray/dp/B00DXO9JRA) [Last accessed August, 2023].
3. Barrett K, Barman S, Yuan J, Brooks H (Eds). Ganong's Review of Medical Physiology, 26th edition. [online] Available from https://www.amazon.com/Ganongs-Review-Medical-Physiology-Twenty/dp/1260122409 [Last accessed August, 2023].
4. Melmed S, Koenig R, Rosen C, Auchus R, Goldfine A. Williams Textbook of Endocrinology, 14th edition. [online] Available from (https://www.elsevier.com/books/williams-textbook-of-endocrinology/bresnahan/978-0-323-55596-8_[Last accessed August, 2023].

CHAPTER 2

Disorders of Pituitary Gland

- Introduction to pituitary gland
  (anatomy and applied embryology; physiology)
  - Pituitary gland
  - Developmental anatomy
- Pituitary disorders
  - Hyperpituitarism
  - Hypopituitarism
- Posterior pituitary disorders
  - Diabetes insipidus
  - Syndrome of inappropriate antidiuresis
- Pituitary incidentaloma

The Chapter 2 is about Pituitary Gland, begin with an introduction to applied anatomy and physiology. It covers hypofunctioning states—hypopituitarism, diabetes insipidus; and hyperfunctioning states—hyperpituitarism, SIAD. This chapter contains 12 Figures, 8 Tables, and 6 Flowcharts to illustrate its text. This chapter ends with how to deal with incidentalomas of pituitary.

INTRODUCTION TO PITUITARY GLAND (ANATOMY AND APPLIED EMBRYOLOGY; PHYSIOLOGY)

Pituitary Gland

Gross Anatomy

An adult pituitary gland weighs approximately 0.5 g and is pea sized. It has two parts: (1) Anterior pituitary or adenohypophysis and (2) posterior pituitary—neurohypophysis. The anterior pituitary constitutes roughly 80% of the pituitary and produces most hormones peptide in nature and collectively called tropic hormones. The posterior pituitary is constituting of fibers (axons) of nerve cells in the supraoptic and paraventricular nuclei of the hypothalamus.

The hormones of anterior pituitary are under control of hypothalamic neurohormones. Neurohormones are secreted from the median eminence, and they reach the gland via a portal venous system. The posterior pituitary hormones are synthesized by the neurons of supraoptic and paraventricular nuclei, and they reach the gland through axonal transport of the pituitary stalk. The hormones are released into the systemic circulation.

The pituitary gland is situated in the sella turcica of a bone called the sphenoid. It has a saddle-shaped depression. The inferior, anterior, and posterior aspects of the pituitary gland are in contact of this depression. The superior aspect of the gland is covered by a fold of dura mater, which is called diaphragma sellae. It separates the cerebrospinal fluid-filled subarachnoid space from the pituitary. The pituitary is connected to the hypothalamus by the infundibulum, which pierces the diaphragma sellae.

The right and left sides of the pituitary are adjacent to the cavernous sinuses. There are five cranial nerves within the cavernous—from above down oculomotor (III), trochlear (IV), abducens (VI), ophthalmic branch of trigeminal nerve, and maxillary branch of trigeminal nerve. Just medial to these nerves, the internal carotid artery passes through the cavernous sinus **(Fig. 1)**.

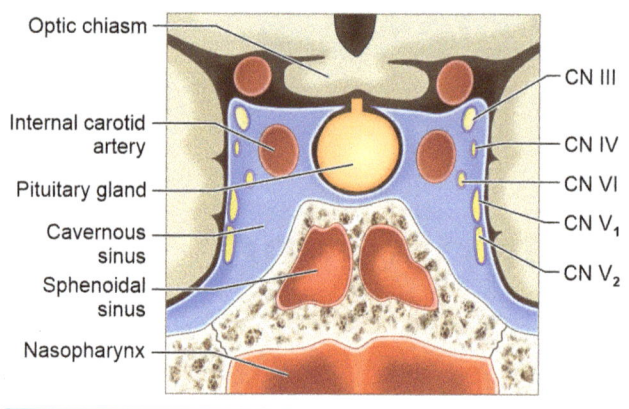

Pituitary gland and adjacent structures

FIG. 1: The cavernous sinuses lies on right and left side of pituitary, five cranial nerves [III, IV, VI, V₁ (ophthalmic branch of trigeminal nerve) and V₂ (maxillary branch of trigeminal nerve)] from above down and the internal carotid artery passe through it medial to these nerves.

Pituitary Gland Microscopic Structure

Histologically, the anterior pituitary, a typical ductless endocrine gland. Secretory cells are cuboidal and arranged in cords and clusters, contain hormones stored in cytoplasmic granules. Hormones are released into the sinusoidal capillaries by exocytosis.

According to histochemical staining, there are three types of pituitary cells: (1) Acidophils, (2) basophils, and (3) chromophobes. Acidophilic cells and basophilic cells contain polypeptide and glycoprotein hormones, respectively but chromophobes have no hormone.

The most abundant cell is acidophilic, situated in the lateral regions of the gland are somatotrope. They secrete growth hormone (GH). There are some acidophilic cells scattered throughout the gland. They are lactotropes, which secrete prolactin (PRL).

The basophilic cells are also of three types: (1) Thyrotropes, (2) corticotropes, and (3) gonadotropes. Thyrotropes lie in the pars distalis, and they secrete thyroid-stimulating hormone (TSH). Corticotropes secrete polypeptides adrenocorticotropic hormone (ACTH) hormones as a precursor hormone pro-opiomelanocortin (POMC). Gondal hormones follicle-stimulating hormone (FSH) and luteinizing hormone (LH) are secreted from gonadotropes.

The posterior pituitary consists of unmyelinated axons of cell bodies of the hypothalamus. Two hormones, oxytocin and antidiuretic hormone (ADH) synthesized in the hypothalamus, are transported and stored at the terminal ends of axons. The ends of the axons are swollen and called Herring bodies. There is a rich network of capillaries that surrounds the Herring bodies to facilitates the uptake of released the hormones into the blood **(Flowchart 1)**.

■ Developmental Anatomy

The developmental origin of the anterior pituitary is from surface ectoderm and posterior pituitary origins from neural ectoderm. During development, the boundary epithelial ectoderm in the roof of the pharynx forms a pocket (Rathke's pouch) that comes into contact with the ectoderm of developing brain. Sequence of events are as follows: At 4 weeks: hypophysial pouch, Rathke's pouch, and diverticulum from roof. At 5 weeks: elongation, contacts infundibulum, and diverticulum of prosencephalon. At 6–8 weeks: connecting stalk between pouch and oral cavity degenerates. The cells of the anterior wall of Rathke's pouch undergo extensive proliferation to form the anterior lobe while the posterior wall proliferates more slowly to form the vestigial intermediate lobe.

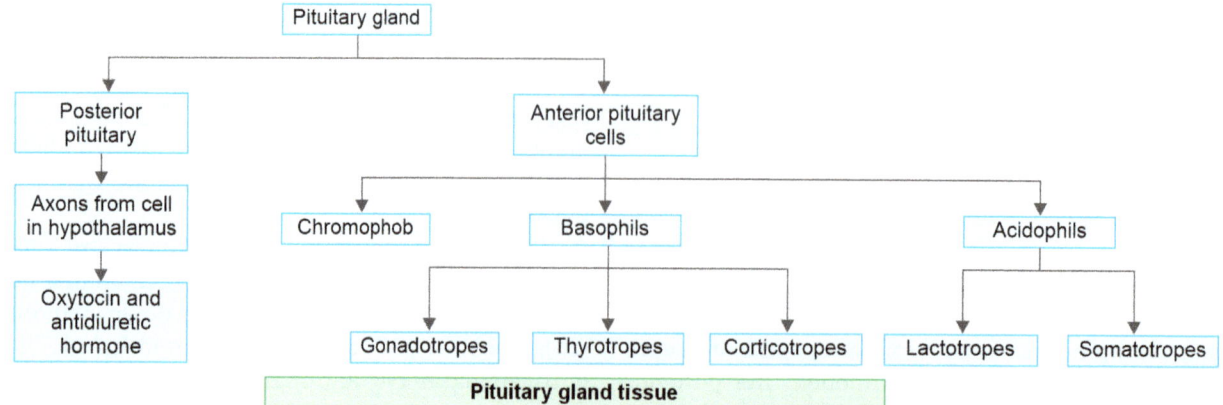

FLOWCHART 1: Histology of pituitary gland tissue. (A) Anterior pituitary: somatotropes and lactotropes; (B) Anterior pituitary: corticotropes, thyrotropes, and gonadotropes; (C) Posterior pituitary oxytocin and antidiuretic hormone in Herring bodies.

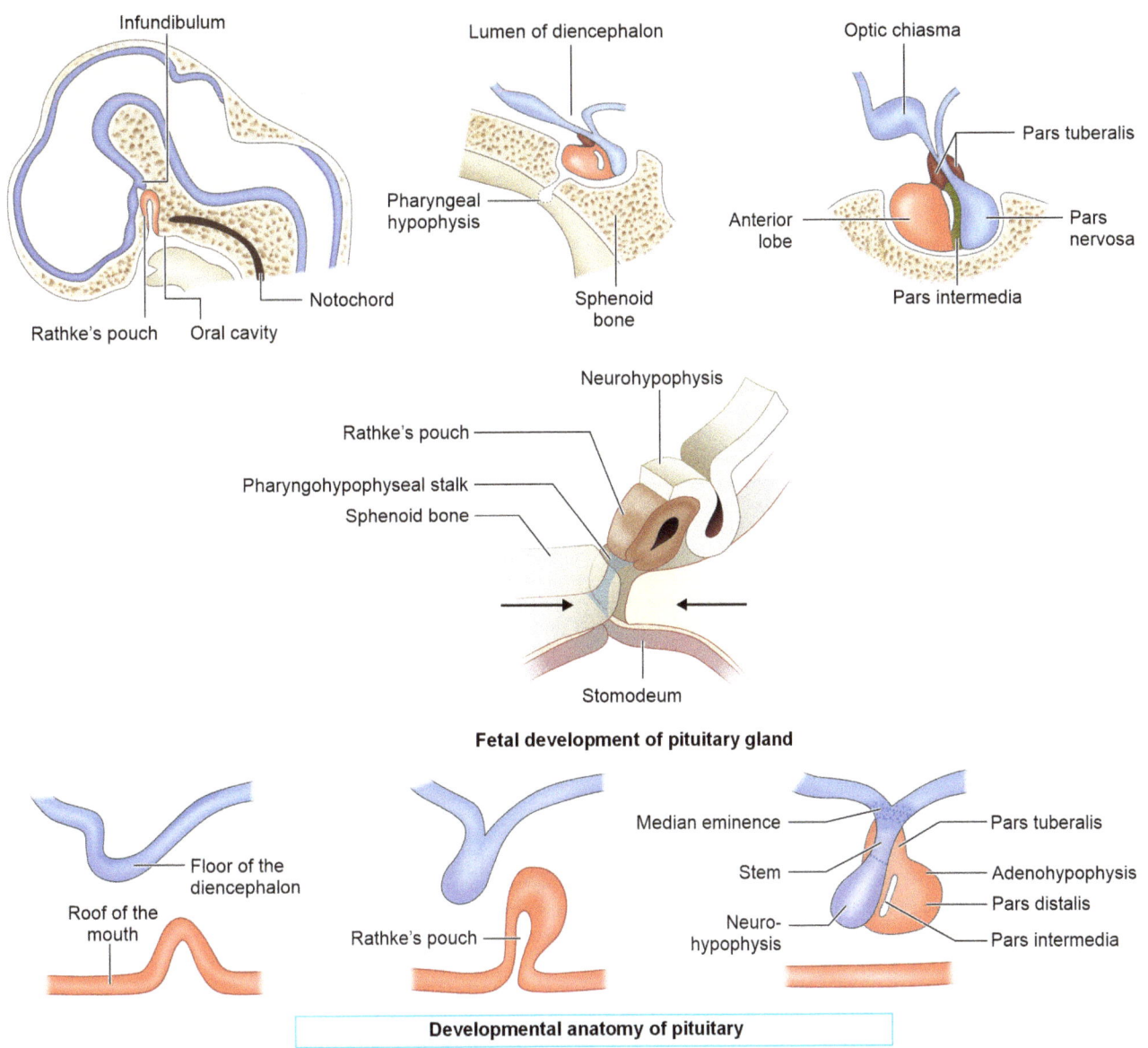

FIG. 2: At 4 weeks: Rathke's pouch, a diverticulum from roof, starts developing. At 5 weeks: Elongation, contacts infundibulum, diverticulum of prosencephalon. At 6–8 weeks: Connecting stalk between pouch and oral cavity degenerates. At 10 weeks: Start producing growth hormone and adrenocorticotropic hormone (ACTH).

Cell patterning and terminal differentiation occurs within the anterior lobe to form the five principal specialized endocrine cell types in different but specific areas of the pituitary gland. The anteromedial area for TSH-producing cells, dorsomedial area, is occupied by nerve terminal of posterior pituitary, ACTH-producing cells in between this two. Two anterolateral areas for GH-producing cells and two posterolateral areas for PRL-producing cells. At 10 weeks: Start producing GH and ACTH **(Fig. 2)**.

PITUITARY DISORDERS

The hormones secreted by pituitary play crucial role in maintaining regulated and synchronized hormonal activities of the body. So, this gland is also leveled as the master endocrine gland. Deranged functional status of the gland is expressed by either excess or deficiency of one or more hormone mediated by it. **Table 1** summarized hormone, cell producing it, factor regulating, target tissue, and disease involved.

TABLE 1: Hormonal source, regulator, target organ/tissue, and disorders of pituitary.				
Hormone	Cells producing	Regulator	Target organ/tissue	Disease (excess/deficiency)
GH	Somatotropes	GHRF/GHIF	Liver	Acromegaly/GHD
PRL	Mamalotropes	PRLIF	Breast/Testes	Galactorrhea
TSH	Thyrotropes	TRH	Thyroid	Hyperthyroidism/Hypothyroidism
ACTH	Ophiocorticotropes	CRF	Adrenal cortex	Cushing's disease/Secondary adrenal failure
FSH	Gonadotropes	GnRH	Ovary/Testes	Hypergonadism/Hypogonadism
LH	Gonadotropes	GnRH	Ovary/Testes	Hypergonadism/Hypogonadism
ADH	Nerve terminals		Kidney	SIAD/CDI
OT	Nerve terminals		Breast/Uterus	Contraction disorders

(ACTH: adrenocorticotropic hormone; ADH: antidiuretic hormone; CDI: cranial diabetes insipidus; CRF: corticotropin-releasing factor; FSH: follicle-stimulating hormone; GH: growth hormone; GHD: growth hormone deficiency; GnRH: gonadotropin-releasing hormone; GHRF: growth hormone-releasing factor; GHIF: growth hormone inhibitory factor; PRLIF: prolactin inhibitory factor; LH: luteinizing hormone; PRL: prolactin; SIAD: syndrome of inappropriate ADH secretion; TSH: thyroid-stimulating hormone)

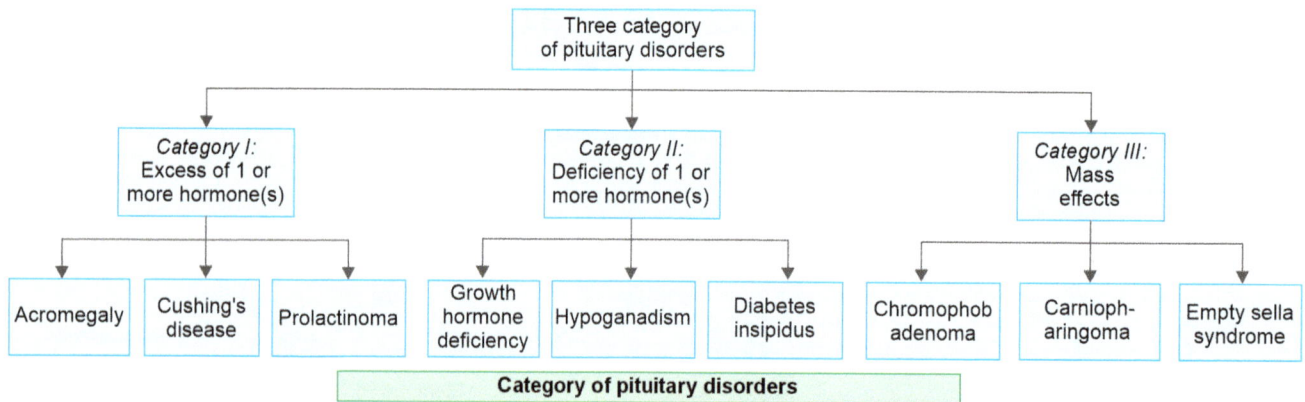

FLOWCHART 2: Category I: Pituitary gland produces excess of one or more hormone(s). Category II: Pituitary gland produces less of one or more hormone(s). Category III: Mass effect producing hormonal imbalance.

Diseases that affect the pituitary gland directly can be divided into three main categories:
- *Category I*: Pituitary gland produces excess of one or more hormone(s). Examples include:
  o Acromegaly/gigantism due to excess GH
  o Cushing's disease due to excess ACTH and
  o Hyperprolactinemia due to excess PRL secretion
- *Category II*: Pituitary gland produces little of one or more hormone(s). Examples include:
  o Adult GH deficiency due to deficiency of GH
  o Diabetes insipidus (DI) due to deficiency of ADH
  o Hypogonadism due to deficiency of LH and FSH
  o Panhypopituitarism due to deficiency of multiple hormones
- *Category III*: Conditions that alter the size and/or shape of the pituitary gland. Examples include:
  o Lesion with mass effect due to chromophob adenoma, prolactinoma, somatotropic adenoma, craniopharyngioma [rarely carotid aneurysm, basal encephalocele, primary central nervous system (CNS) tumors, etc.]
  o Empty sella syndrome (**Flowchart 2**)

Clinical parameters (signs and symptoms) may be obvious in full-blown cases of category I and II disorders, and intensity of the parameters is likely to be proportionate to the severity of abnormality of the particular hormonal (excess or lack). On the other hand, clinical parameters of category III disorders the mass effects (headache and visual disturbance) become dominant over the hormonal features and empty sella syndrome, usually no frank symptoms, is marked and identified during imaging study.

In general, a rational management approach consists of stepped diagnostic workup, treatment/therapy, and then follow-up protocol.
- *Step 1*: Clinical suspicion (signs and symptoms recording)
- *Step 2*: Ophthalmological evaluation (visual field and fundus)

- *Step 3*: Imaging study [(X-ray/computed tomography (CT)/magnetic resonance imaging (MRI)/positron emission tomography (PET) scan]
- *Step 4*: Hormone study

Steps 1 and 4 are mandatory to all case while others should not be skipped because of their potentiality of great informative.

Principle modalities of treatment in category I disease include surgery (including microsurgery), radiation therapy (including Gamma Knife), and drugs; while for category II deficiency replacement, and category III surgery for mass lesions and replacement when required but for empty sella syndrome replacement of particular hormone(s) reserve is poor.

Regarding follow-up: Replacement therapies are lifelong. Follow-up protocols for postsurgery and radiation cases are structured, so that early detection of deficiencies and initiation of replacement can be done keeping cured cases apart.

Disease-specific protocol will be describing in appropriate place.

Hyperpituitarism

Hyperpituitarism belongs to category I. Pituitary disorders due excess production of one or more hormone(s). Example are: (1) Acromegaly, (2) gigantism, (3) prolactinoma, etc. Each of these can clinically present singly or even in combinations **(Flowchart 3)**.

Acromegaly and Gigantism

Both are chronic disfiguring and disabling disorders with increasing morbidity and mortality due to prolong hypersecretion of GH. Adult onset/onset after the closer of epiphysis of long bones shows characteristic enlargement of peripheral (acral) parts of the body (hands and feet including head) are termed as *Acromegaly*. On the other hand, onset before after the closer of epiphysis of long bones results in excessive tallness giving rise to gigantic appearance termed as *Gigantism*.

Clinical Stigmata of Acromegaly

Physical changes in peripheral parts of the body—head, face, hands, and legs—occur insidiously, therefore may remain unnoticed in early states but with time there is:
- Prominent or enlarged nose and supra orbital ridge
- Coarse and puffy face
- Enlarge mandible (*Prognathism*)—lower teeth arch is outer to that of upper one; gap between teeth is increased.
- Large thicken spade-like fingers and toes due to soft tissue enlargement (*acral enlargement*). A bulky sweaty handshake may initiate a diagnostic workup and history of increase in shoe, ring, and hat size may support it **(Figs. 3A to C)**.

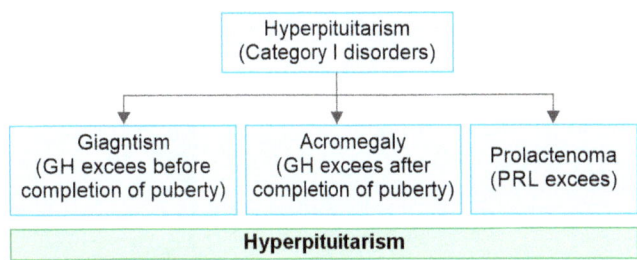

FLOWCHART 3: Category I: Pituitary disorders due to excess production of one or more hormone(s). For example, (1) acromegaly, (2) gigantism, (3) prolactinoma, etc.

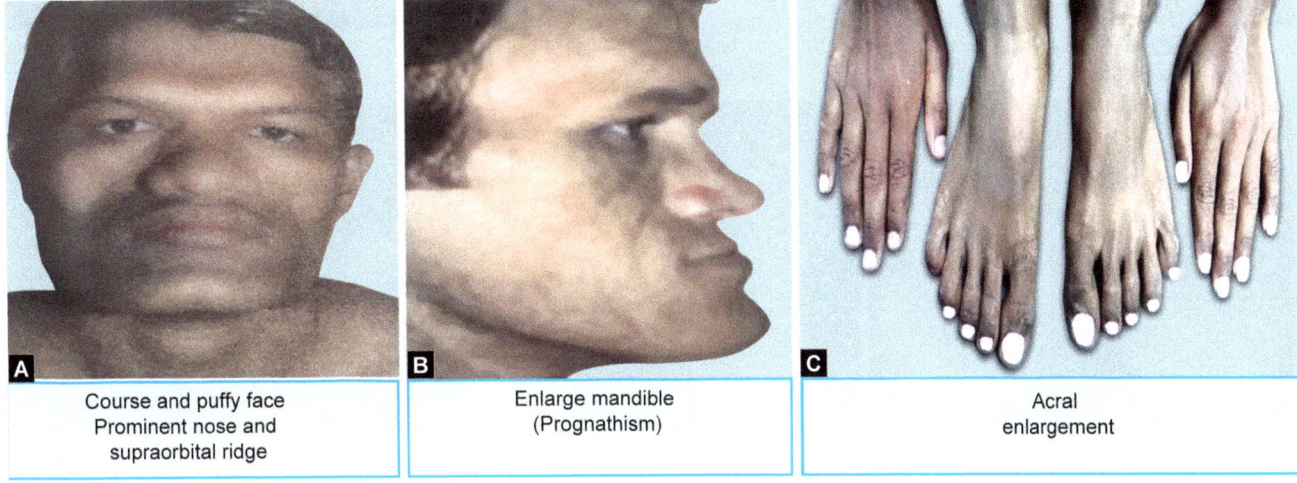

FIGS. 3A TO C: Physical features of acromegaly.

- Other physical stigmata may include:
  - Skin may show increased sweating and oiliness.
  - Acne, sebaceous cysts, and excess body hair are common.
  - Moderate weight gain, fatigue, and lethargy are common complaints.
  - Paresthesia due to entrapment of nerves (e.g., Carpel Tunnel syndrome) is common.
  - Arthralgia and degenerative arthropathies are common in long-standing cases.
  - In adolescence/childhood-onset cases, the person become very tall (*giant*) due to high growth velocity and limb length larger than the body (*eunuchoid*) due to delayed puberty.
- Other stigmata may include:
  - Features of mass lesion in pituitary fossa, such as visual disturbance and headache.
  - Other medical conditions, such as diabetes mellitus, hypertension, renal calculi, and enlarge thyroid.
- Radiological changes are also considered important stigmata for the disease which include:
  - Skull films: (1) Sellar size increase due to mass effect. (2) Other changes due to GH excess: (i) thickened calvarium, (ii) prominent nuchal protuberance, (iii) enlarger paranasal air sinus (maxillary and frontal), and (iv) enlarged mandible with increased interdental space.
  - Hand and leg films: Changes due to GH excess (1) increased soft tissue, (2) increased width of intra articular cartilage, (3) "Arrowhead" tufting of distal phalanges, (4) cystic change in the carpal/tarsal bones, and (5) "Heel pad sign" increased thickening of the heel pad (>18 mm for male and >22 mm for female) (**Figs. 4A to F**).

Three Steps of Diagnostic Workup for Acromegaly/Gigantism

Initial step: Clinical suspicions. It is based on physical (with history) + Radiological stigmata.

Step II: Biochemical documentation of excess secretion of GH secretion and action.

List of endocrine test include:
- Serum somatomedin C [insulin-like growth factor-1 (IGF-1)] level assay (an elevated level virtually establish diagnosis of active acromegaly)
- Serum GH level: Basal level/glucose suppression test for GH

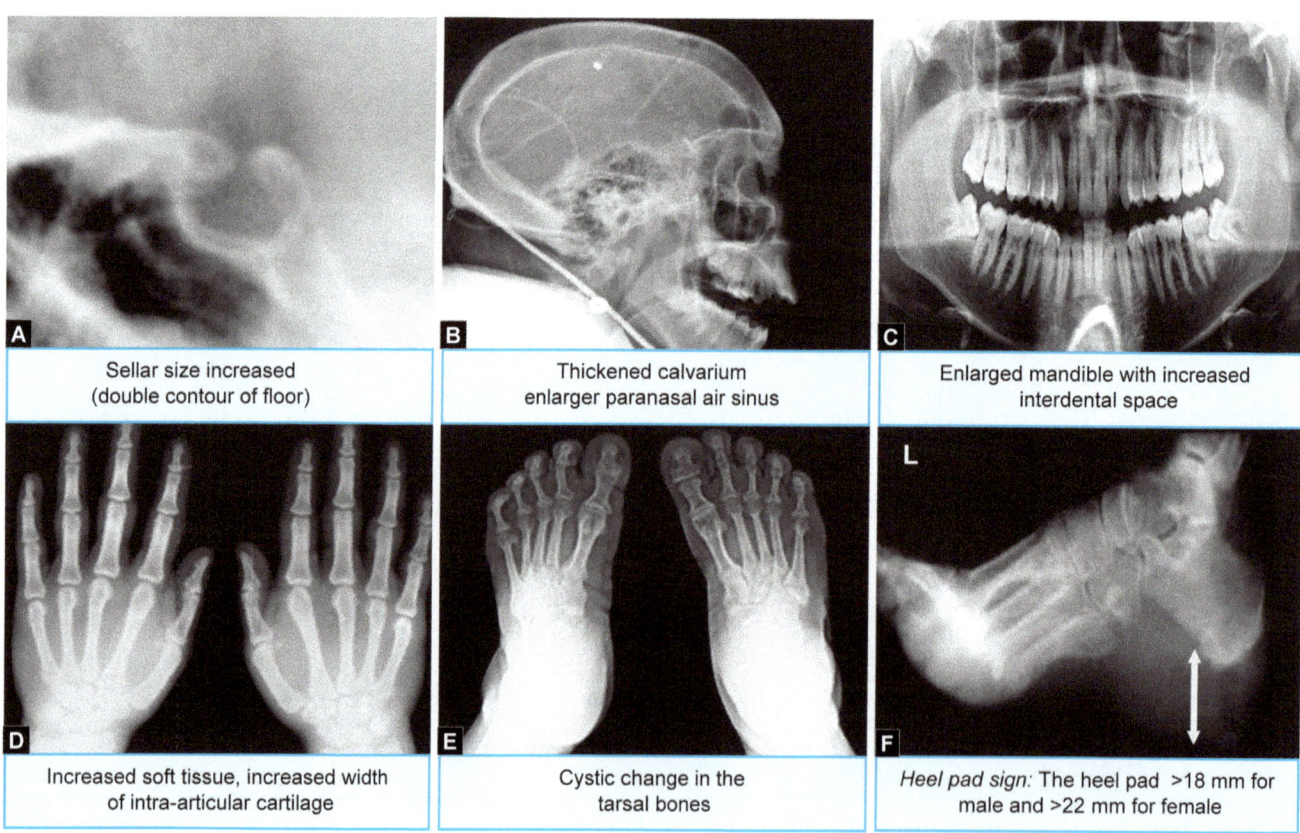

FIGS. 4A TO F: Skull, hand, and leg films of acromegaly.

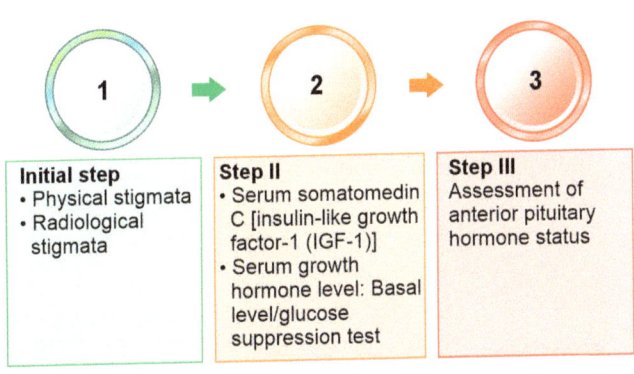

FIG. 5: Three steps diagnosis of acromegaly.

Step III: Assessment of anterior pituitary hormone status.

It is required for diagnostic plus treatment follow-up.

A significant proportion of acromegaly cases will have hyperprolactinemia. Mass effect of somatotropic/somatomamaltropic macroadenoma can produce hypofunction other pituitary tropic hormone(s) **(Fig. 5)**.

Treatment and Follow-up for Acromegaly/Gigantism

Aim of treatment are:
- To halt the disease process by bringing GH secretion to normal
- To relieve the mass effect of a growing pituitary tumor
- To preserve normal pituitary function or treat hormone deficiencies
- To improve the symptoms of acromegaly
  Modalities of treatment for acromegaly/gigantism are: (1) Surgery; (2) radiotherapy, and (3) medicine.

Surgical treatment

Surgery is the first option recommended for most people with acromegaly, as it is often a rapid and effective treatment. The transsphenoidal surgery, where the surgery is done on reaching the pituitary via an incision through the nose or inside the upper lip and removes the tumor tissue, is the preferred method of choice because of its low incidence postoperative hypopituitarism **(Fig. 6)**.

In one study postoperative GH levels <3 ng/mL has documented 90% remission of condition. Some authors consider GH levels <1 ng/mL and IGF-I within 2 standard deviation (SD) of reference range as biochemical cure. After a successful surgery, facial appearance and soft tissue swelling improve within a few days.

Complications of surgery are:
- Damage to the surrounding normal pituitary tissue causing other hormone(s) deficiencies requiring lifelong replacement therapy
- DI usually temporarily but rarely may be permanent.
- Other potential problems include cerebrospinal fluid leaks and, rarely, meningitis.

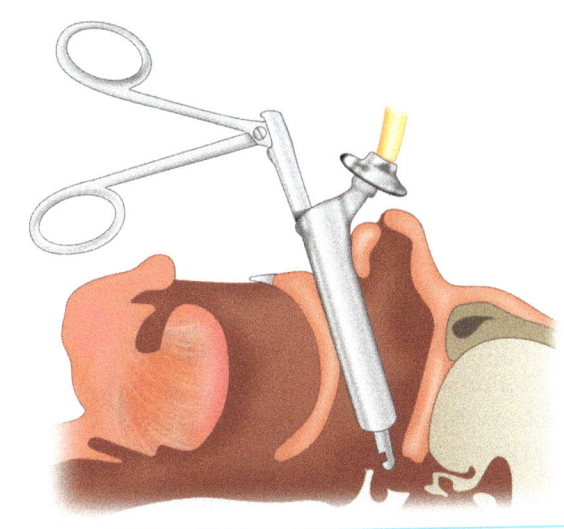

FIG. 6: Transsphenoidal surgery of acromegaly.
(*Successful surgery*: Postoperative growth hormone (GH) levels <3 ng/mL have documented 90% remission of condition. GH levels <1 ng/mL and insulin-like growth factor-1 (IGF-1) within 2 SD of reference range are considered biochemical cure. After surgery, facial appearance and soft tissue swelling improve within a few days).

Follow-up of pituitary surgery cases: Even after a successful surgery with return of hormone levels to normal, people with acromegaly must be carefully monitored for years, because there is chance of recurrence of the disease. Commonly hormone levels improve, but do not return to normal; therefore, additional treatment may be required particularly steroid coverage during stress.

Radiotherapy

In general, radiation therapy is recommended if GH hypersecretion is not normalized with surgery. Radiation prevents further growth of the tumor in >99% of patients after surgical resection.

Conventional super voltage irradiation of total 4,500 to 5,000 rads are given in divided dose (usually five times a week over 4–6 weeks). In general, radiation treatment takes very long time to bring down GH/IGF-I level to their target. In one series, at 2, 5, and 10 years after radiation 38%, 73%, and 81%, respectively were found to have a normal GH. A significant proportion of cases will ultimate become panhypopituitarism/hypoadrenalism/hypogonadism. Some studies suggest that radiation is associated with the development of secondary tumors.

Local irradiation by heavy particle implantation (Yttrium 99 or Iridium 192) may bring remission relatively early (approximately 80% by 5 years). But the drawback of this include (1) local radiation narcosis and (2) procedure involve all faculties of microsurgery plus implantation material handling.

Stereotactic radiosurgery/stereotactic radiation therapy

After determination of location and amount of the tissue to be destroyed by use of CT/MRI, the total radiation dose is calculated and delivered in a single session (radiosurgery) or in few sessions (radiotherapy). There are two types of machine of this purpose. One that produce hundreds of weak beams converge at the tumor to give a higher radiation dose, e.g., Gamma Knife. And other ones continuously produce beams by a linear accelerator and moves around the head, e.g., X-Knife, CyberKnife, Clinac, etc. Tumors with irregular shape does not respond well with such treatment. This therapy is also avoided if the tumor is very close to the optic nerves **(Fig. 7)**.

Therapy with proton beam radiation

In this form of treatment, a beam of protons is used instead of X-rays. Protons are positive parts of atoms; they cause little damage to tissues; they pass through and only release their energy after traveling a desire distance. So, it has the advantage of focusing the radiation more precisely on the tumor cell. This therapy is still under investigation if it is proven safer or more effective than stereotactic radiosurgery or stereotactic radiotherapy, and may become the future modality for the purpose **(Fig. 8)**.

Medical therapy

Medical therapy is the least promising modality. There are three groups of drugs—(1) Somatostatin analogs, (2) GH antagonists, and (3) dopamine agonist.

- *Somatostatin analogs*: They blocks GH (somatotropin) production by adenomas. Short acting-octreotide (Sandostatin) is given subcutaneously three times daily; while long-acting lanreotide (Somatuline Depot) and pasireotide (Signifor LAR) are given as injection

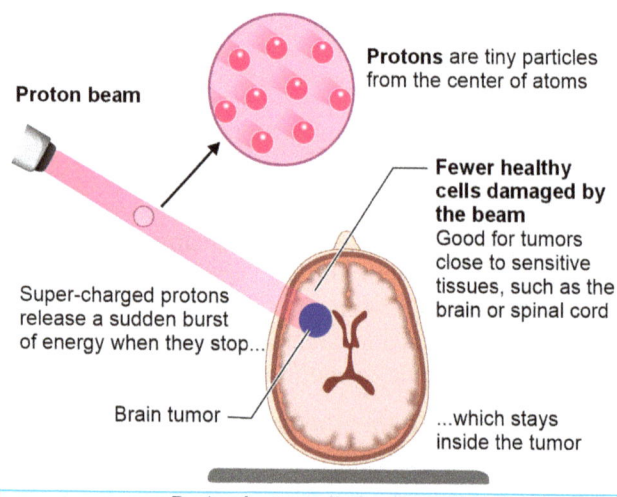

Proton beam radiation therapy

FIG. 8: Protons are positive parts of atoms; they cause little damage to tissues they pass through and only release their energy after traveling a certain distance. Like stereotactic radiation, it has the advantage of focusing the radiation more precisely on the tumor cell. It is likely to become the future modality for the purpose.

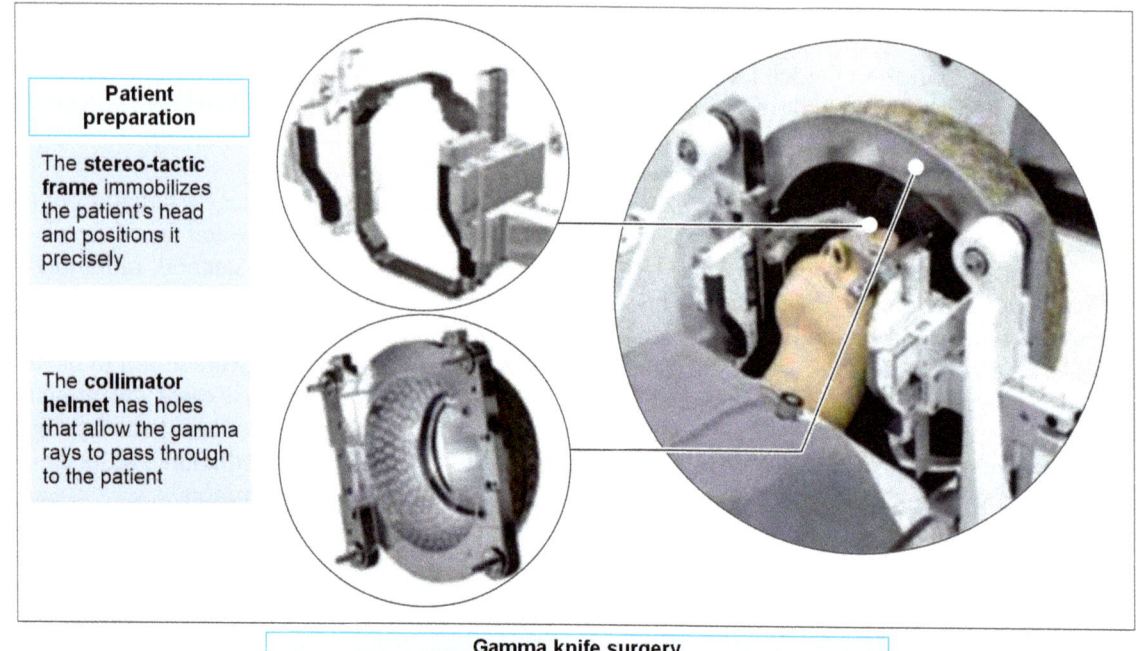

Gamma knife surgery

FIG. 7: Hundreds of weak beams converge at the tumor to give a higher radiation dose.

once in every 4 weeks. Serum GH and IGF-1 levels drop down slowly and are monitored periodically. Tumors size shrinks very slowly. Side effects of them include bradycardia, nausea, vomiting, diarrhea, stomach pain, dizziness, headache, and pain at the site of injection.
- *Growth hormone antagonists*: Pegvisomant (Somavert®) works by blocking the action of GH on target cells. It can effectively lower blood IGF-1 levels, but cannot block GH secretion by the pituitary gland or shrink pituitary tumors. Its side effects include hypoglycemia and may cause mild liver damage in some people. It is administered daily by subcutaneous injection.
- *Dopamine agonists*: Cabergoline or bromocriptine can reduce GH levels in about 20% patients. Usually higher doses are needed for these tumors than for prolactinomas. Some patients have trouble with their side effects. An advantage of these drugs is that they are taken orally.

Prolactinomas

Hypersecretion of PRL by mamalotrophs of anterior pituitary from an adenoma (macro- or microadenoma) or hyperplasia. Clinically in women, it usually presents with amenorrhea and galactorrhea, and in men decreased libido, infertility, and rarely galactorrhea. Women seek medical attention earlier due to menstrual disturbance, but in men prolactinoma may remain unnoticed till a mass effect of a huge lesion become obvious.

Causes of hyperprolactinemias include diseases and drugs. **Table 2** summarizes the cause list.

Three Step of Diagnostic Workup for Hyperprolactinemia

Step I: Clinical suspicion depends on (1) galactorrhea, (2) oligomenorrhoea or amenorrhea, (3) decreased libido of male and female, (4) signs and symptoms of estrogen (in female) or androgen (in male) deficiency, (5) delayed or arrested puberty, or (6) suspected pituitary tumor.

Step II: Hormone assay:
- Serum PRL
- TSH and (other when indicated by clinical clue)

Step III: Assessment of adenoma size/effect:
- Sellar imaging (X-ray/CT/MRI)
- Visual fields/evoked potential study **(Figs. 9 and 10)**

Treatments and Drugs

Goals in the treatment of prolactinoma include:
- Return the production of PRL to normal levels
- Restore normal pituitary gland function
- Reduce the size of the pituitary tumor
- Eliminate any signs or symptoms from tumor pressure, such as headaches or vision problems
- Improve quality of life

Sl. no	Class/group	Disease/drugs
	TABLE 2: Cause list of hyperprolactinemias.	
1	Pituitary cause	Prolactinoma, acromegaly
2	Hypothalamic disease	Craniopharyngioma, meningioma, sarcoidosis, dysmeningiomas, eosinophilic granuloma, stalk lesion, etc.
3	Neurogenic cause	Nipple stimulation, spinal cord lesions, and chest wall lesions
4	Medication	*Antipsychotics*: Haloperidol chlorpromazine, thioridazine, thiothixene, risperidone, amisulpride, molindone, and zotepine
		Antidepressants: *Tricyclic*—amitriptyline, desipramine, clomipramine, and amoxapine
		SSRI: Sertraline, fluoxetine, and paroxetine
		MAO-I: Pargyline and clorgyline
		Other psychotropics: Buspirone and alprazolam
		Prokinetics: Metoclopramide and domperidone
		Antihypertensive: Alpha-methyldopa, reserpine, and verapamil
		Opiates: Morphine
		H_2 *antagonists*: Cimetidine and ranitidine
		Other drugs: Fenfluramine, physostigmine, and chemotherapeutics
5	Other cause	Pregnancy, primary hypothyroidism, cirrhosis of liver, and chronic renal failure
6	Idiopathic	

Prolactinoma treatment consists of two main therapies: medications and surgery.

1. *Medical therapy*: It is the most promising modality. They are the dopamine agonists which are capable to decrease PRL production and reducing the tumor of most prolactinoma. (1) Bromocriptine and (2) cabergoline are mostly used. Other drugs are lisuride and quinagolide. Cabergoline is preferred than bromocriptine, because it is more effective and has less side effects. Both the drugs are considered safe in early pregnancy, but their safety throughout pregnancy is not yet established. Common side effects of the drugs are nausea and vomiting, nasal stuffiness, headache, and drowsiness. The drugs may be tapered if the tumor size reduces significantly and PRL level remains normal at least for 2 years but follow-up is recommended.
2. *Surgery for prolactinoma*: It is preserved for (1) medically nonresponsive cases and (2) pregnancy planning in women with large tumor having pressure/mass effect. The surgery is usually *transsphenoidal surgery*; rarely large tumor or has spread to nearby brain tissue may require *transcranial surgery*.

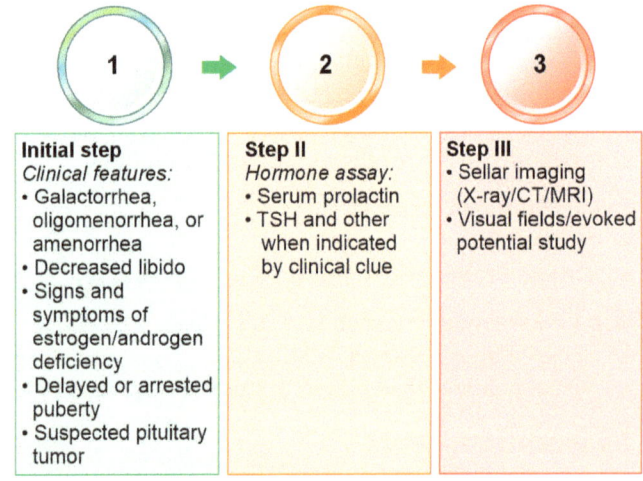

FIG. 9: Three steps of diagnosis of hyperprolactinemia.

Hypopituitarism

Hypopituitarism is defined by recognizable failure (either clinically or by laboratory tests) of secretory functions

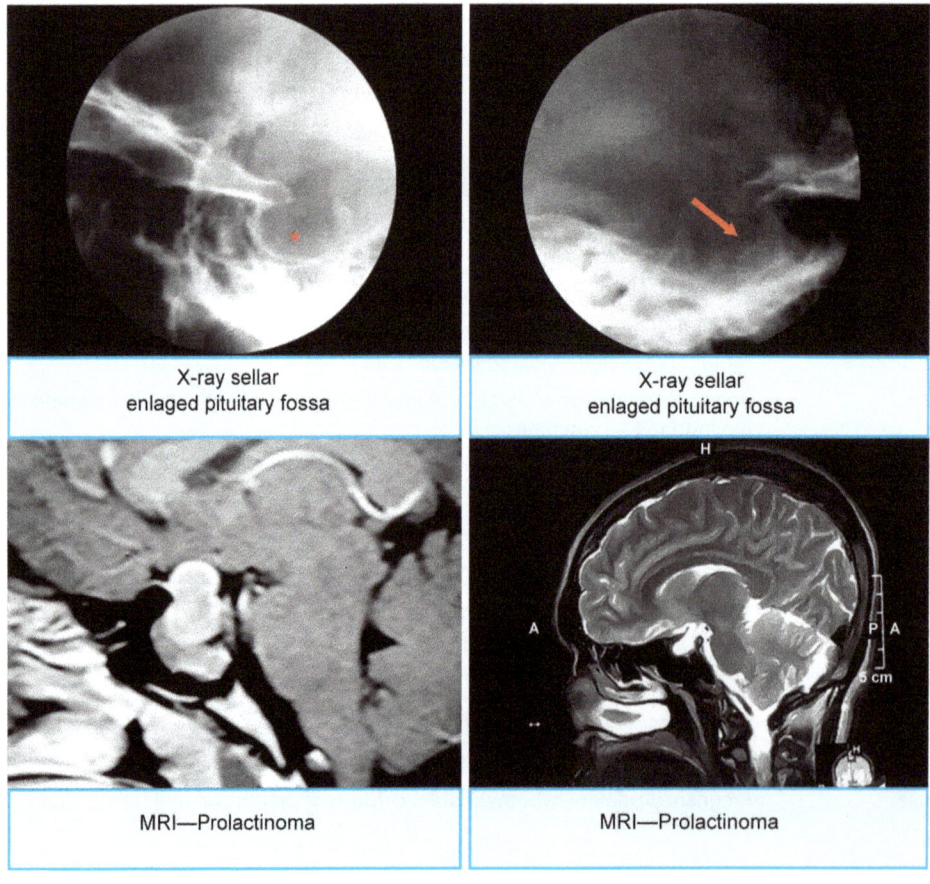

FIG. 10: Imaging (X-ray/MRI) features of case with hyperprolactinemias.

of one/more hormones of anterior pituitary (isolated/panhypopituitarism). Onset of pituitary insufficiency is often gradual. Clinical features are related to lack of individual pituitary hormone and their target gland deficiency.

Causes of hypopituitarism: Nine I's *Invasive, Injury, Immunologic, Infection, Infarction, Infiltrative, Iatrogenic, Isolated,* and *Idiopathic*.

Table 3 summarizes the cause list.

Sheehan's Syndrome

Hypopituitarism is a result of ischemic damage of anterior pituitary in postpartum period, following hemorrhage and vascular collapse.

The pituitary is one of the highly vascularized tissues in the body. Its volume increases twofolds during pregnancy, mostly due to the massive hyperplasia of lactotrophs as a result of elevated estrogen secretion. Enlarged pituitary gland is vulnerable to ischemia and does not have the ability to regenerate. Scar tissue substitutes the necrotic cells. The presence of 50% of pituitary gland is sufficient for the maintenance of normal functions. Clinical picture of a Sheehan's syndrome is determined by the extent of the pituitary damage. Clinical features are usually not seen until 75% of the cell mass is destroyed.

Clinical presentation of Sheehan's syndrome with their relative frequencies (as per some old large studies) is given in **Table 4**.

Diagnostic Work up for Sheehan's Syndrome

Step I: Clinical suspicion
(see clinical features in **Flowchart 4**).

Step II: Hormone assay:
- Serum PRL
- *Paired tests*: TSH and FT_4; FSH, LH, and estrogen; ACTH and cortisol
- *Stimulation test*: Triple stimulation test [A sequential pituitary *stimulation test*, consisting of (1) insulin-induced hypoglycemia followed by (2) stimulation of gonadotropin-releasing hormone (GnRH), and (3) thyroid-releasing hormone].

Hormone study result will document deficiencies of hormones are due to anterior pituitary deficiency disorder.

TABLE 3: Cause list of Sheehan's syndrome.

Sl. no	Class/group	Diseases
1	Invasive	Craniopharyngioma, large pituitary tumors, carotid aneurysm, basal encephalocele, CNS tumors, e.g., meningioma, chordoma, optic glioma, epidermoma, dermoid, and pineal tumors
2	Injury	Head injury and child abuse
3	Immunologic	Lymphocytic hypophysitis
4	Infection	Tuberculosis, syphilis, and mycosis
5	Infarction	Postpartum necrosis (Sheehan's syndrome), pituitary apoplexy
6	Infiltrative	Histiocytosis, sarcoidosis, and hemochromatosis
7	Iatrogenic	Surgery and radiation
8	Isolated	Growth hormone deficiency, gonadotropin hormone deficiency, ACTH hormone deficiency, and TSH hormone deficiency
9	Idiopathic	Familial

(ACTH: adrenocorticotropic hormone; CNS: central nervous system; TSH: thyroid-stimulating hormone)

TABLE 4: Symptoms of Sheehan's syndrome in relation to pituitary hormone deficiency.

Due to gonadotropin deficiency	Due to ACTH deficiency	Due to TSH deficiency
• Failure to lactate after giving birth (90%) • Failure to start menstruation again (90%) • Atrophy of breast, vagina and uterus (superinvolution) (80%) • Loss of libido (95%) • Loss of body hairs—pubic hairs do not grow after shave of at the time of delivery (95%)	• Hypotension (90%) • Asthenia, lethargy (100%) • Anorexia (90%) • Weight loss (80%) • Pale skin, lack of pigmentation, absence of sun tan (80%) • Loss of pigmentation from nipples and areola (80%)	• Delayed relaxation of ankle jerk (90%) • Dry skin (80%) • Cold intolerance (80%) • Myxedematous face (30%)

Note: If hypopituitarism is unrecognized or untreated death may result from adrenal crisis or profound hypoglycemia.

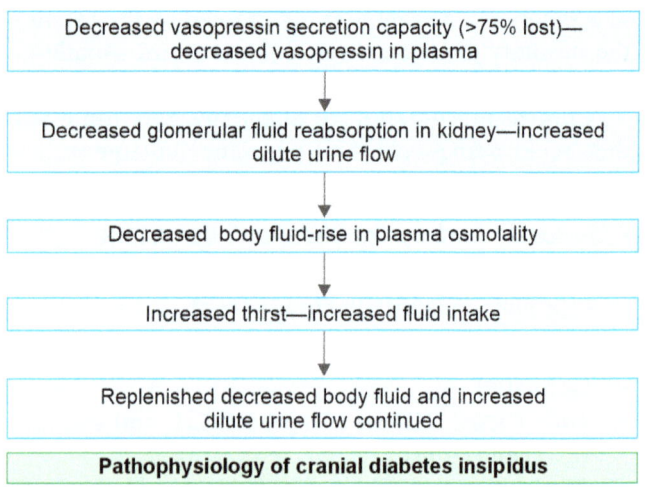

FLOWCHART 4: Cranial diabetes insipidus is due to deficiency of vasopressin.

Treatment of Sheehan's Syndrome

Principle: Replacement of target gland hormone deficiencies for all and GH and ovulation induction is considered in some cases when needed. Steroid and thyroid replacements are life-saving while others are considered for improvement of quality of life.
- *For ACTH deficiency*: Glucocorticoid–hydrocortisone (30 mg/day), prednisolone (7.5 mg/day) or cortisone (35 mg/day) in two divided doses with morning:evening = 2:1 ration is the maintenance dose. Doses have to be increased for stress coverage.
- *For TSH deficiency*: Free thyroxine (FT_4) replacement is started with a low dose, after glucocorticoid replacement is established, and the dose is titrated to reach its serum level at or around the median of the normal reference range.
- *For gonadotropin deficiency*: Estrogen and progesterone replacement therapy is done with same protocol for a hormone replacement therapy (HRT) for a postmenopausal woman (HRT). But if wants fertility should undergo ovulation induction with assisted reproductive technique (ART).
- *For GH and PRL deficiency*: Growth hormone replacement with recombinant human growth hormone (hGH) can be done to maintain a serum IGF-1 level normal, but yet it is not popular. Treatment for PRL deficiency is still not tried by anybody.

POSTERIOR PITUITARY DISORDERS

Hormones of the posterior pituitary: Vasopressin/ADH and oxytocin and important diseases include:
- DI
- Syndrome of inappropriate ADH secretion (SIAD).

Diabetes Insipidus

Definition: Diabetes insipidus is characterized by the excretion of abnormally large amount of dilute urine due to lack or ineffectiveness of vasopressin. Quantitatively, DI may be defined as 24-hour urine volume >2.5 L and specific gravity <1.010 or osmolality <300 mOsmol/kg of water.

Signs and Symptoms

The predominant manifestations of DI are as follows: (1) Polyuria: The daily urine volume is relatively constant for each patient but is highly variable between patients (3–20 L), (2) polydipsia, and (3) nocturia. The most common form is central DI after trauma or surgery to the region of the pituitary and hypothalamus, which may exhibit either as transient or permanent.

In infants with DI, the most apparent signs may be the following: (1) Crying, (2) irritability, (3) growth retardation, (4) hyperthermia, (5) weight loss, etc.

In children, the following manifestations typically predominate: (1) Enuresis, (2) anorexia, (3) growth failure, and (4) fatigability.

Physical findings vary with the severity and chronicity of DI; they may be entirely normal or may include the following: (1) Hydronephrosis, with pelvic fullness, flank pain or tenderness, or pain radiating to the testicle or genital area, (2) bladder enlargement in some patients, and (3) dehydration if the thirst mechanism is impaired or access to fluid is restricted **(Table 5)**.

On the basis of causes, nonosmotic polyuria or abnormally large volume of dilute urine is subgrouped into three categories. The nomenclatures are:
- *Category I*: Cranial diabetes insipidus (CDI). Other names: Neurogenic, hypothalamic, or vasopressin sensitive DI
- *Category II*: Nephrogenic diabetes insipidus (NDI). Other names: Vasopressin insensitive DI
- *Category III*: Primary polydipsia (PP). Other names: Potomania, dipsogenic DI, or compulsive water drinking

The cause list of nonosmotic polyuria varies according to the category as described in **Table 6**.

TABLE 5: Symptoms of diabetes insipidus (DI) according to age.		
In adult	In neonate	In children
• Polyuria • Polydipsia • Nocturia	• Crying • Irritability • Growth retardation • Hyperthermia • Weight loss, etc.	• Enuresis • Anorexia • Growth failure • Fatigability

CHAPTER 2: Disorders of Pituitary Gland

TABLE 6: The cause list of nonosmotic polyuria.

Sl. no	Category	Causes
1	*Category I*: Cranial diabetes insipidus (CDI)	Traumatic such as head trauma, surgery at or around hypothalamus
		Vascular injury such as Sheehan's syndrome, aneurysm, coronary artery bypass, etc.
		Granulomatous diseases: Histiocytosis-X, sarcoidosis, etc.
		Infection: Meningitis and encephalitis
		Pituitary hypothalamic tumor, benign or metastatic, from breast and lung
		Idiopathic or unknown, approximately 50% of cases are idiopathic
2	*Category II*: Nephrogenic diabetes insipidus (NDI)	Drugs such as lithium, demeclocycline, and methoxyflurane
		Metabolic disorders such as hypocalcemia and hypercalcemia
		Vascular: Sickle cell disease
		Granulomatous: Sarcoidosis
		Infection: Cystitis, pyelonephritis
		Idiopathic
		Familial (sex-linked recessive)
3	*Category III*: Primary polydipsia (PP)	*Psychogenic*: Schizophrenia and mania
		Granulomatous: Sarcoidosis
		Metabolic: Hypocalcemia
		Infection: Tuberculous meningitis
		Vasculitis
		Drug: Lithium
		Other: Multiple sclerosis

Pathophysiology of Nonosmotic Polyuria

Pathophysiology of nonosmotic polyuria in the three categories is different.

The initial event are (1) Decreased vasopressin secretion capacity, (2) renal insensitivity to vasopressin, and (3) compulsive water/fluid intake in CDI, NDI, and PP, respectively. Sequences of events are described in **Flowcharts 4 to 6**.

Diagnosis of the three conditions of increased dilute urine flow:
- *Category I*: CDI depends on documentation of inability to produce vasopressin in the face of hyperosmolality of plasma.
- *Category II*: NDI depends on documentation of inability vasopressin to concentrate urine due to resistance at kidney.
- *Category III*: PP depends on documentation of low plasma osmolality (Posm) and intact urine concentrating capacity after normalization of Posm.

Diagnostic approach is a five-step process:
Step 1: To ascertain nonosmotic polyuria measurement of:
- Urine specific gravity and/or osmolality
- Urine volume per day and/or urine flow rate during sleeping

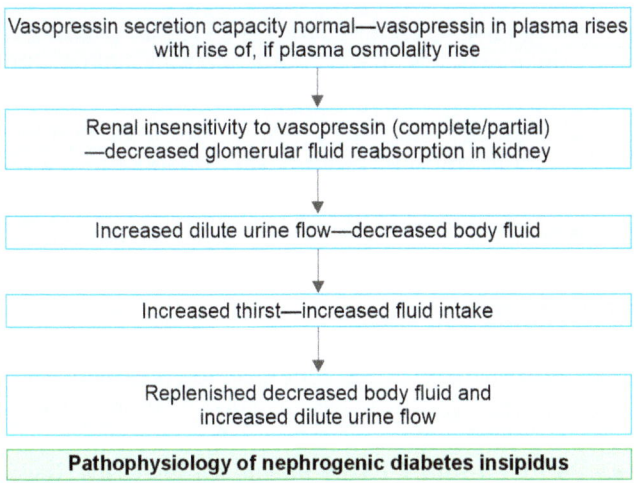

FLOWCHART 5: Nephrogenic diabetes insipidus is due to insensitivity of vasopressin.

Positive result means urine specific gravity <1.010 and/or osmolality < Posm, and urine volume per day >3 L and/or urine flow rate during sleeping >1.5 mL/min. Severity is also scaled as mild, moderate, and severe for volume per day <4.5, 4.5–9 and >9 L.

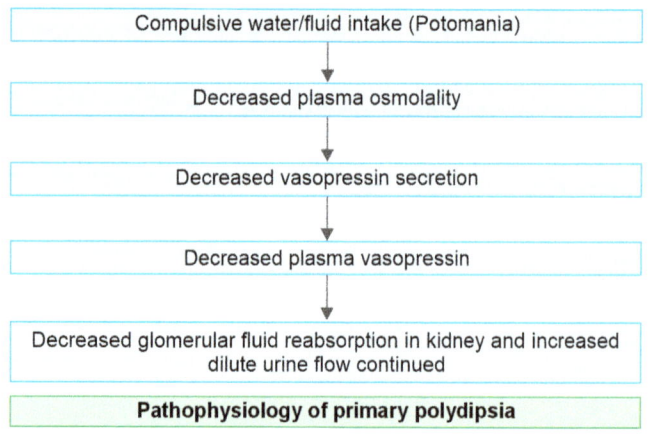

FLOWCHART 6: Primary polydipsia is due to decreased serum vasopressin level in response to excess water intake.

Step 2: For spot identification of DI at ad libitum water intake:
- Posm and/or serum sodium
- Corresponding urine osmolality (Uosm)

Positive result means Posm > 296 mOsm/L and/or serum sodium > 143 mEq/L, and Uosm < Posm.

Step 3: To differentiate between DI and PP measurement of Posm and Uosm during water deprivation.
- Urine osmolality and volumes are measured at an interval of 1–2 hours
- Posm and serum sodium are measured at midpoint of urine volume measurements.

Positive result for DI means a high urine flow rate with Posm > 296 mOsm/L and/or serum sodium > 143 mEq/L, and Uosm < Posm.

Positive result for PP means a low urine flow rate (about 0.5 mL/min) with Posm < 296 mOsm/L and/or serum sodium < 143 mmol/L, and Uosm > Posm (usually >1.5 times).

Step 4: To differentiate between CDI and NDI vasopressin sensitivity test for DI cases.

After initiating fluid intake restriction for 2–3 hours, a test dose of 5–10 units desmopressin (dDAVP) nasal spray or 2 µg subcutaneous injection is given. Urine flow rate, Uosm, and Posm are measured serially or hourly.
- Positive result for CDI means a progressive lowering urine flow rate (about 0.5 mL/min) with Posm < 296 mOsm/L and/or serum sodium < 143 mmol/L, and Uosm > Posm (usually >1.5 times). There will be improvement of patient due to prompt and complete abolishment of the thirst, polydipsia, and polyuria.
- Positive result for NDI means no such changes.

Step 5: Look for causes **(Table 6)**

Water Deprivation Test

A test to measure how much urine is made and how concentrated it becomes when no water is given to a patient for a certain amount of time.

The patient is allowed fluids overnight. The patient is deprived of fluids for 8 hours or until 5% of the body mass has been lost. The patient needs to be weighed hourly. Posm is measured 2 hourly and urine volume and osmolality every hour.

The test will last for around 6–8 hours. You will be required to stay at the hospital for the duration of the test to give regular blood and urine samples. It helps to bring something to read or listen to as there will be periods of waiting.

dDAVP Challenge Test

- Inject 2 µg of dDAVP subcutaneously
- Ask patient to empty bladder at 1 and 2 hours after the injection and measure the osmolality of these samples.
- If either sample has an osmolality >50% higher than the value immediately before dDAVP was given, the patient probably has complete (severe) neurogenic DI.
- If the rise in Uosm after dDAVP is <50%, then complete (severe) nephrogenic DI is very likely.

Syndrome of Inappropriate Antidiuresis

Features associated with hypoosmolality with normal extracellular fluid volume (euvolemia) due to inappropriate (abnormal) secretion of ADH is called syndrome of inappropriate antidiuresis. SIAD is the most common causes of hyponatremia. It is a disorder of sodium and water balance. There is a big list of causes of SIAD, and they can be grouped into categories as summarized in **Table 7**.

Clinical Features of Syndrome of Inappropriate Antidiuresis

Clinical manifestation of SIAD is from hypoosmolality and mostly of neurological due to brain edema. Significant symptoms do not occur until serum sodium falls <125 mEq/L. Severity of symptoms can be roughly correlated with the degree of hypoosmolality and ran rapidity of its development. Features of SIAD are leveled as either essential or supplementary. There are five essential and three supplementary shown in **Table 8**.

Management of Syndrome of Inappropriate Antidiuresis

Management depends on type of presentation. Presentation may be (A) acute onset (<24 hours or coma, seizure),

TABLE 7: Cause list of syndrome of inappropriate antidiuresis (SIAD).

Category	Group	Disease
1	Neoplastic disorders	(A) Carcinoma (e.g., CA lung), (B) Lymphoma, (C) Leukemia, (D) Mesothelioma, (E) Sarcoma, (F) Thymoma, etc.
2	Respiratory disorders	(A) Asthma, (B) Empyema, (C) Pneumonia, (D) Positive pressure ventilation, (E) Pneumothorax, (F) Tuberculosis, etc.
3	Central nervous system disorders	(A) Acute intermittent porphyria, (B) Brain abscess or tumor, (C) Cerebral thrombosis, (D) Encephalitis, (E) Guillain–Barré syndrome, (F) Head injury, (G) Meningitis, (H) Subarachnoid hemorrhage
4	Drugs	(A) Carbamazepine, (B) Chlorpropamide, (C) Clofibrate, (D) Cyclophosphamide, (E) Monoamine oxidase inhibitors, (F) Nicotine, (G) Oxytocin, (H) Thiazide diuretics, (I) Vasopressin, (J) Vinblastine, (K) Vincristine, etc.
5	Others	(A) Adrenal insufficiency, (B) Hypothyroidism, (C) Idiopathic, (D) Postoperative, (e) Psychosis

TABLE 8: Clinical features of syndrome of inappropriate antidiuresis (SIAD).

Five essential features

1. Decreased effective osmolality of extracellular fluid

    Posm < 127 mOsm/kg H_2O

2. Inappropriately concentrated urine

    Uosm > 100 mOsm/kg with normal renal function

3. Normal fluid volume (euvolemia)

    Absent—*hypervolemia* (subcutaneous edema or ascites) *or hypovolemia* (orthostasis, tachycardia, decreased skin turgor, dry mucous membrane)

4. Elevated urinary sodium excretion (with normal salt and water intake)

5. Absence of other causes of euvolemic hypoosmolality

    Not on diuretic, inadequately treated or untreated hypothyroid and adrenal insufficiency

Supplementary features

1. Abnormal water load test

    4-hour urine collection after a 20 mL/kg water drinking: Urine volume < 90% of water volume and/or Uosm <100 mOsm/kg

2. Inappropriate elevated plasma vasopressin (in relation to corresponding Posm)

3. Fluid restriction improve plasma osmolality

(B) moderate symptoms (duration is uncertain), or (C) asymptomatic **(Figs. 11A to C)**.

- *Acute onset (<24 hours or coma, seizure)*: Start immediate correction by (1) 3% saline infusion at 1-2 mL/kg body weight per hour; (2) injection furosemide 20 mg intravenous with an aim of increasing serum sodium 2 mmol/L/h. Check serum sodium 2 hourly to adjust infusion rate. Stop infusion after symptoms improve. Begin diagnostic evaluation.
- *Moderate symptoms (duration is uncertain)*: Begin diagnostic evaluation to rule out extracellular fluid volume depletion (CT/MRI). If volume depletion is present, use only 0.9 saline otherwise add 20 mg of furosemides with an aim to raise serum sodium 0.5-2 mmol/L/h. Stop when serum sodium raises 8-10 mmol/L in first 24 hours. Check serum sodium 4 hourly to adjust infusion rate.
- *Asymptomatic*: Begin diagnostic evaluation and restrict fluid intake.

For all three types, diagnostic evaluation consists of rule out or address correctable factors.

For chronic hyponatremia, restrict fluid intake and encourage dietary intake of salt and protein. If hyponatremia still persists, demeclocycline, urea, or vasopressin receptor agonist may be considered.

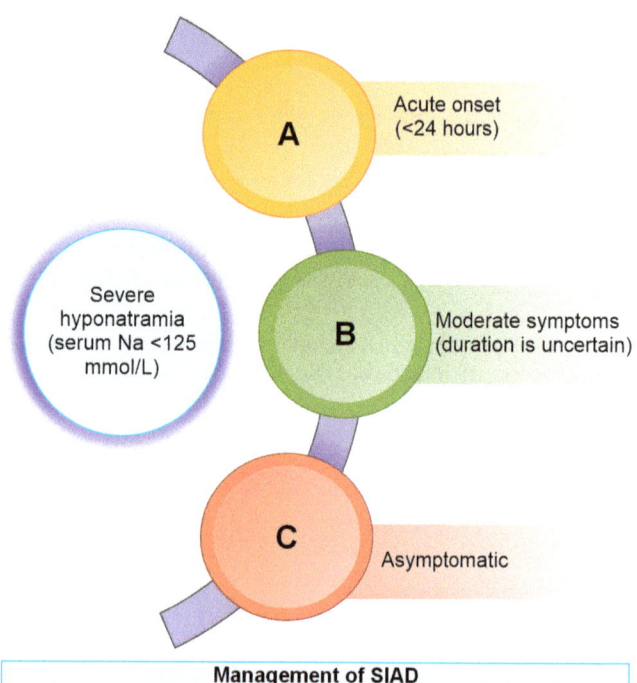

FIGS. 11A TO C: Management according to type of presentation. Presentation may be: (A) Acute onset (<24 hours or coma, seizure), (B) Moderate symptoms (duration is uncertain), or (C) Asymptomatic.

PITUITARY INCIDENTALOMA

A pituitary lesion that is discovered on imaging study in a person with no obvious symptoms to suggest pituitary disease is called "Pituitary Incidentaloma." Studies documented the incidence of such lesion vary from 10% to 20% of the population. A pituitary lesion detected on imaging study most commonly a pituitary adenoma (either functional or nonfunctional), but it may also be a Rathke cleft cyst, craniopharyngioma, meningioma, hypophysitis, or metastasis.

Functioning pituitary adenomas are less common than the nonfunctioning. Functional tumors may show sign and symptoms related to the hormone(s) secreted by the lesion. The nonfunctional pituitary tumors can present with symptoms of the pressure effect such as difficulty of vision, headache, and specific hormone(s) deficiency. Microincidentalomas (size <10 mm) are usually a benign in character, but macroincidentalomas (≥10 mm) carried the risk for hormone abnormalities and mass effects.

Management of such a lesion requires a five-step process: (1) Clinical and imaging (with/without ophthalmological) evaluation; (2) Hormonal study for deficiency disease(s); (3) Hormonal study for hypersecretion(s); (4) Treatment if indicated, or (5) Follow-up of incidentaloma.

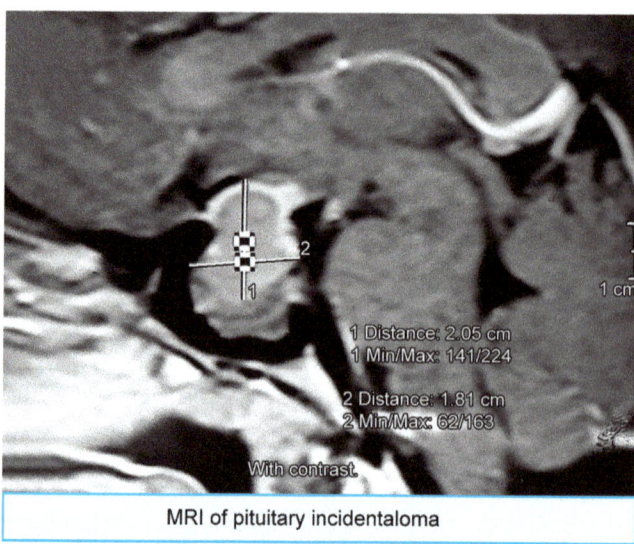

FIG. 12: MRI is to be done in all cases that were initially diagnosed by CT. If there is compression of the optic chiasm, visual field assessment by perimetry is to be done.

1. Patients with pituitary incidentaloma are to be evaluated initially by followings steps:
   i. A detailed medical history and physical examination
   ii. Hormonal laboratory investigation to evaluate pituitary hormone excess or deficiency
   iii. If initially diagnosed by computed tomography than MRI in all cases
   iv. If MRI documents presence of a tumor abutting the optic nerves or chiasma than visual field assessment **(Fig. 12)**.
2. Screening tests for hormonal deficiency in pituitary incidentaloma are of two types:
   i. Initial test should include:
      a. Paired measurement of FT_4 and TSH (thyrotropin)
      b. Cortisol, IGF-1
      c. LH and FSH in men and postmenopausal women and total testosterone in adult men
   ii. Stimulation tests should include:
      a. ACTH and GH deficiency by TRH for TSH, GnRH for GH or hypoglycemia for both. These are done in cases where baseline cortisol and IGF-1 test results are not confirmatory.

In microincidentalomas, significant hypopituitarism is very rare. Asymptomatic pituitary hormone deficits are likely to occur with larger lesions. So, test for hypopituitarism recommended to be done in all macroincidentalomas and also in larger microincidentalomas (size 6–9 mm).

3. Screening tests for hormonal excess in pituitary incidentaloma are of the following types:
   Investigation should include measurements for PRL, GH, and ACTH.
   i. Approximately 50% of pituitary incidentalomas are likely to be nonfunctional. Prolactinomas are the most common functional mass. Elevated PRL may be due to pituitary tumor or stalk dissection by a large nonfunctioning pituitary mass.
   ii. For GH excess, it is recommended to measure of IGF-1 level and to treat to stop long-term complications.
   iii. For high ACTH, laboratory screening for glucocorticoid excess is to be done.
4. *Treatment options*:
   i. Surgical intervention is recommended for cases with:
      a. Hypersecreting tumors except prolactinomas
      b. Pituitary apoplexy cases with visual disturbances
      c. Lesions compressing the optic nerves or chiasm on MRI, or in the presence of visual field deficit due to the lesion
   ii. Surgical resection is not recommended for nonfunctioning microadenomas.
   iii. Dopamine agonist therapy is recommended for patients with prolactinoma.
   iv. Somatostatin analogs may be used in some cases of pituitary incidentaloma, but yet it is not approved.
   v. Replacement therapy for deficient hormones(s) may be required. It is to be done as per protocols for adult deficiency states.
5. *Follow-up*: Schedule for follow-up testing of pituitary incidentaloma for micro- and macroincidentaloma are different.
   i. *For macroincidentaloma*:
      a. First follow-up pituitary MRI along with clinical and biochemical testing for hypopituitarism is to be done at 6 months after the initial diagnosis.
      b. Thereafter yearly follow-up for several years, with visual field assessment.
      c. If the tumor enlarges and tends to compress the optic nerves or chiasm, surgical intervention is advocated.
   ii. *For microincidentaloma*: First follow-up MRI should be performed at 12 months after the initial diagnosis. There is no need to test for hypopituitarism if there was no change in the clinical and radiographic features.

FURTHER READINGS

1. OpenStax. Anatomy and Physiology. Rice University; 2017.
2. Susan S (Ed). Gray's Anatomy: The Anatomical Basis of Clinical Practice, 41st edition. UK: Elsevier Health; 2015.
3. Barrett K, Barman S, Yuan J, Brooks H (Eds). Ganong's Review of Medical Physiology, 26th edition. India: McGraw-Hill Education/Medical; 2019.
4. Melmed S, Koenig R, Rosen C, Auchus R, Goldfine A (Eds). Williams Textbook of Endocrinology, 14th edition. Elsevier: 2019.
5. Gardner D, Shoback D (Eds). Greenspan's Basic and Clinical Endocrinology, 10th edition. McGraw Hill; 2017.
6. Freda PU, Beckers AM, Katznelson L, Molitch ME, Montori VM, Post KD, et al. Pituitary incidentaloma: an endocrine society clinical practice guideline. J Clin Endocrinol Metab. 2011;96(4):894-904.
7. Bevan JS. Pituitary incidentaloma. Clin Med JR Coll Physicians London. 2013;13(3):296-8.
8. Ezzat S, Asa SL, Couldwell WT, Barr CE, Dodge WE, Vance ML, et al. The prevalence of pituitary adenomas: a systematic review. Cancer. 2004;101(3):613-19.
9. Scangas GA, Laws ER. Pituitary incidentalomas. Pituitary. 2014;17(5):486-91.
10. Boguszewski CL, de Castro Musolino NR, Kasuki L. Management of pituitary incidentaloma. Best Pract Res Clin Endocrinol Metab. 2019;33(2):101268.
11. Esposito D, Olsson DS, Ragnarsson O, Buchfelder M, Skoglund T, Johannsson G. Non-functioning pituitary adenomas: indications for pituitary surgery and post-surgical management. Pituitary. 2019;22(4):422-34.
12. Fernández-Balsells MM, Murad MH, Barwise A, Gallegos-Orozco JF, Paul A, Lane MA, et al. Natural history of nonfunctioning pituitary adenomas and incidentalomas: a systematic review and meta-analysis. J Clin Endocrinol Metab. 2011;96(4):905-12.

CHAPTER 3

Disorders of Thyroid Gland

- ❑ Introduction to the thyroid gland (anatomy and applied embryology; physiology)
  - ➢ Thyroid gland
  - ➢ Physiology of thyroid
- ❑ Thyroid disorders
  - ➢ Thyroid function test
  - ➢ Hypothyroidism
  - ➢ Hyperthyroidism
  - ➢ Graves' disease
  - ➢ Thyrotoxic crisis
  - ➢ Thyromegaly (goiter)
  - ➢ Thyroid nodule
  - ➢ Thyroid malignancy
- ❑ Thyroid incidentaloma

This chapter is about Thyroid Gland, begin with an introduction to applied anatomy and physiology. It covers hypofunctioning states, hyperfunctioning states, goiter/nodule, and thyroid malignancy. This chapter consists of 18 Figures, 5 Flowcharts, 16 Tables, and 2 Boxes to illustrate its text. This chapter ends with how to deal with incidentalomas of thyroid.

INTRODUCTION TO THE THYROID GLAND (ANATOMY AND APPLIED EMBRYOLOGY; PHYSIOLOGY)

■ Thyroid Gland

The thyroid gland is a typical endocrine gland. It is located in front of the neck, from the level fifth cervical (C5) to the first thoracic (T1) vertebrae. It is deep to the platysma, sternothyroid, and sternohyoid muscles. The gland consists of two lobes (left and right), connected by a thin isthmus at the level of the second to fourth tracheal rings. It looks like "H", "U", or "Butterfly". In adult average weight of a thyroid gland is 20–25 g, but slightly heavier in women, enlarges during menstruation and pregnancy. The thyroid has a capsule. The capsule extends into the substance of the gland forming septae.

The septae divide the gland into lobes and lobules. Each lobule is composed of follicles, which are the structural units of the lung. Each lobule consists of 20-40 follicles. A follicle is a cavity lined with single layer of simple epithelium filled with colloid. This colloid contains the precursor to thyroid hormones called iodothyroglobulin. The size of a follicle varies in size. The follicles are surrounded by dense plexuses of capillaries, lymphatic vessels, and sympathetic nerves.

There are two types of epithelial cells: follicular and parafollicular cells. Follicular cells are responsible for formation of the colloid (iodothyroglobulin), and parafollicular cells produce the calcitonin hormone. Parafollicular cells lie adjacent to the follicles within the basal lamina **(Figs. 1A to C)**.

Blood supply: The thyroid is a highly vascularized.

Arterial supply: The superior and inferior thyroid arteries are two main arteries supplying the thyroid gland. These vessels lie between the fibrous capsule and the pretracheal layer of deep cervical fascia. Two superior thyroid arteries (right and left) supply the upper half of the thyroid gland. Each artery divides into anterior and posterior branches to supply right and left sides of the thyroid. Two inferior thyroid arteries (right and left) supply the lower half of the thyroid.

CHAPTER 3: Disorders of Thyroid Gland

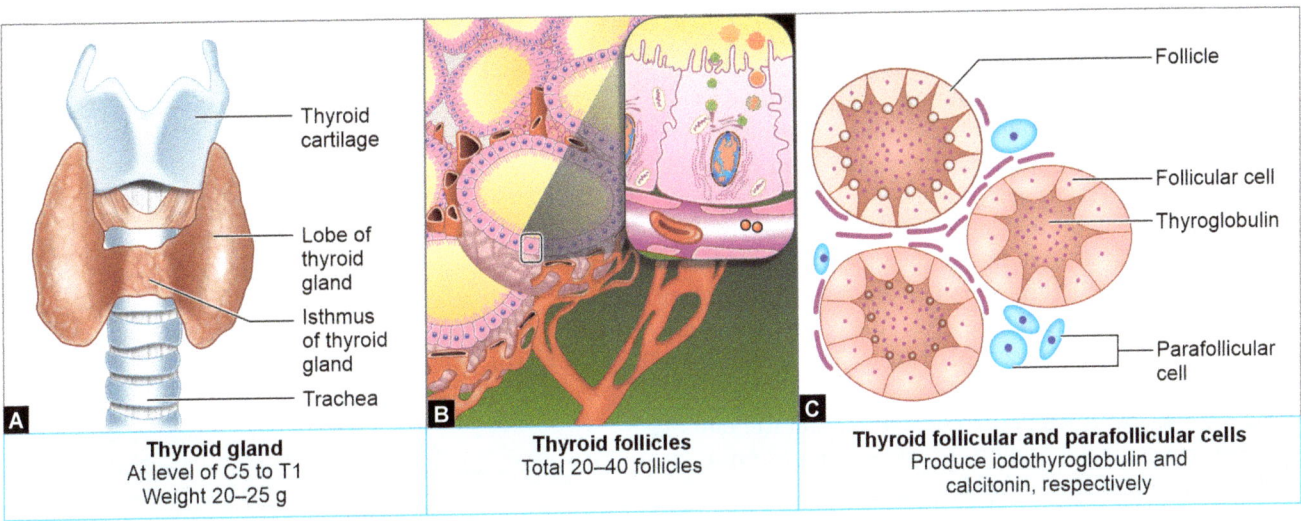

FIGS. 1A TO C: Thyroid gland anatomy.

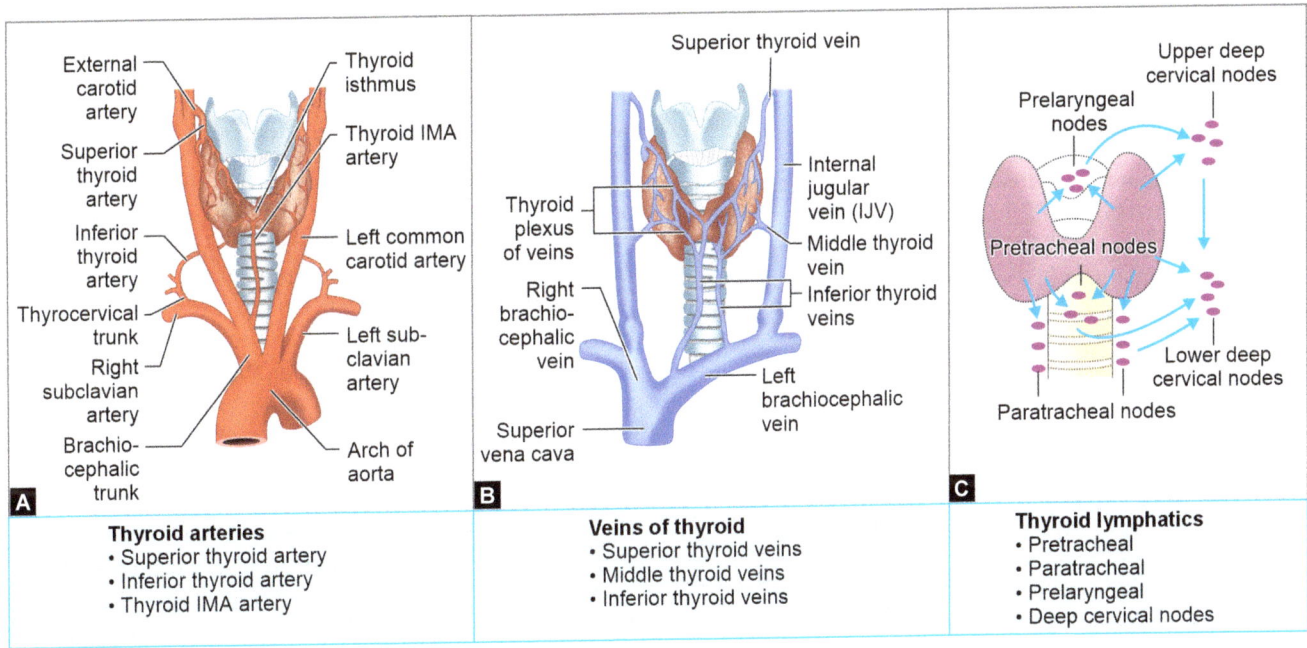

FIGS. 2A TO C: Thyroid gland arteries, veins, and lymphatics.

Venous drain: There are three main veins that drain the thyroid gland. The veins arise from the venous plexus on the anterior surface of the thyroid. Their names are: the superior, middle, and inferior thyroid veins. They drain upper, middle, and lower portion of the thyroid, respectively. The superior and middle thyroid veins drain into the internal jugular veins, and the inferior thyroid vein drains into the brachiocephalic veins, behind the manubrium of the sternum.

Lymph drainage: Lymphatic drainage of the thyroid gland is extensive. Immediate drainage flows first to the periglandular nodes. Subsequently to the prelaryngeal, pretracheal, and paratracheal nodes along the recurrent laryngeal nerve, and then finally to the mediastinal lymph nodes.

Nerve supply: The thyroid gland gets nerve supply from the autonomic nervous system. These nerves reach the thyroid gland by coursing with the blood vessels—superior and inferior thyroid periarterial plexuses; sympathetic fibers from superior, middle, and inferior cervical ganglia and parasympathetic fibers from the vagus nerves **(Figs. 2A to C)**.

Embryology of the Thyroid Gland

The thyroid gland appears at 3–4 weeks' gestational age. Initially, it appears as an epithelial proliferation. The site is the base of the tongue in between the tuberculum impar and the copula linguae. The copula soon becomes covered over by the hypopharyngeal eminence. The point is later indicated by the foramen cecum. The thyroid then descends in front of the pharyngeal gut through the thyroglossal duct. By the next few weeks by passing in front of the hyoid bone, it migrates to the base of the neck. The thyroid remains connected to the tongue by a narrow canal called the thyroglossal duct during the migration process. The thyroglossal duct degenerates at the end of the fifth week. The detached thyroid continues on to its final position over the next 2 weeks **(Fig. 3)**.

Developmental anomalies of the thyroid gland are: (1) Agenesis (failure to formation), (2) lingual thyroid (failure to descent), (3) aberrant thyroid (retrosternal goiter)—descent into thorax, (4) thyroglossal cyst (persistent part of thyroglossal duct), (5) thyroglossal fistula (thyroglossal duct opens to skin), etc. **(Fig. 4)**.

Physiology of Thyroid

The thyroid gland produces the hormones L-thyroxine/L-tetraiodothyronine (T_4) and L-triiodothyronine (T_3). Major functions of T_4 and T_3 include: (1) metabolic processes regulation, (2) cell respiration, (3) expenditure of energy, (4) tissue growth and maturation, and (5) hormones, substrates, and vitamins turnovers.

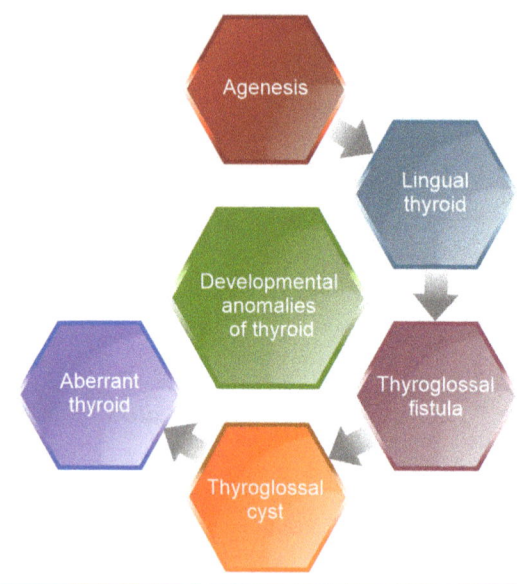

Developmental anomalies of thyroid gland

FIG. 4: Anomalies of thyroid gland are: (1) Agenesis (failure to formation), (2) lingual thyroid (failure to descent), (3) aberrant thyroid (retrosternal goiter)—descent into thorax, (4) thyroglossal cyst (persistent part of thyroglossal duct), (5) thyroglossal fistula (thyroglossal duct opens to skin), etc.

Iodine contributes 58% and 65% of weight of T_3 and T_4, respectively. Diet is the principle source of body iodine. The iodine circulates within the blood as iodide (I^-). It is actively transported into the follicular cells by Na^+/I^- symport in the basal membrane. This pump concentrates iodine in the colloid at a level up to 250 times greater than the plasma level. This process is called iodide trapping. The pump is regulated by thyroid-stimulating hormone (TSH) of the pituitary gland. Thyroperoxidase (TPO) is the principle enzymes produced in the endoplasmic reticulum of the thyroid cell that oxidizes iodine for T_3 and T_4 production. The majority (90%) of hormone produced by the follicular cells is T_4. T_3 is three times the metabolic potent than T_4, so T_4 is considered a prohormone that broken down to form T_3 in the tissues **(Fig. 5)**.

Release of the T_3 and T_4 into the bloodstream is regulated by a negative feedback system. These feedbacks operate between hypothalamic, pituitary, and thyroid gland. In case there is a low level of serum T_3 and/or T_4, it signals the hypothalamus to secrete thyrotropin-releasing hormone (TRH), which travels to the anterior pituitary gland and stimulates secretion of TSH. TSH, in turn, stimulates the thyroid gland to manufacture and release stored T_3 and T_4 until the metabolic rate is normalized. An elevated T_3 and T_4 serum levels inhibit the release of TRH and TSH, and thereby reduce production and release of T_3 and T_4. In a recent study we documented in euthyroid

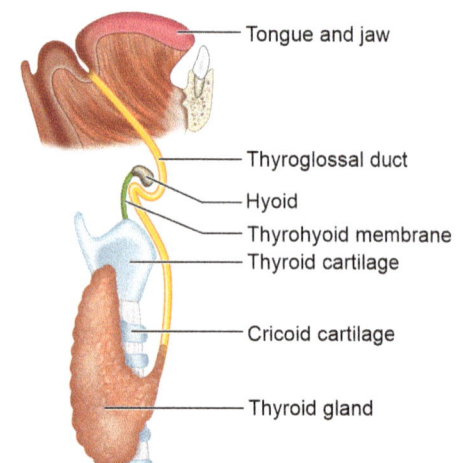

Embryology of the thyroid gland

FIG. 3: (1) Thyroid gland appears at 3–4 weeks' gestational age at base of tongue; (2) Covered over by the hypopharyngeal eminence; (3) Descends in front of the pharyngeal gut as a bilobed diverticulum (through the thyroglossal duct); (4) Migrates to the base of the neck to its final position, passing in front of the hyoid bone.

Structure of thyroid hormones

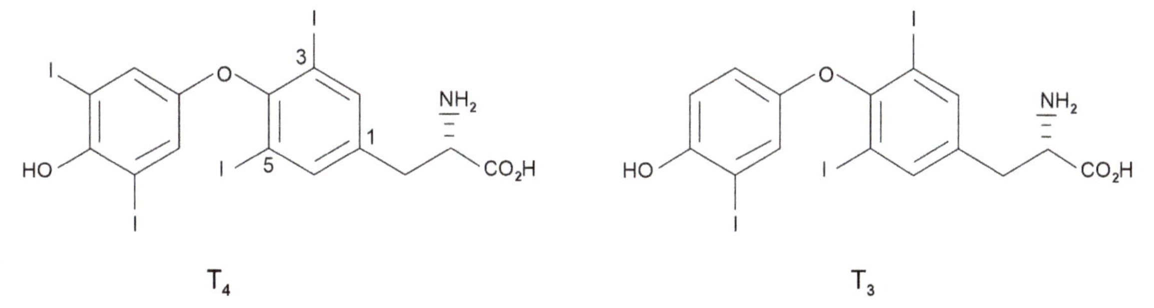

FIG. 5: (1) L-thyroxine/L-tetraiodothyronine (T_4) and L-triiodothyronine (T_3) are two thyroid hormones; (2) Iodine constitutes 58% and 65% of weight of T_3 and T_4, respectively; (3) Thyroxine-binding globulin (TBG) to T_3 and T_4 in the plasma called Total T_3 and T_4, respectively; (4) Free hormones (FT_3 and FT_4) are metabolically active; (5) Molecular weight of FT_3 and FT_4 is 650.98 g/mol and 776.87 g/mol, respectively.

A negative feedback system between hypothalamic, pituitary, and thyroid

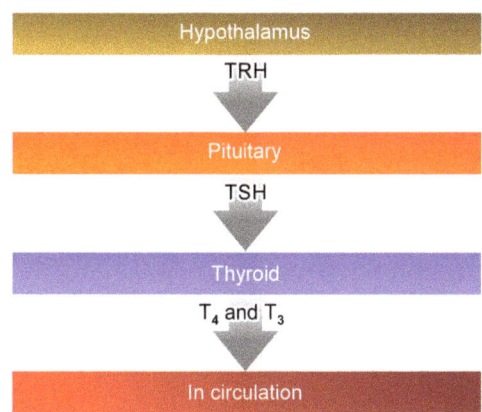

FIG. 6: The hypothalamic-pituitary-thyroid axis includes roles of thyrotropin-releasing hormone (TRH), thyroid-stimulating hormone (TSH), thyroxine (T_4), and triiodothyronine (T_3). A decrease in serum T_3 and/or T_4 levels signals the hypothalamus to secrete TRH, which travels to the anterior pituitary gland and stimulates secretion of TSH. Elevated T_3 and T_4 serum levels inhibit release of TRH and TSH.

or metabolically equilibrium state the negative feedback control between TSH and free thyroxine (FT_4), which remains temporarily silent.

L-triiodothyronine and T_4 in the plasma mostly (>90%) bind to thyroxine-binding globulin (TBG) and serve as temporary reserve pool. Only free hormones (FT_3 and FT_4) are metabolically active at tissue and are not affected any change of TBG concentration blood **(Fig. 6)**.

THYROID DISORDERS

Thyroid disorders may involve either disturbance of thyroid hormones or structural disturbances of the gland or both. Hormonal disorders are of two major categories: (1) Hyperthyroidism if serum thyroid hormone levels (T4 and T3) are increased and (2) hypothyroidism if serum thyroid hormone levels (T4 and T3) are decreased. Thyroid disease is generally subclassified based on etiologic factors, physiologic abnormalities, etc. The presentation of diseases is also determined by age at onset of the disorder. A simplified approach for classification of disorders depending on functional status includes hypothyroidism (deficiency of hormone) and hyperthyroidism (excess of hormone) or depending on structural abnormalities, goiter (enlargement of gland) and thyroid nodule(s) with/without malignancy **(Flowchart 1)**.

Thyroid Function Test

For assessment of functional status of thyroid, we use paired FT_4 and TSH test. This tool classifies functional status of thyroid into total nine classes—one normal or euthyroid, four with abnormality only at thyroid, and four abnormalities at thyroid and pituitary. The nomenclature (biochemical definition) of them is as follows: (1) Euthyroid (FT_4 and TSH normal); (2) Primary hypothyroid (FT_4 low and TSH high); (3) Primary hyperthyroid (FT_4 high and TSH low); (4) Compensated hypothyroid (FT_4 normal and TSH high); (5) Compensated hyperthyroid (FT_4 normal and TSH low); (6) Secondary hypothyroid (FT_4 low and TSH low); (7) Secondary hyperthyroid (FT_4 high and TSH high); (8) Isolated hypothyroximia (FT_4 low and TSH normal); and (9) Isolated hyperthyroximia (FT_4 high and TSH normal). Four abnormal classes (primary and compensated hypo-/hyperthyroids) are having intact pituitary-thyroid negative feedback and rest four (secondary hypo-/hyperthyroids and isolated hypo/hyperthyroximias) lost their pituitary-thyroid feedback.

In our institute, we used Chemiluminescent Microparticle Immunoassay (CIMA) for FT_4 with reference range of 9.14–23.18 pmol/mL and TSH with reference

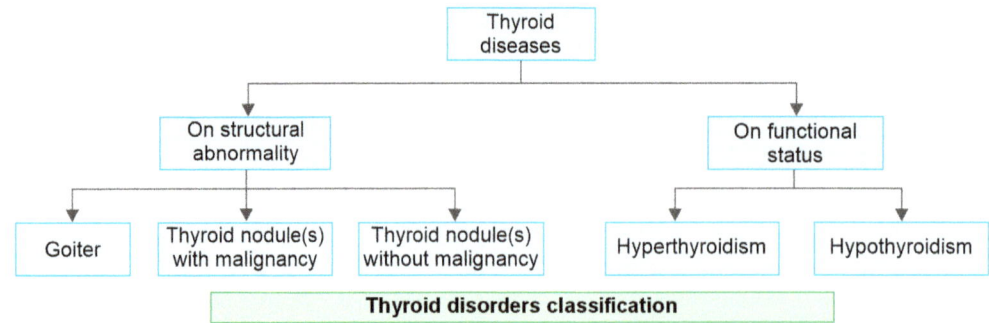

FLOWCHART 1: (1) On functional status—hypothyroidism and hyperthyroidism; (2) On structural abnormality—goiter, nodule(s), and nodule(s) with malignancy.

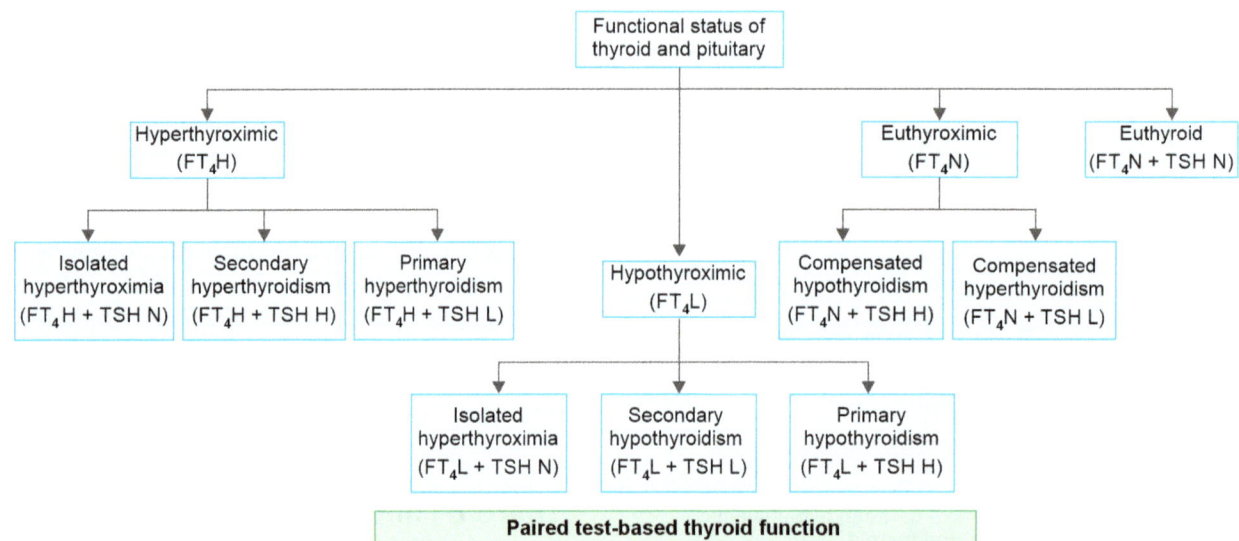

FLOWCHART 2: Total nine classes. One normal or euthyroid, four classes (primary and compensated hypo-/hyperthyroids) having intact pituitary–thyroid feedback, and four classes (secondary hypo-/hyperthyroids and isolated hypo-/hyperthyroximias) lost pituitary–thyroid feedback.
(FT_4: free thyroxine; TSH: thyroid-stimulating hormone)

ranges for (1) neonate 1.30–16.0; (2) infant 0.52–16.0; (3) children 0.37–6.0, and (4) adult 0.47–5.01 IU/mL. In an analysis of a series of 58,166 paired tests, there were 43,242 euthyroid cases. FT_4 and TSH levels of this euthyroid class were 14.65–14.70 pmol/mL and 2.44–2.46 IU/mL, respectively as 95% of confidence interval (CI). There was no correlation between its two hormones (r -.049; sig. 000).

The four classes with abnormality at thyroid and pituitary is normal had significant correlation (sig. 0.00) between their FT_4 and TSH (Class 2–5). The rest four classes (where pituitary–thyroid axis were inactive) had nonsignificant (sig. > 0.251) correlation between their FT_4 and TSH (Class 6–9). According to Cohen's standard of r values euthyroid and compensated hypothyroid (r -.049; sig. 000) have no correlation ($r < 0.1$); primary hypothyroid (r -.490; sig. 000) and primary hyperthyroid (r -.349; sig. 000) have moderately negative correlation ($r > 0.3–0.5$) and compensated hyperthyroid (r -.211; sig. 000) has mild negative correlation ($r > 0.1–0.3$) between their FT_4 and TSH.

We used paired FT_4 and TSH test at diagnostic setting. The cases of rare classes (class 5–9) require special attention to complete their diagnostic workups for rare diseases such TSHomas, resistance to FT_4, etc. in hyperthyroximia states (class 7 and 9) or thyroid–pituitary dissociated states either from mass lesion at hypothalamic–pituitary region or of other causes like Sheehan's syndrome/head injuries, etc. in hypothyroximia states (class 6 and 8) **(Flowchart 2)**.

There is no correlation between FT_4 and TSH hormones; therefore, in follow-up/treatment monitoring setting we used only FT_4 test to check its value with the 95% CI of FT_4 of euthyroid class **(Fig. 7)**.

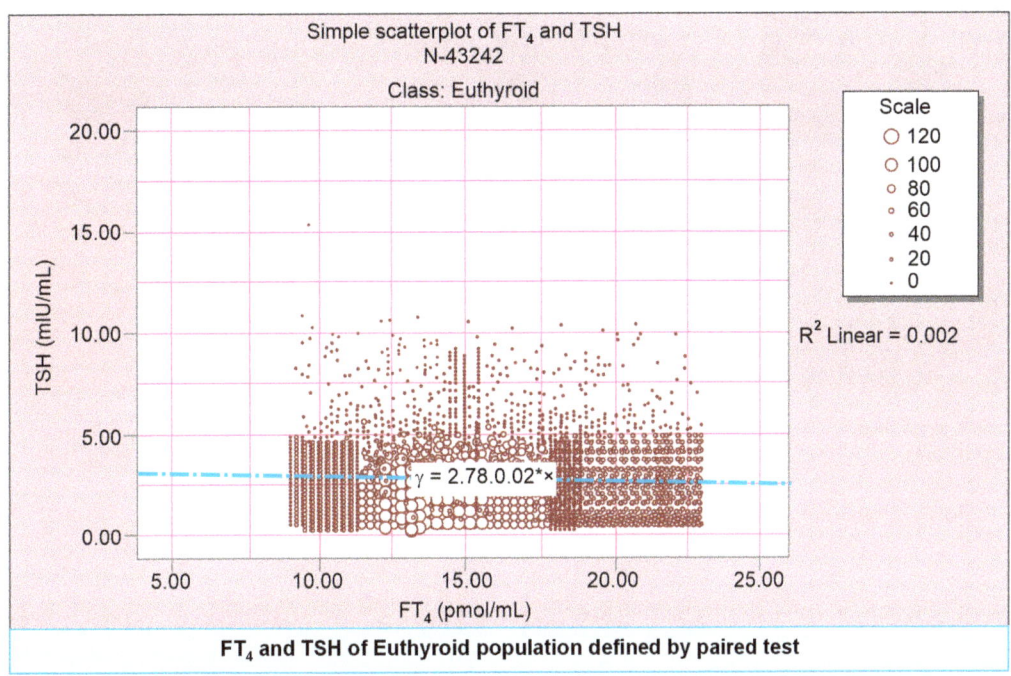

FIG. 7: Euthyroid population has both FT$_4$ and TSH within normal range. 95% of confidence interval of them in a study was 14.65–14.70 pmol/mL and 2.44–2.46 IU/mL, respectively. There was no correlation between its two hormones (r -.049; sig. 000).
(FT$_4$: free thyroxine; TSH: thyroid-stimulating hormone)
Source: Ahmed T et al. Thyroid function status by paired test.

Hypothyroidism

Hypothyroidism is a clinical syndrome due to deficiency of thyroid hormones, which results in generalized slowing down of metabolic processes. Clinical features are mostly determined by age and severity of deficiency.
- Age at onset is prime determinant of the clinical features. Infantile/congenital and childhood hypothyroidism affects growth and development, producing serious permanent consequences (including mental retardation); extreme cases called *Cretinism*.
- Adult-onset hypothyroidism slows down all metabolism, deposits glycosaminoglycan in the intracellular spaces, particularly in skin and muscle; extreme cases called *Myxoedema* **(Fig. 8)**.

For description of hypothyroidism, we will categorize it in three clinical scenarios:
1. Hypothyroidism in neonate/infant
2. Hypothyroidism in childhood and adolescences
3. Hypothyroidism in adult **(Figs. 9A to C)**

Congenital Hypothyroidism (Hypothyroidism in Neonate/Infant)

Congenital hypothyroidism is a partial or complete loss of function of the thyroid that affects infants from birth

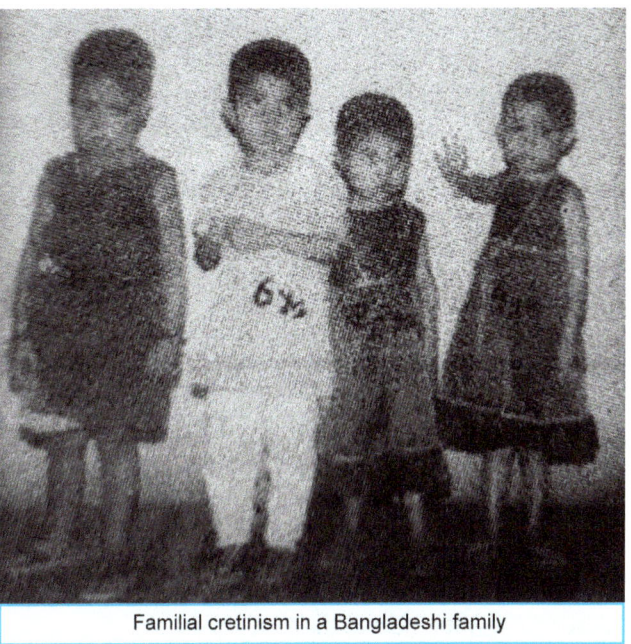

Familial cretinism in a Bangladeshi family

FIG. 8: Four cretins in a family. The incidence of cretinism in 2007 was estimated to be 31.5 per 100,000 individuals in the United States. Cretinism is more in the Asian and Hispanic races than the White and Black races. Cretinism affects the females more than males.

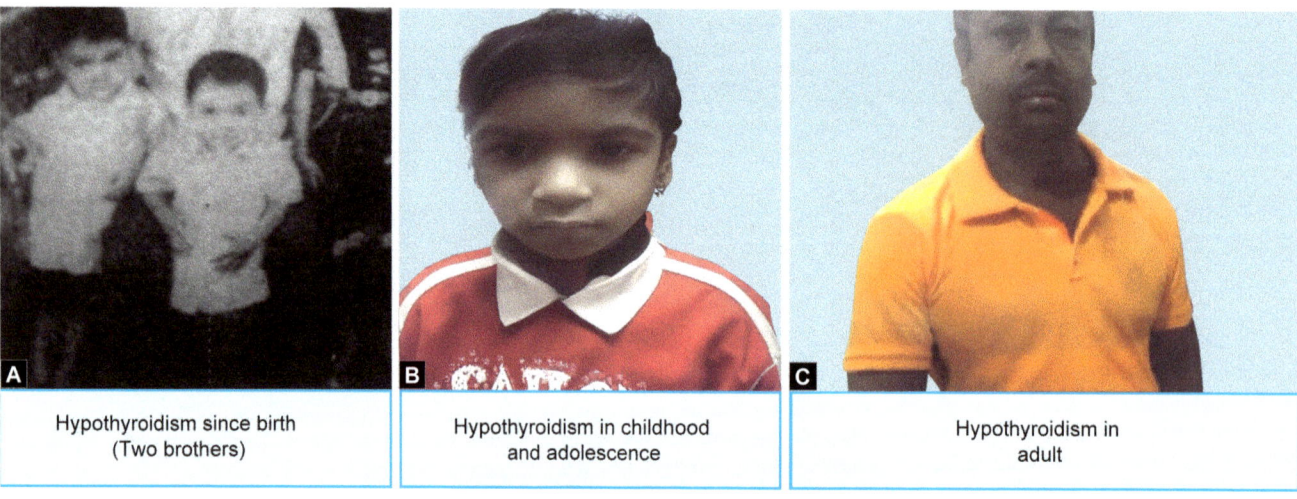

FIGS. 9A TO C: Features of hypothyroidism vary with age at presentation.

TABLE 1: Cause list of congenital hypothyroidism.	
Permanent hypothyroidism	
Developmental defects	Absent gland (agenesis)
	Gland severely reduced in size (hypoplastic)
	Abnormally located (ectopic)
Functional defects	Hereditary hormone synthesis disorder (dyshormonogenesis)
	Hypothalamic–pituitary (secondary/tertiary) hypothyroidism
Transient hypothyroidism	
	Transmission of maternal medications or maternal blocking antibodies (if mother is suffering from Graves' disease)
	Iodine deficiency (in endemic goiter zone)
	Iodine excess (amniofetography, painting cervix or umbilical stump with iodine)
	Prematurity

TABLE 2: Sign and symptoms of congenital hypothyroidism.			
Symptoms	Incidence	Signs	Incidence
Prolong jaundice	33%	Macroglossia	27%
Constipation	32%	Large fontanels	25%
Cutis marmarata	33%	Hypotonia	20%
Umbilical hernia	31%	Distended abdomen	20%
Lethargy	30%	Hoarse cry	20%
Feeding difficulty	22%	Jaundice	20%
Cool body surface	08%	Dry skin	10%
		Hypothermia	08%

Source: Oregon Health Science University, USA 1993.

(congenital). Congenital hypothyroidism affects an estimated 1 in 2,000–4,000 newborns. Female are affected more than twice than males. Causes are grouped into two: permanent and transient. In 80–85% of cases, hypothyroid state is a permanent one, due to either developmental or functional defects of the thyroid gland, rest are transient. These are summarized in **Table 1**.

Therapy is initiated within 2 weeks of birth. Infants whose mothers have hypothyroidism and undertreated during pregnancy have significant impairment of mental development despite early treatment. If untreated for several months after birth, severe congenital hypothyroidism can lead to growth failure and permanent intellectual disability who are called *Cretins*.

Clinical Features

Screening (universal) test is the tool to identify congenital hypothyroidism. Most infants with congenital hypothyroidism appear unaffected at birth, probably because of placental transfer of thyroid hormone. Less than 5% infants may have symptoms of hypothyroidism. Multiparous mother may notice less movement of the baby in utero. Approximately one-third babies are postmature for 2 weeks. Birth size is usually at 50th percentile for length and weight but head circumference approximately at 70th percentile. Sign and symptoms in newborns (with their incidence rate from an old large series) are as follows **(Table 2)**.

Congenital abnormalities associated with congenital hypothyroidism: Approximately 10% of congenital hypothyroidism cases may have associated anomalies like atrial septal defect (ASD), ventricular septal defect (VSD), pulmonary stenosis, subluxation of hip, and club foot.

Diagnosis

Thyroid deficiency may cause brain damage in neonate. Most of the newborns with congenital hypothyroidism escape severe brain damage because of transplacental transfer of maternal hormone. So, its diagnosis and prompt treatment are a pediatric emergency.

- *Hormone study*: Classically, there will be high TSH and low FT_4 in blood. Because of nonspecific and subtle features, ideally it may be a routine test for neonate or newborn screenings for hypothyroidism (heel prick/cord blood TSH and followed by TSH and FT_4 for high TSH subset).
- *Other test for congenital hypothyroidism are*:
  - A technetium-99m (Tc-99m pertechnetate) thyroid scan is performed to detect a structurally abnormal gland.
  - A radioactive iodine (RAIU) examination will help differentiate developmental defect and dyshormonogenesis.
  - X-ray of the knee may document absences of ossification points at lower end of femur and upper end of tibia, indicating prenatal severe hypothyroidism **(Table 3)**.

Treatment

The treatment of congenital hypothyroidism is early diagnosis and optimum T_4 replacement.

Criteria of optimum T_4 replacement include:
- Rapidity of correction of serum FT_4 level
- Avoidance of over treatment
- Continued biochemical euthyroidism [normal thyroid function test (TFT)]
- Continued clinical euthyroidism (normal growth and development)
- Similar psychometric outcome to genetic potential

For correction of serum FT_4 and TSH levels: A start dose of 10–15 µg/kg/day of levothyroxine orally in single dose (e.g., a 50-µg tablet for a full-term 4 kg baby) in most cases rapidly brings FT_4 level above the middle of the reference range and TSH down within range.

- *For avoidance of over treatment*: The initial recheck is to be done at the end of first week and first month to avoid over treatment.
- *For continued biochemical euthyroidism*: TFT for an infant with congenital hypothyroidism may be as follows:
  - Once in every 1–2 months during the first 6 months of life
  - Once in every 3 months between 6 months and 3 years of age
  - Once in every 4–6 months until growth is complete:
    - More frequent testing is suggested when nonadherence to treatment is suspected.
    - A repeat test is advised after 4 weeks after any change in levothyroxine dose.
- *For continued clinical euthyroidism*: Growth and development for an infant with congenital hypothyroidism must be recoded in his/her height, weight, and puberty chart.
- *For psychometric outcome*: Assessment of the infant with congenital hypothyroidism should be recorded by scoring for verbal IQ, performance IQ, and full scale IQ periodically.

Hypothyroidism in Childhood and Adolescence

Children suffer from thyroid dysfunction—hypothyroidism commonly from autoimmune thyroiditis (primary hypothyroidism) and also rarely from hypothalamic-pituitary disease (central hypothyroidism). The primary hypothyroidism may be either *overt* or *subclinical form*. The overt one may have classical features with high serum TSH and low serum FT_4 concentrations, and a *subclinical* one may have high serum TSH and normal serum FT_4 with minimum clinical feature.

A hypothyroidism in children is affected on their growth, pubertal development, and academic performance. The causes of hypothyroidism in children are grouped into nine. They are summarized in **Table 4**.

Clinical Manifestations

The most common manifestation of hypothyroidism in children is short stature. The growth velocity is declined and may be insidious in onset. So, any child with declining growth velocity should be evaluated for hypothyroidism.

Other common feature includes declining school performance, become less active, sluggishness, lethargy, cold intolerance, constipation, dry skin, brittle hair, facial puffiness, muscle aches and pains, etc. If hypothyroidism is a part of hypothalamic or pituitary disease, the child may have others headaches, visual symptoms, or manifestations of other pituitary hormone deficiencies also.

TABLE 3: Stomata of congenital hypothyroidism.		
Hormone study	**Technetium scan**	**X-ray of the knee**
High TSH and low FT_4 screenings for hypothyroidism (heel prick/cord blood TSH and followed by TSH and FT_4 for high TSH subset)	Tc-99m Na pertechnetate thyroid scan: No thyroid gland in pretracheal area	X-ray: No ossification points at lower end of femur and upper end of tibia

(FT_4: free thyroxine; Tc-99m: technetium-99m; TSH: thyroid-stimulating hormone)

TABLE 4: Cause list of hypothyroidism in childhood and adolescences.

Autoimmune thyroid disease (AITD)	
Late-onset congenital hypothyroidism	Ectopic or hypoplastic thyroid gland
	Dyshormonogenesis
Goitrogen exposure	Drugs blocking organification of iodine—propylthiouracil (PTU), methimazole (MMI)
	Iodine—antitussive agents, amiodarone, iodinated radiopaque dyes, topical iodine containing cleansing agents
	Perchlorate, thiocyanate
	Lithium, arsenic, cobalt
	Para-aminosalicylic acid, aminoglutethimide, phenylbutazone
Postthyroidectomy	
Postradiation	I^{131} ablation for thyrotoxicosis or cancer
	External radiation—Hodgkin's disease
Iodine deficiency	
Infiltrative diseases	Cystinosis
	Histiocytosis X
Central hypothyroidism	
TRH/TSH deficiency	Isolated
	Associated with growth hormone, prolactin, FSH, LH deficiency

(FSH: follicle-stimulating hormone; LH: luteinizing hormone; TRH: thyrotropin-releasing hormone; TSH: thyroid-stimulating hormone)

Physical examination findings may revel:
- Thyroid enlarge (goiter approximate 40%; likely autoimmune)
- *Height*: Below the mean for age (may be short statue)
- *Weight*: Above the mean for height (more for fluid retention than obesity)
- Osseous maturation (dentation) delayed
- *Face*: Hypothyroid face (dull, puffy, and placid expression)
- *Muscle*: Bulky (?pseudohypertrophy)
- *Pulse*: Slow
- *Tendon (ankle) jerk*: Delayed deep reflexes
- *Other features*: Lethargy, decreased energy, dry skin, sleep disturbance, cold intolerance, and constipation
- *Rare/occasion feature*:
  - Iso-sexual precocity—central type: Pubertal maturity in a short boy/girl (FSH and LH in pubertal range and High TSH) known as *Van Wyk and Grumbach syndrome*.
  - Children with myopathy and very high serum creatine kinase levels, known as *Kocher-Debre-Semelaigne syndrome*.

Diagnosis
- Clinical suspecting
- *Hormone study*:
  - Paired hormone test: FT_4 coupled with TSH is the initial hormone test for all children and adolescents with clinical features suggestive of hypothyroidism.
  - A high TSH and low FT_4 are confirmatory of diagnosis—primary hypothyroidism (1°).
  - There is a subset of primary hypothyroidism defined by a raised TSH and normal FT_4 called subclinical hypothyroidism. In contrary the name subclinical this group may have some important clinical features like slow growth, infertility, difficulty in losing weight, etc.
  - TRH stimulation test: A minimally raised or normal or low TSH and low or low normal FT_4 needs a TRH stimulation test to differentiate between pituitary (2°) and hypothalamic (3°) hypothyroidism. A marked raise in TSH is noted after administration of TRH in hypothalamic (3°) but no or minimal in pituitary (2°) hypothyroidism.
- *Other tests*:
  - Antithyroid antibodies for autoimmune thyroid diseases (AITDs)
  - An RAIU and scan of thyroid gland to developmental defect and dyshormonogenesis
  - X-ray for bone age determination.

Treatment

The treatment of hypothyroidism in children and adolescent is prompt initiation and lifelong optimum T_4 replacement and monitoring growth and development.
- Biochemical target of T_4 is to keep FT_4 in between the median and the upper limit of reference value for normal or within the 95% CI value of FT_4 of the population with normal FT_4 and TSH.
- TFT for hypothyroidism in children and adolescent may be as follows:
  - Once in every 2 months during the first 6 months of start of treatment
  - Once in every 3 months until growth is complete
  - Once in every 4–6 months thereafter:
    – More frequent testing is suggested when nonadherence to treatment is suspected.
    – A repeat test is advised after 6–8 weeks after any change in levothyroxine dose.
- *Monitoring of growth and development*: Each patient must have his/her height, weight, and puberty chart and is to be recorded till growth is complete.

Hypothyroidism in Adult

Hypothyroidism, a state of thyroid hormone deficiency in adult, is very common one. Prevalence and incidence of primary hypothyroidism are much higher in women than men. In one study (The Whickham survey), it was found female versus male were (prevalence: 18 per 1,000 and 4.1 per 1,000 per year) versus (prevalence: 1 per 1,000 and 0.6 per 1,000 per year).

Raised serum TSH (>2 mU/L) and positive thyroid antibodies are two independent risk factors of developing overt hypothyroidism. People with both raised serum TSH and positive antibodies develop hypothyroidism 4.3% per year, with only raised TSH or positive antibodies 2.6% and 2.1% per year, respectively. A 20-year follow-up of the survey documented hypothyroidism in 55%, 33%, and 27% of the three respective groups but only in 4% in the control (people without the two risk factors).

Causes of hypothyroidism in adult: There are differences in causes of different types of hypothyroidisms in adult. **Table 5** summarizes the causes of hypothyroidism in adult.

Clinical Manifestations of Hypothyroidism in Adult

The onset of hypothyroidism in adult is usually insidious, *early symptoms* are variable and often nonspecific; with progression symptoms become prominent and late features are obvious and untreated severe cases called myxedema coma is a life-threatening emergency.

Early features include (1) tiredness and lethargy leading to difficulty in performing a full day's work, (2) constipation may develop, or if present, become worse, (3) sensitivity to cold, (4) loss of libido, and (5) menstrual disturbance and infertility in women.

Features with progression include (1) slowing of intellectual function and motor activity and even drowsiness, (2) loss of interest in work and environment, (3) women often complain of hair loss, dry skin, and brittle nails, and (4) weight gain in spite of reduced appetite.

Late features include (1) husky voice, (2) skin thickened, dry, pale, and cool, (3) pretibial puffiness,

TABLE 5: : Cause list of hypothyroidism in adult.		
Type	**Mechanism**	**Cause**
Primary (thyroprivic) hypothyroidism	Loss of functional thyroid tissue	• Chronic autoimmune thyroiditis • Reversible autoimmune hypothyroidism (silent and postpartum thyroiditis, cytokine-induced thyroiditis) • Surgery and irradiation (^{131}I or external irradiation) • Infiltrative and infectious diseases, subacute thyroiditis • Thyroid dysgenesis
	Functional defects in thyroid hormone biosynthesis and release	• Congenital defects in thyroid hormone biosynthesis • Iodine deficiency and iodine excess • *Drugs*: Antithyroid agents, lithium, natural and synthetic goitrogenic chemicals, tyrosine kinase inhibitors
Central (hypothalamic/ pituitary or trophoprivic) hypothyroidism	Loss of functional tissue	• Tumors (pituitary adenoma, craniopharyngioma, meningioma, dysgerminoma, glioma, metastases) • Trauma (surgery, irradiation, head injury) • Vascular (ischemic necrosis, hemorrhage, stalk interruption, aneurysm of internal carotid artery) • Infections (abscess, tuberculosis, syphilis, toxoplasmosis) • Infiltrative (sarcoidosis, histiocytosis, hemochromatosis) • Chronic lymphocytic hypophysitis • Congenital (pituitary hypoplasia, septo-optic dysplasia, basal encephalocele)
	Functional defects in TSH biosynthesis and release	• Mutations in genes encoding for TRH receptor, TSH-β, pituitary transcription factors (Pit-1, PROP1, LHX3, LHX4, HESX1), or LEPr, IGSF1 • *Drugs*: Dopamine, glucocorticoids, bexarotene, L-T4 withdrawal
Peripheral (extrathyroidal) hypothyroidism	Consumptive	Consumptive hypothyroidism (massive infantile hemangioma)
	Resistance	Mutations in genes encoding for MCT8, SECISBP2, TR-α or TR-β (thyroid hormone resistance)

(TRH: thyrotropin-releasing hormone; TSH: thyroid-stimulating hormone)

TABLE 6: Features of hypothyroidism in adult.			
Early features	**Features with progress**	**Late features**	**Very late feature**
• Tiredness and lethargy • Constipation • Sensitivity to cold • Loss of libido • Menstrual disturbance and infertility in women	• Slowing of intellectual function and motor activity and drowsiness • Loss of interest in work and environment • Women often complain of hair loss, dry skin, and brittle nails • Weight gain	• Husky voice • Skin thickened, dry, pale and cool • Pretibial puffiness • Puffy, edematous face • Thicken tongue • Progressive deafness	Myxedema coma

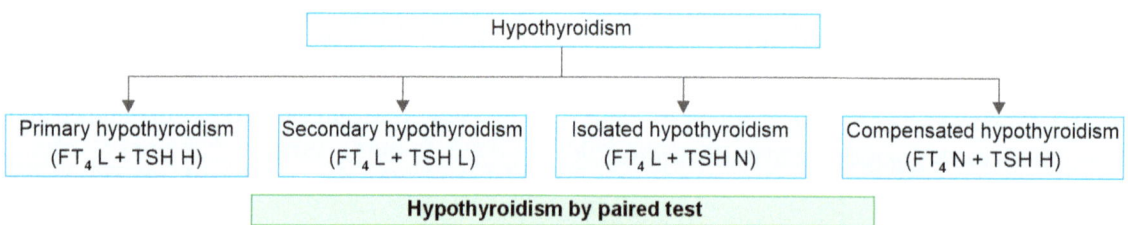

FLOWCHART 3: The four types of hypothyroidism. Thyropituitary axis is likely to be intact in first and fourth but not in rest two.
(N: within reference range for normal; H: above reference range for normal; L: bellow reference range for normal; FT_4: free thyroxine; TSH: thyroid-stimulating hormone)

(4) puffy, edematous face, (5) thicken tongue, and (6) progressive deafness.

Very late feature is call *myxedema coma*—characterized by stupor, hypothermia, hypoventilation, hypoglycemia, hyponatremia, water intoxication, shock, coma, and death **(Table 6)**.

Diagnosis of Hypothyroidism in Adults
- Diagnosis is done by hormone tests as mentioned for children and adolescences.
- The tests to determine the causes such as (1) antithyroid antibodies and (2) RAIU and scan of thyroid gland should also be included routinely.
- Tests to see the systemic manifestations of hypothyroidism may also be required in some cases.

The four types of hypothyroidism on the basis of hormone profile of paired test during diagnosis are as shown in **Flowchart 3**.

Treatment of Hypothyroidism in Adults
The treatment of hypothyroidism in adult is prompt initiation and lifelong optimum T_4 replacement.
- Biochemical target of T_4 is to keep FT_4 in between the median and the upper limit of reference value for normal or within 95% CI of population with normal FT_4 and TSH.
- TFT for hypothyroidism in adult may be as follows: Once in every 3 months and a repeat test is advised after 6–8 weeks after any change in levothyroxine dose.

FT_4 and TSH both should be within in their reference ranges but in cases of discordant in value of FT_4 is to be considered.
- Everyone should know that the treatment is a lifelong one and women during pregnancy need monitoring more frequent to meet the increasing demand of T_4 in time.

Hashimoto's Disease/Chronic Thyroiditis
It is the most common cause of hypothyroidism, resulting from autoimmune destruction of the thyroid gland in the post era of universal iodinization of table salt.
There are three types of clinical presentations:
1. The most common form is mild diffused thyromegaly and variable features of hypothyroidism.
2. Patient at times may present with thyrotoxicosis (hashitoxic phase).
3. Rarely, it is a part of syndrome called Schmidth's syndrome and consist of (A) adrenal insufficiency (?idiopathic) or hypoparathyroidism, (B) type 1 diabetes mellitus, (C) premature ovarian failure, (D) candida infection along with (E) hypothyroidism due to Hashimoto's disease.

Cause: It occurs due to autoimmune destruction of thyroid gland by in genetically susceptible individuals. There is antibody-mediated chronic thyroiditis and glandular destruction.

Diagnosis: Two steps:
- *Step I*: Clinical suspicion
- *Step II*: Investigation:
  - Thyroid function status—hypothyroidism: (1) High TSH and low FT_4 (primary hypothyroidism) or (2) High TSH and Normal FT_4 (compensated hypothyroidism) or normal TSH and normal FT_4 (euthyroidism).
  - Radioiodine uptake status—classically low (may be normal or high).
  - Perchlorate discharge is abnormal.
  - Antithyroid antibodies (antithyroglobulin and antimicrosomal) titer is high but thyroid-stimulating immunoglobulin (TSIg) is absent.
  - Fine-needle aspiration cytology or biopsy material shows Hurthle cells and lymphocytic infiltration.

Treatment of Hashimoto's Disease

According to hormonal status:
- T_4 replacement treatment as in primary hypothyroidism state
- Routine follow-up of euthyroid cases and to start replacement promptly (at compensated hypothyroidism state)
- Beta-adrenergic receptors blocker (propranolol/sotalol) with or without microsomal inducer (phenobarbitone) in hyperthyroid (hashitoxic) state
No treatment is recommended for autoimmunity.

In cases it is part of a syndrome, management protocols is based on components of syndrome.

Hyperthyroidism

Clinical syndrome resulting from excess of thyroid hormones resulting in hypermetabolic state is the hyperthyroidism. There are number of common symptoms and signs of hyperthyroid state. Severe and extreme hyperthyroid states are called "Thyrotoxicosis" and "Thyrotoxic crisis," respectively.

Signs and Symptoms of Hyperthyroidism

Common symptoms of thyrotoxicosis include (1) hyperactivity—nervousness, restlessness, emotional lability/mood swings, (2) decreased attention span—declining school performance, (3) hand writing deterioration, (4) increased appetite, (5) heat intolerance, (6) excessive sweating, (7) sleep disturbance—insomnia, restlessness, enuresis, (8) fatigue—muscle weakness, and (9) frequent loose stools.

Common signs of thyrotoxicosis include (1) restless—short attention span, (2) weight loss despite increased appetite, (3) on cardiovascular examination—tachycardia or atrial arrhythmia (fibrillation), systolic hypertension with wide pulse pressure, (4) on ocular examination—prominence of eye, stare, lid lag, and more advance eye changes called Graves' ophthalmopathy (refer to American Thyroid Association classes), (5) on hand examination—warm, moist, smooth skin with fine tremor, (6) muscle weakness—shoulder, pelvic girdle muscle, and (7) tall stature (in adolescents) **(Table 7)**.

There is variation in presentation of thyrotoxicosis depending on age at presentation.
- Younger patients show symptoms of sympathetic activation such as anxiety, hyperactivity, and tremor.
- Older patients show more cardiovascular symptoms such as dyspnea and atrial fibrillation and unexplained weight loss.
- Neonates show irritability, flashing, poor weight gain, tachycardia, hypertension, goiter, and exophthalmos.

Findings on thyroid examination:
- In thyrotoxicosis due to Graves' disease, the thyroid gland is diffusely enlarged and slightly firm consistency. Sometimes, a thyroid bruit can be heard by osculation.
- In toxic multinodular goiters (MNG), the gland is often soft, but individual nodules can occasionally be palpated.
- In subacute, painful, or granulomatous thyroiditis, thyroid gland is classically enlarged and painful. But degeneration or hemorrhage into a nodule and supportive thyroiditis may also have these findings.

TABLE 7: Signs and symptoms of hyperthyroidism of thyrotoxicosis.

Common symptoms	Common signs
Hyperactivity—nervousness, restlessness, emotional lability/mood swings	Restless—short attention span
Decreased attention span—declining school performance	Weight loss despite increased appetite
Hand writing deterioration	Cardiovascular examination—tachycardia or atrial arrhythmia (fibrillation), systolic hypertension with wide pulse pressure
Increased appetite	Ocular examination—prominence of eye, stare, lid lag, and more advance eye changes called Graves' ophthalmopathy
Heat intolerance	Hand examination—warm, moist, smooth skin with fine tremor
Excessive sweating	Muscle weakness—shoulder, pelvic girdle muscle
Sleep disturbance—insomnia, restlessness, and enuresis	Tall stature (in adolescents)
Fatigue—muscle weakness	
Frequent loose stools	

TABLE 8: Causes of hyperthyroidism.	
Group	Disease
Excess secretion of hormone by the gland	• Graves' disease (diffuse toxic goiter) • Pulmmer disease (toxic adenoma) • Marine—Lenhart syndrome (multinodular toxic goiter) • Hashitoxicosis (Hashimoto's thyroiditis) • De Quervain's disease (subacute thyroiditis)
Exogenous intake of hormone	• Iatrogenic • Factitious
Other (rare) forms	• Placental TSH/hCG—choriocarcinoma/hydatiform mole • TSH-secreting pituitary adenoma • Following iodine ingestion/injection/radiation

(hCG: human chorionic gonadotropin; TSH: thyroid-stimulating hormone)

Findings on eye and skin examination:
- In thyrotoxicosis, presence of thyroid ophthalmopathy and dermopathy is due to Graves' disease.

The causes of hyperthyroidism can be either due to (1) excess secretion of hormone by the gland, or (2) exogenous intake of hormone or (3) other (rare) forms. **Table 8** summarizes the causes of hyperthyroidism.

Diagnosis of Hyperthyroidism

Hormone study includes:
- *Coupled hormone test*: FT_4 and FT_3 coupled with TSH is the hormone test for all people with clinical features suggestive of hyperthyroidism.
- A suppressed TSH (<.01 IU/mL) plus high FT_4 and FT_3 is the hallmark of primary hyperthyroidism. There are more two subset of hyperthyroidism:
  o One is called T_3 *thyrotoxicosis*: Here TSH is suppressed (<.01 IU/mL), FT_4 is normal but FT_3 is high. These are more prevalent in regions with low levels of iodine and Graves' disease, toxic nodular goiter, and thyroid adenoma. The treatment striges are same as for the overt hyperthyroidism.
  o Second one is called compensated hyperthyroidism (previously called *subclinical hyperthyroidism*): Here TSH is low (usually 0.01–0.10 IU/mL) and FT_4 and FT_3 are normal. Etiologically, cases are linked with nodular goiter and toxic adenomas, hyperemesis gravidarum, excessive thyroid hormone replacement, excessive iodine ingestion, or pituitary adenoma; however, the most common cause is Graves' disease. There is evidence of increased health risks (arrhythmias, reduction of bone density) among the group and but benefits of any specific treatment modalities are not yet established. So, regular follow-up is still the practical tool for their management.

Other tests that are necessary to establish etiology of hyperthyroidism include:
- *Antithyroid antibodies study*:
  o TSIgG—positive in Graves' disease
  o Peroxidase/antimicrosomal antibody (AMA) and antithyroglobulin antibody (ATA) are positive both in Hashimoto's disease and Graves' disease. Titer of AMA is much higher in Hashimoto's disease.

An RAIU and scan of thyroid gland is an important investigation in hyperthyroidism.
- A high uptake (40–100% at 24 hour) with rapid turnover with uniform scan in enlarged thyroid is the feature of Graves' disease.
- Mild-to-moderate uptake (25–60% at 24 hour) with multiple hot nodules in an enlarged thyroid is the feature of Marine–Lenhart syndrome (multinodular toxic goiter).
- Mild-to-moderate uptake (25–60% at 24 hour) with single hot nodule in a normal/enlarged thyroid is the feature of Pulmmer disease (toxic adenoma).
- Mild-to-moderate uptake (25–60% at 24 hour) with a normal thyroid is the feature of pituitary tumors producing TSH.
- A variable uptake (25–100% at 24 hour) with a normal/enlarge thyroid is the feature of human chorionic gonadotropin (molar pregnancy/choriocarcinoma).
- Very low or absent uptake is the feature of (1) de Quervain thyroiditis, (2) Hashitoxicosis, (3) factitious thyrotoxicosis, struma ovarii, (4) iodide-induced thyrotoxicosis, and (5) metastatic thyroid carcinoma **(Figs. 10A to D)**.

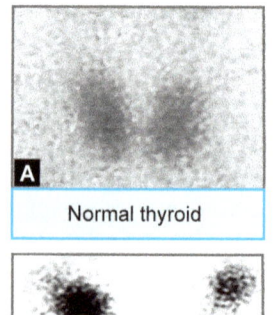
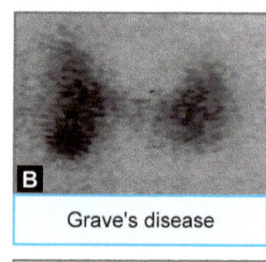
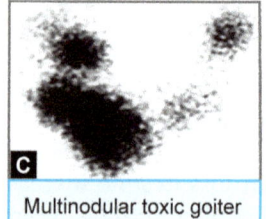
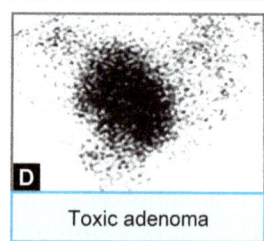

FIGS. 10A TO D: Radioiodine scan of thyroid in normal and three hyperthyroid disorders.

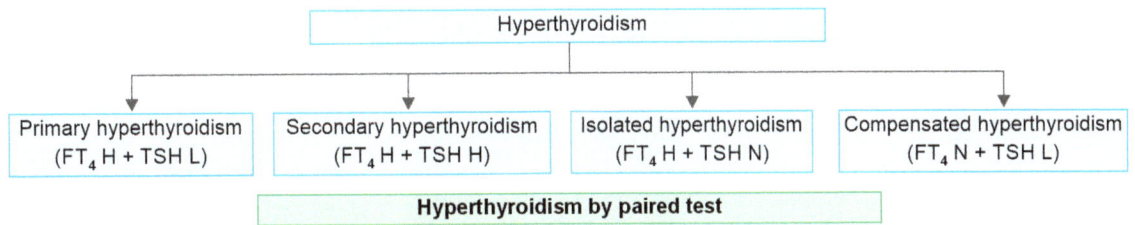

FLOWCHART 4: The four types of hyperthyroidism. Thyropituitary axis is likely to be intact in first and fourth but not in rest two.
(N: within reference range for normal; H: above reference range for normal; L: bellow reference range for normal; FT_4: free thyroxine; TSH: thyroid-stimulating hormone).

The four types of hyperthyroidism on the basis of hormone profile paired test during diagnosis are as in **Flowchart 4**.

Treatment for Hyperthyroid States

There are three modalities of treatment for hyperthyroid states—(1) antithyroid drugs, (2) radioablation, and (3) surgery.

1. *Antithyroid drugs*: Drugs either decrease the synthesis and release of thyroid hormone or reduce the symptoms of thyrotoxicosis.
   i. *Carbimazole and propylthiouracil (PTU)*: These are two commonly used antithyroid drugs. These drugs decrease the synthesis and release of thyroid hormone. They can work only when the gland has uptake of iodine. They are started in divided doses till hormone come within normal range and then can be maintained with single dose until disease undergoes spontaneous remission.
   ii. *Beta blocker*: Hyperthyroid state is associated with an increased number of beta-adrenergic receptors, and therefore use of beta blocker relives thyrotoxicosis like palpitations, tachycardia, tremulousness, anxiety, and heat intolerance. If there is no contraindication they should be started patients as soon as the diagnosis of hyperthyroidism is made and continued until resolution of hyperthyroidism.
   iii. *Phenobarbitone*: In cases with very high FT_4 level, this drug is used initially to reduce its load as microsomal inducer.
2. *Radioablation*: Generally, the ^{131}I is administered orally. The dose calculation is done by 75–200 μCi/g of estimated thyroid tissue divided by the percent of ^{123}I uptake in 24 hours. This dose is intended to make the patient hypothyroid. Radioactive iodine therapy is the most common treatment for Graves' disease in adults in some countries. It is effective and safe.
3. *Surgery*: Thyroidectomy may be considered for debulking of MNG with toxicities, and there is no extra benefit over antithyroid drug/radioablation for other cases of hyperthyroidism.

For description of hyperthyroidism, we will do it in four clinical scenarios:
1. Graves' disease
2. Toxic adenoma
3. Multinodular toxic goiter
4. Subacute thyroiditis

■ Graves' Disease

Definition: *Graves' disease*, also known as *toxic diffuse goiter*, is an autoimmune disease. It is a very common cause of hyperthyroidism. In addition to hyperthyroidism, *Graves' disease* in most cases presents with diffuse thyroid enlargement, in some cases with specific eye (Graves' ophthalmopathy) and skin (dermopathy) changes—all these three together constitutes clinical triad of *Graves' disease* **(Fig. 11)**.

Mechanism of development of hyperthyroidism in *Graves' disease*: TSIg binds to the thyrotropin receptor (TSH receptor) of the gland and stimulates synthesis and secretion of T_4 and T_3. The high levels of circulating thyroid hormones suppress the TSH secretion of pituitary.

Diagnosis of hyperthyroidism of Graves' disease is two steps.
- *Step I*: Clinical suspicion (features of hyperthyroidism with/without Graves' ophthalmopathy and dermopathy).
- *Step II*: Investigations:
  ○ *Hormone study*: FT_4 and FT_3 coupled with TSH—classically primary hyperthyroidism is the finding of *Graves' disease* but rarely T_3—hyperthyroidism or compensated hyperthyroidism may found.
  ○ *Antithyroid antibodies study*: In Graves' disease, TSIg is positive; in *Graves' disease* and Hashimoto's disease both peroxidase/AMA and ATA may be positive but titer of ATA is much higher than Hashimoto's disease.
  ○ *RAIU and scan of thyroid gland*: A high uptake (40–100% at 24 hour) with rapid turnover with uniform scan in enlarged thyroid is a feature of Graves' disease.

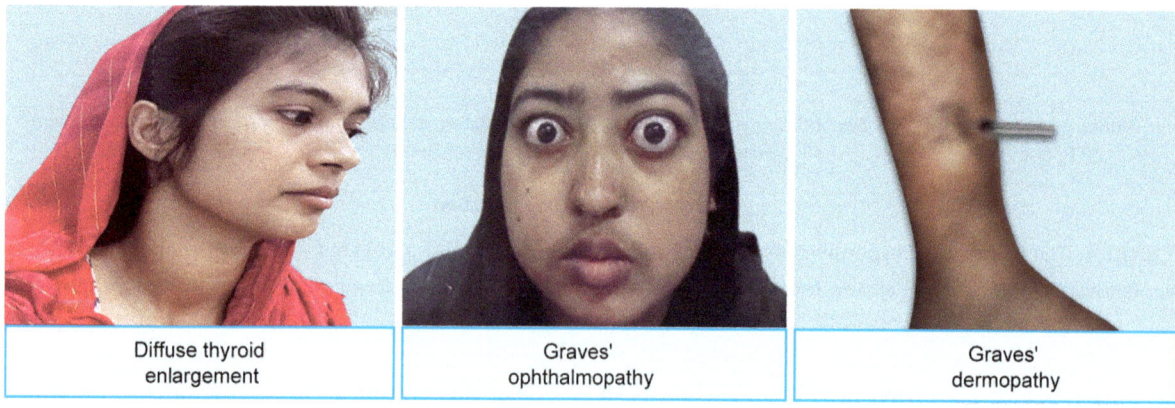

FIG. 11: Clinical triad of Graves' disease.

TABLE 9: The American Thyroid Association classification of Graves' ophthalmopathy.

American Thyroid Association class	Severity	Mnemonic	Definition
0	Mild	N	No sign and symptoms
1		O	Only sign, no symptoms (signs limited to upper lid retraction, stare and lid lag)
2		S	Soft tissue involvement (signs + symptoms)
3	Moderate	P	Proptosis (measured by exophthalmometer)
4		E	Extraocular muscle involvement
5	Severe	C	Corneal involvement
6		S	Sight loss (optic nerve involvement)

Management of Graves' Disease

Of the three modalities of treatment for hyperthyroid states, antithyroid drugs and radioablation are in use because no extra benefit from surgery.

- Antithyroid drugs are used to control hyperthyroidism till remission occurs. There are two antithyroid drugs commonly used: (1) Carbimazole (CMZ) and (2) PTU. The first choice of drug is CMZ. If this is not tolerated, PTU is used. Usually, the dose of CMZ is 15–30 mg daily and that of PTU is 200–400 mg daily in divided dose. Both drugs can cause minor side effects, such as altered taste sensation or nausea. Other significant side effect of both drugs is a rash, which is usually a generalized itchy redness. It clears up if the drug is stopped. Rare but most serious potential side effect of both drugs is bone marrow depression—called *agranulocytosis*. In that case drug is withdrawn. Radioablation is offered for hyperthyroidism after managing agranulocytosis.
- Radioablation is used in cases where drugs fail to bring sustained remission or contraindicated for side effect like agranulocytosis.

Graves' Ophthalmopathy

Definition

Ophthalmopathy due to Graves' disease is also called Graves' orbitopathy. It is the common cause of bilateral exophthalmos. It is a progressive lesion features and may range from minor stare, lid lags to permanent sight loss.

Classification: American Thyroid Association classified Graves' ophthalmopathy into seven classes on the basis of the signs and symptoms **(Table 9 and Fig. 12)**.

Management of Graves' Ophthalmopathy

General measures include:
- Hyperthyroid patient is to made euthyroid.
- Regular follow-up of TFTs to ensure minimum or no fluctuation of TSH level. Rapid rise of TSH deteriorates Graves' ophthalmopathy and is marked in (1) postradio ablation hypothyroidism and (2) nonwithdrawal of antithyroid drugs during remission phase.

Measures required for specific manifestations: There are number of treatment options for individual manifestations of Graves' ophthalmopathy. **Table 10** summarizes those treatment options.

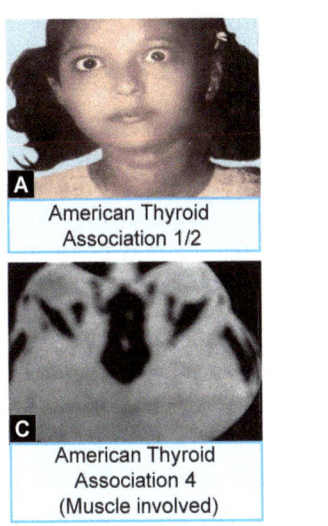
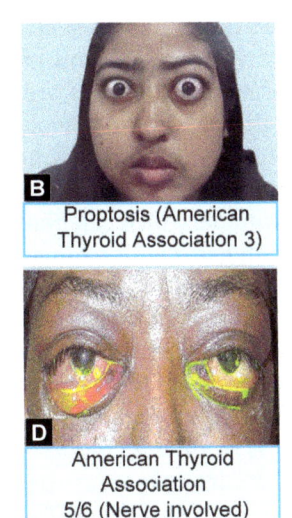

FIGS. 12A TO D: Graves' ophthalmopathy.

TABLE 10: Treatment options/modes of Graves' ophthalmopathy.	
Manifestations	**Treatment options/modes**
Edema—periorbital and lid	Head end of the bed is elevated
Eye lids close normally, but with gritty, sandy sensation	Artificial tears—eye drops (1% methyl cellulose)
Mild exophthalmos with imperfect eye closure due to lid retraction	Pressure dressing at night, Muller's muscle section, scleral graft insertion in eyelid or lateral tarsorrhaphy
Severe exophthalmos with imperfect eye closure	Glucocorticoid trail, orbital decompression, or retro-orbital irradiation
Severe inflammation (chemosis, ingestion, pain)	Steroid systemic or retrobulbar, super voltage X-ray therapy
Intermittent diplopia	Await for remission or prism use
Persistent diplopia	Glucocorticoid trail, extra ocular muscle surgery with/without decompression
Optic neuropathy, corneal ulcer, severe discomfort	Orbital decompression, super voltage X-ray therapy

Thyrotoxic Crisis

Definition: It is a medical emergency arise as an extreme accentuation of thyrotoxicosis. It is commonly associated with Graves' disease, multinodular toxic goiter, and subtotal thyroidectomy (in patients with inadequate preoperative preparation). Common precipitating factors include radiation thyroiditis, diabetic ketoacidosis, toxemia of pregnancy, and parturition.

Clinical features of thyrotoxic crisis can be grouped into:
- Dominant
- Early features
- Late features

TABLE 11: Features of thyrotoxic crisis.		
Dominant features	**Early features**	**Late features**
• Hyperthermia (usually >40°C) • Marked prostration • Tachycardia (sinus/ectopic) • Pulmonary edema or congestive heart failure (CHF)	• Tremulousness or restlessness with/without delirium or psychosis • Nausea, vomiting, and abdominal pain	• Apathy, stupor, and coma • Blood pressure drops suddenly and collapses

Dominant features include (1) hyperthermia (usually >40°C), (2) marked prostration, (3) tachycardia (sinus/ectopic), (4) pulmonary edema or congestive heart failure (CHF).

Early features include (1) tremulousness or restlessness with/without delirium or psychosis and (2) nausea, vomiting, and abdominal pain.

Late features include (1) Apathy, stupor, and coma and (2) blood pressure drops suddenly and collapses **(Table 11)**.

Management of Thyrotoxic Crisis

The outcome of the condition is often fatal. Any delay in management is ominous. So, treatment should be initiated without waiting for laboratory reports in all cases with clinical features suspicious of crisis, particularly in a known case of hyperthyroidism or a person with stigma of Graves' ophthalmopathy.

Aim of treatment:
- To control thyrotoxicosis
- To identify the precipitating illness and treat simultaneously
- To provide general supportive measures

Control of thyrotoxicosis: Medical treatment is based on three principles:
1. Counteracting the peripheral effects of thyroid hormones
2. Inhibition of thyroid hormone synthesis
3. Treatment of systemic complications:
   i. *Large dose of antithyroid drug*: Carbimazole or PTU to inhibit synthesis and release of hormones, e.g., carbimazole 40 mg or PTU 200 mg 4 hourly orally or by stomach tube.
   ii. *Iodine therapy*: To stop acute release of hormone from the gland, five drops of SSKI (saturated solution of potassium iodide) every 6 hourly or sodium iodide intravenously may be given followed by antithyroid drugs.

iii. *Dexamethasone therapy*: Large dose of dexamethasone, e.g., 2 mg orally 6 hourly is given to inhibit conversion of T_4 to T_3.
iv. *Propranolol*: If there is no cardiac insufficiency 20–40 mg of propranolol is given 6 hourly.
v. *Supportive measures include*: Cooling and fluids managements.

De Quervain's Thyroiditis/Subacute Thyroiditis

Definition: Subacute (de Quervain's) thyroiditis is a transient inflammatory thyroid disease due to viral infection. Classically, it is associated with:
- Pain and tenderness over the gland; pain may radiate to ear or teeth.
- Generalized somatic symptoms such as fever, weakness, and fatigue along with other symptoms of thyrotoxicosis/hyperthyroidism such as nervousness, heat intolerance, weight loss, sweating, diarrhea, tremor, palpitations, etc.

Positive laboratory investigations for de Quervain's thyroiditis in early phase include:
- High erythrocyte sedimentation rate (ESR) (>60 mm in firs hour)
- High serum thyroglobulin level
- Low/no RAIU uptake
- Hyperthyroidism (low TSH and High FT_4 level)
- Ultrasonographic images are generally characterized by heterogeneous hypoechoic areas of the affected tissue with lack of flow on color Doppler ultrasound.

Classically, a case of de Quervain's thyroiditis passes through three different phases as shown in **Table 12**.

Management

Management of subacute thyroiditis is aimed at two different aspects—(1) pain management and (2) management of thyroid dysfunction.

Pain management: For severe pain the first-line agents used are nonsteroidal anti-inflammatory drugs (NSAIDs)—such as such as ibuprofen (800–1,200 mg/day in divided doses) and naproxen (1–1.5 g/day in divided doses). The dosages are tapered as the pain subsided. High-dose aspirin is avoided, because it can competitively displace thyroid hormone from its binding protein and increase the free, or bioactive, fraction of thyroid hormone, which can make patients feel more thyrotoxic.

In cases with stronger pain steroids may be included with narcotic analgesics. In the most extreme cases, high-dose steroids such as prednisone 40–60 mg/day is administered for short time say 4/5 days. It is highly effective, and relief of pain is quick and dramatic.

Thyroid dysfunction management:
- *Hyperthyroid phase*:
    ○ Ipodate may be administered to inhibit the conversion of T_4 to T_3 in patient with very high level of hormones. An ipodate dose of 1,000 mg in two divided doses daily usually provides a rapid reduction in T3 levels and symptoms.
    ○ Patients with mildly high levels of thyroid hormone can be managed with beta blocker drugs.
- *Hypothyroidism phase*: It is usually mild and transient; typically does not require treatment. Symptomatic cases or with high TSH should be treated with replacement of levothyroxine (the starting dose can be 25–50 µg/day). In some cases, the hypothyroidism may become permanent, with the patient requiring lifelong replacement therapy.

Thyromegaly (Goiter)

Abnormal enlargement of the thyroid gland is term "goiter." A goiter may extend into the retrosternal space, with or without substantial anterior enlargement. Functional status of a goiter may be normal (nontoxic goiter), hypofunctioning (hypothyroid goiter), or hyperfunctioning (toxic goiter). The enlargement of the gland is usually either diffuse or nodular. It is common condition more seen in female than in male. There are a number of systems for goiter grading or classification of

TABLE 12: Phases of de Quervain's thyroiditis.		
Phase 1 (Destruction)	**Phase 2 (Resolation)**	**Phase 3 (Recovery)**
Charecterized by: • Low/no radioactive iodine uptake • Thyrotoxicosis—high FT_4 and very low TSH • Very highy ESR (>60 mm in first hour) • Mild transient rise of antibodies (AMA and ATA) (last up to ~2 months)	• It is a transient phase of hypothyroidism • It is cherecterized by— low/normal FT_4 and high TSH following a short perod normal FT_4 and TSH (last up to few weeks)	• If there is no repeated thiroditis, majority (~95%) of cases become normal *Showing*: • Normal radioactive iodine uptake • Euthyroid—normal FT4 and TSH • Normal ESR A person with repeated thyroiditis may endup with hypothyrodism permanently
(AMA: antimicrosomal antibody; ATA: antithyroglobulin antibody; ESR: erythrocyte sedimentation rate; FT_4: free thyroxine; TSH: thyroid-stimulating hormone)		

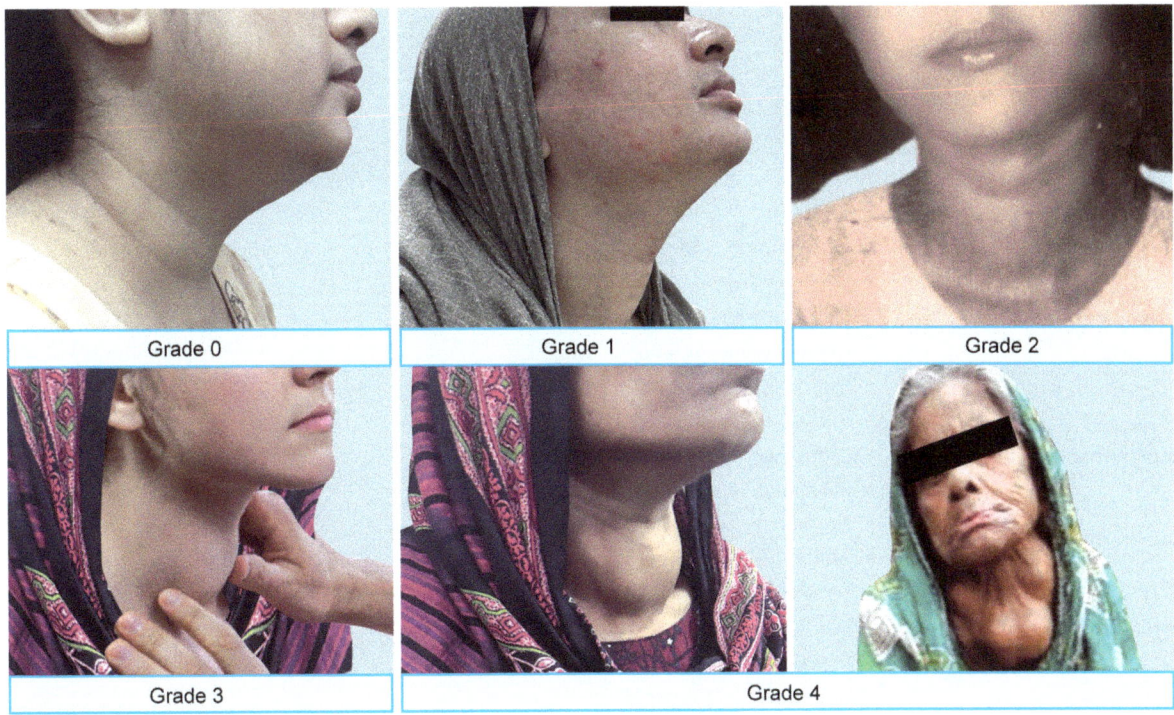

FIG. 13: Grade of goiter.

nontoxic goiter—one of them has 5 grade—0 to 4 with following description.
- *Grade 0*: Not visible (even in neck extension) and not palpable (persons without goiter)
- *Grade 1*: Not visible but palpable
- *Grade 2*: Visible only in neck extension and on swelling
- *Grade 3*: Visible in all positions
- *Grade 4*: Monstrous/large goiter **(Fig. 13)**

Causes of Goiter

There are wide variety of causes of goiter, which can be grouped into nine—(1) endemic goiter, (2) physiological goiter, (3) goitrogens in diet, (4) AITD, (5) dyshormonogenesis, (6) cyst, (7) thyroiditis, (8) tumors, and (9) others. A cause list is given in **Table 13**.

Evaluation and Management of Goiter

In addition to the history and physical examination other investigations such as (1) hormone test (TSH and FT_4), (2) imaging (ultrasonogram, radionuclear scan), (3) antithyroid antibody test, and (4) fine needle cytology (FNC) may be required for evaluation of goiter.

Management modality of goiter depends on cause, grade, and functional status of the goiter. **Table 14** summarizes the management of goiter.

TABLE 13: Cause list of goiter.

Group	Disease
Endemic goiter	Iodine deficiency goiter
Physiological goiter	(1) Pubertal and (2) pregnancy
Dietary	Goitrogens in diet
Autoimmune thyroid disease	(1) Graves' disease and (2) Hashimoto's disease
Enzymatic disorders	Dyshormonogenesis
Cystic change	Cyst
Thyroiditis	(1) Subacute and (2) chronic fibrotic (Riedel's)
Tumors	(1) Adenoma, (2) carcinoma, and (3) lymphomas
Others	(1) Sarcoidosis and (2) tuberculosis

Thyroid-stimulating Hormone Suppression Therapy for Diffuse Nontoxic Goiter

Oral administration of T_4 at a dose that suppress the serum TSH level below its lower limit (0.4 to 0.1 mU/L) can decrease the size of diffuse nontoxic goiter.

Originally, TSH suppression therapy was introduced to prevent differentiated thyroid cancer growth or spread

TABLE 14: Management modalities of goiter.		
Goiter (depending on cause)	**Features**	**Management modality**
Simple goiter	• Diffuse (scan) • RIU normal • Hormone—euthyroid • Antibody—negative	TSH suppression therapy
Pubertal goiter	• Onset during puberty • Other features as "simple goiter"	TSH suppression therapy
Iodine deficiency/endemic goiter	• *Size*: Any grade • Urinary iodine excretion—low • Hormone—euthyroid/hypothyroid • Antibody—negative	TSH suppression therapy and iodine supplement after the goiter regressed
Goiter of dyshormonogenesis	• Diffuse with calcification • Perchlorate discharge test—abnormal • Hormone—hypothyroid • Antibody—negative • Family history—positive	Thyroxine replacement
Goiter due to goitrogen in diet	• *Size*: Any grade • *Diet*: Goitrogen positive • Hormone—hypothyroid • Antibody—negative	Restrict goitrogen and TSH suppression therapy
Multinodular goiter (MNG)	• *Size*: Grade > 2 with multiple nodules (cold/warm/hot) • Euthyroid/hypothyroid/hyperthyroid • Antibody—negative	Surgery and thyroxine replacement
Post-thyroidectomy	• History of thyroid surgery • No supplement/replacement of thyroxine • Hormone—normal	TSH suppression therapy
Postradiation	• History radiation for malignancy/hyperthyroidism • Hormone—normal	TSH suppression therapy
Goiter with hypothyroidism		Thyroxine replacement
(RIU: radioactive iodine uptake; TSH: thyroid-stimulating hormone)		

in late 40s of last century. Regular follow-up should have done to adjust the dose of T_4, because aggressive suppression (TSH < 0.1 mU/L) has some potential long-term risks, such as (1) decrease bone density, (2) abnormal hepatic enzyme, (3) cardiac arrhythmia, etc.

Thyroid Nodule

A thyroid nodule is a discrete lesion within the normal thyroid. Such nodules are a common occurrence in the general population and a frequent incidental finding on computed tomography (CT) and magnetic resonance imaging (MRI). But ultrasound has most important role in the assessment of thyroid nodules. It is highly sensitive for detecting nodules, and the sonographic features of the nodules can be used to determine the need for further investigation. Nowadays sonographic features of thyroid nodules are utilized as a reliable guideline to specifically target nodules that require biopsy or not. There is scoring system on (1) composition, (2) echogenicity, (3) shape, (4) margin, and (5) echogenic foci in addition to the size of the nodule **(Flowchart 5)**.

Table 15 shows the score distribution of nodule on sonographic data.

Table 16 shows the score-based grouping and selection for fine needle aspiration cytology (FNAC) study.

Thyroid Malignancy

Malignant lesions of thyroid include:
- Papillary carcinoma
- Follicular carcinoma
- Medullary carcinoma
- Anaplastic carcinoma
- Miscellaneous—lymphoma, metastatic thyroid cancer, etc.

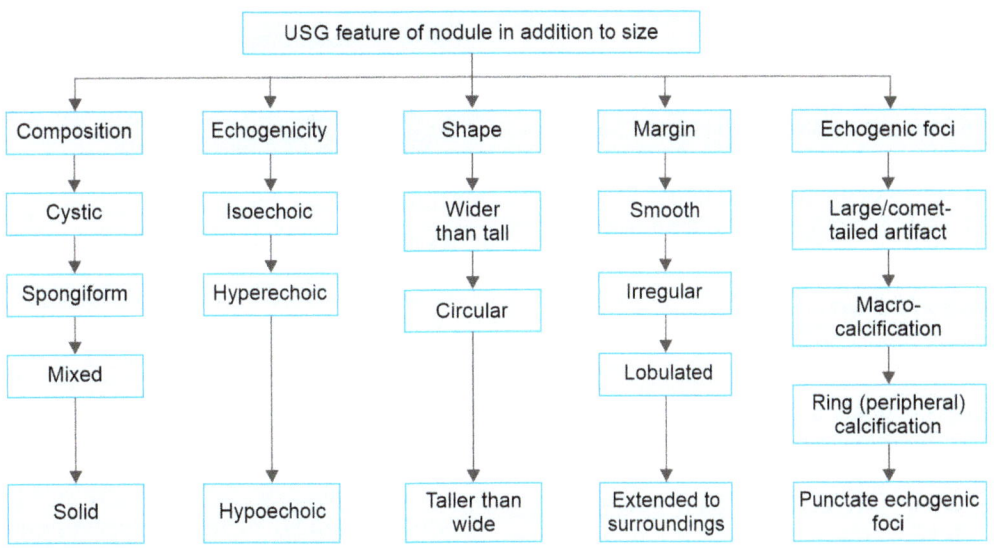

FLOWCHART 5: Sonographic feature of thyroid nodule.

TABLE 15: Score distribution of nodule on sonographic data.				
	Score			
Data on	**0**	**1**	**2**	**3**
Composition	Cystic/spongiform	Mixed (cystic and solid)	Solid	
Echogenicity	Anechoic	Hyperechoic/isoechoic	Hypoechoic	Very hypoechoic
Shape	Wider than tall			Taller than wide
Margin	Smooth/ill-defined		Lobulated/irregular	Extrathyroidal extension
Echogenic foci	Large/comet-tailed artifact	Macrocalcification	Ring (peripheral) calcification	Punctate echogenic foci

TABLE 16: Total score-based group and suggested strategies of fine needle aspiration cytology (FNAC) of nodule.				
Total score 0	**Total score 2**	**Total score 3**	**Total score 4–6**	**Total score >7**
Benign group	Not suspicious group	Mildly suspicious group	Moderately suspicious group	Highly suspicious group
No FNAC	No FNAC	• FNAC if >2.5 cm • Follow if >1.5 cm	• FNAC if >1.5 cm • Follow if >1.0 cm	• FNAC if >1.0 cm • Follow if >0.5 cm
			Molecular diagnosis may be done if available and patient party agree	

Papillary Carcinoma of Thyroid

Papillary thyroid carcinoma (PTC) is the most common form of well-differentiated thyroid cancer, accounts for 80–90% all thyroid cancers. It commonly results from exposure to radiation.

Papillary thyroid carcinoma appears as an irregular solid or cystic mass or nodule in a normal thyroid parenchyma. Presenting features are summarized in **Box 1**.

BOX 1: Presenting features of papillary carcinoma of thyroid.

- Usually presents as a solitary solid nonfunctional thyroid nodule during ultrasound and radioiodine
- May be as the dominant nodule in a multinodular goiter (MNG)
- As a cervical lymph node (in children)—lymph node metastasis
- On histopathological examination of thyroidectomy specimen

Microscopic Features of Papillary Carcinoma of Thyroid
- Single layer of thyrocytes arranged in vascular stalk
- The nuclei of the cells are large and pale
- *Psammoma bodies*—laminated calcified spears may be seen at the tip of papillary projection.
- Lesion is very slow growing—may remain confined in the gland or lymph node for many years **(Fig. 14)**.

Treatment and Follow-up
Treatment
- *Surgery*:
  - Lobectomy for small nodule (<1.5 cm)
  - Near total thyroidectomy for large nodule and/or lymph node metastasis
- *Thyroxine therapy*: It is lifelong; TSH is targeted to be kept at or near lower limit.
- *Radioiodine therapy*: For cases under went near total thyroidectomy (high-risk population).

Follow-up: Serum thyroglobulin assay and ultrasound of neck should be done in 6–12 months' interval for 3–5 years. If there is rise in thyroglobulin level or any sign of recurrence, repeat radioiodine therapy +/– ve additional surgery.

Follicular Carcinoma of Thyroid
Follicular carcinoma of thyroid (FCT) is the second most common cancer of the thyroid, after papillary carcinoma comprise 6–10% carcinoma of thyroids. Dietary iodine insufficiency is a risk factor. On radionuclide scan FCT are usually solitary "cold" nodule.

Presentation of FCT is usually as a painless thyroid nodule identified by ultrasonogram and FNAC examinations.

Presenting features are summarized in **Box 2**.

> **BOX 2: Presenting features of papillary carcinoma of thyroid.**
> - Presentation of follicular carcinoma of thyroid (FCT) is usually as a painless irregular firm nodule
> - Solitary solid nodule like that in papillary carcinoma of thyroid
> - On scan (radioactive iodine and ultrasonogram) area is surrounded by solid or mixed tumor
> - Features of blood born metastasis to lungs, lungs, bone, or other tissue

Ultrasonographic Features of Follicular Carcinoma of Thyroid
- Nodule(s) are characterized by thick, irregular, and/or interrupted halo with or without satellite nodule(s).
- *Echogenicity*: Hypoechoic or markedly hypoechoic with predominantly solid pattern, cluster of grapes sign, micro- or macrocalcifications, and rim calcifications are independent risk factors of FCTs.
- Satellite nodule(s) with or without halo ring are specific sonographic features for FCTs **(Fig. 15)**.

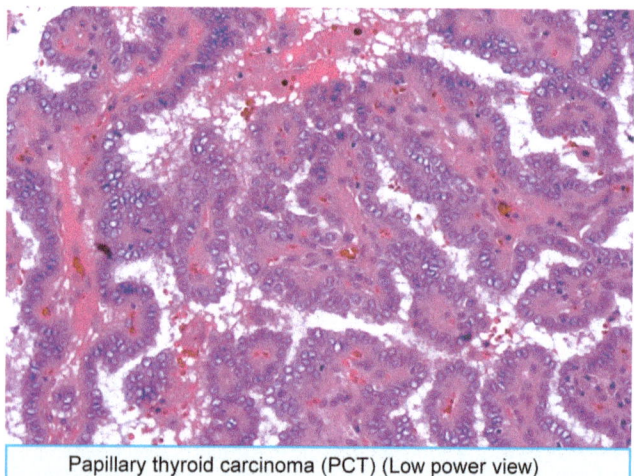

Papillary thyroid carcinoma (PCT) (Low power view)

FIG. 14: Distinctive nuclear features: (1) Nuclear enlargement, elongation, and overlapping; (2) Chromatin characteristics: chromatin clearing, margination, and glassy nuclei; (3) Nuclear membrane irregularity: irregular nuclear contour, nuclear groove, and nuclear pseudoinclusion.
Courtesy: Professor Masud Parvez.

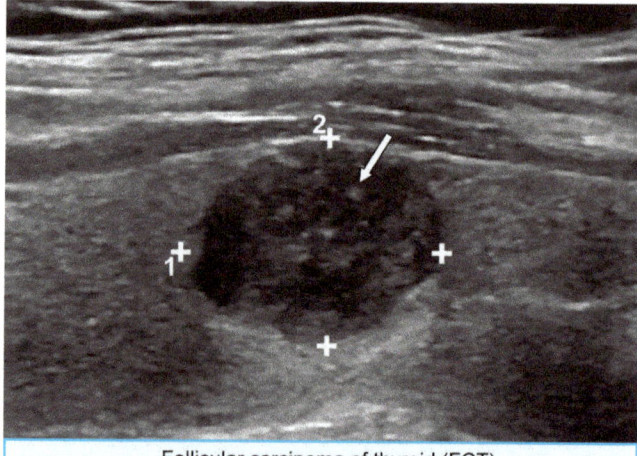

Follicular carcinoma of thyroid (FCT)

FIG. 15: Ultrasonographic features: Thick, irregular and/or interrupted halo with or without satellite nodule(s), hypoechoic or markedly hypoechoic echogenicity, a predominantly solid pattern, cluster of grapes sign, micro- or macrocalcifications, and rim calcifications are independent risk factors of FCTs. And an interrupted halo and satellite nodule(s) with or without halo ring are specific sonographic features for FCTs.

Microscopic Features of Follicular Carcinoma of Thyroid

- Adenocarcinoma in follicles of different size
- Follicular differentiation but there is no nuclear features of papillary carcinoma.
- *Three subtypes*:
    i. Minimally invasive follicular carcinoma—with capsular invasion only
    ii. Encapsulated angioinvasive—tumors with limited vascular invasion (<4) have a better prognosis than those with extensive vascular invasion
    iii. Widely invasive—extensive invasion of thyroid and extrathyroidal soft tissue **(Fig. 16)**

Treatment and Follow-up

Treatment: Depends on the stage of FCT at presentation.
- For minimally invasive FCT, thyroid lobectomy and isthmectomy are recommended.
- For invasive FCT, near total/total thyroidectomy followed by radioiodine ablation and thyrotropin suppressing medications are recommended.
- For patients with metastasis to bones and soft tissues of FCT either radiotherapy or chemotherapy or both are indicated after the total thyroidectomy. Chemotherapy that has been reported to control tumor progression and prolong progression-free survival includes tyrosine kinase inhibitors such as sorafenib, lenvatinib, vandetanib, and cabozantinib. Thyroglobulin levels are measured to monitor for recurrence.

Prognosis:
- Prognosis of noninvasive follicular carcinoma is same as normal person.
- For invasive carcinoma, 50% survival is drooped to about 17 years only.

Anaplastic Carcinoma of Thyroid

Anaplastic or undifferentiated carcinoma of thyroid is characterized by:
- It usually occurs in seventh to eighth decade of life.
- It is the most aggressive form of thyroid carcinoma.
- Patients usually have long standing goiter.
- There may be sudden enlargement of thyroid and pressure symptoms such as dysphasia or vocal cord paralysis.
- More than 50% cases show distances metastasis at diagnosis.

Computed tomography scan of neck features of anaplastic carcinoma of thyroid (ACT) are:
- Usually with a large neck mass with necrosis an extrathyroidal extension
- Calcification of tumor mass
- Lateral compartmental lymphadenopathy with necrosis and cysts
- There is contrast enhancement.

Histological features of ACT are small cell, giant cell, and spindle carcinoma **(Fig. 17)**.

Treatment: ACT is very resistant to treatment. The best option is complete surgical removal. Even those patients with potentially resectable disease will usually have invasion into surrounding structures like the trachea, esophagus, large blood vessels, and often growth into the chest and complete resection is seldom possible.

Life expectancy is 6–30 months after diagnosis.

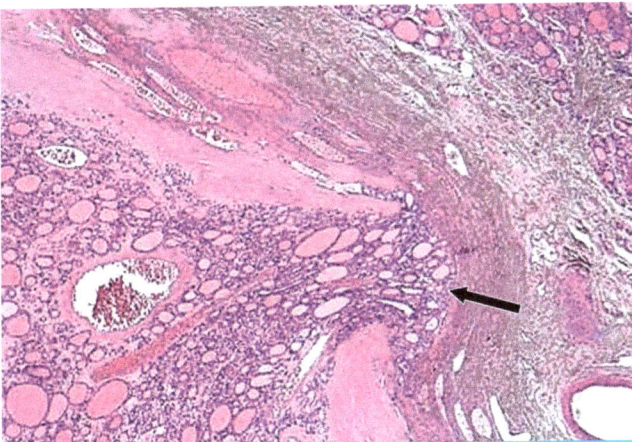

FIG. 16: Histopathological features: Follicular differentiation but no papillary nuclear features. Three subtypes: (1) Minimally invasive follicular carcinoma—with capsular invasion only; (2) Encapsulated angioinvasive—tumors with limited vascular invasion (<4) have a better prognosis than those with extensive vascular invasion; (3) Widely invasive—extensive invasion of thyroid and extrathyroidal soft tissue.
Courtesy: Professor Masud Parvez.

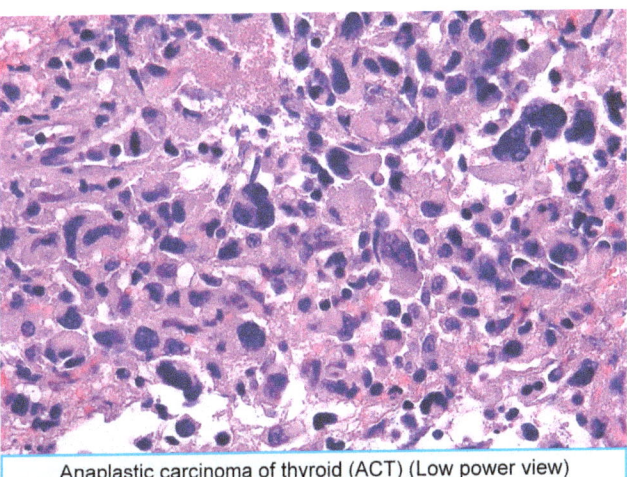

FIG. 17: Histopathological features of ACT: Small cell carcinoma and giant cell, and spindle carcinoma.
Courtesy: Professor Masud Parvez.

Medullary Carcinoma of Thyroid

Medullary carcinoma of thyroid (MCT) is characterized by:
- Most versatile carcinoma of thyroid.
- It arises from parafollicular cells; it is frequently multifocal.
- It spread both locally and distally.
- It secretes calcitonin and carcinoembryonic antigen (CEA).
- It has strong genetic association and associated with other cancer.

Cancer associations of MCT are described as following syndromes:
- Multiple endocrine neoplasia IIa (MEN-IIa) having (1) medullary carcinoma or C-cell hyperplasia, (2) pheochromocytoma (bilateral), (3) adrenal medullary hyperplasia, and (4) hyperparathyroidism (four-gland hyperplasia).
- MEN-IIb having (1) medullary carcinoma, (2) pheochromocytoma (bilateral), and (3) marfanoid appearance with multiple mucosa neuroma.
- Familial medullary carcinoma having with positive family history without pheochromocytom and hyperparathyroidism.

Histological features of MCT are nuclei with neuroendocrine features (round nuclei with salt-and-pepper chromatin), +/–amyloid deposits (fluffy appearing acellular eosinophilic material), and +/–C-cell hyperplasia **(Fig. 18)**.

Treatment: Complete resection of the thyroid tumor and any locoregional metastases can cured MCT. If there is residual, recurrent disease after initial surgery or those with distant metastases because most patients even with metastatic disease have slow progression for several years. Radioactive iodine therapy or TSH suppression are not effective. Recently, two tyrosine kinase inhibitors (TKIs) are approved for use in patients with advanced, metastatic or progressive MCT they are vandetanib and cabozantinib.

THYROID INCIDENTALOMA

A thyroid incidentaloma is defined as an asymptomatic thyroid tumor identified during the investigation of an unrelated condition. Prevalence rate of incidentaloma of thyroid varies depending on the investigating tool. In the absence of history of external beam radiation or familial medullary thyroid cancer, the risk of malignancy of incidentaloma of thyroid ranges between 5 and 13% when discovered with ultrasound, CT, or MRI, but is rises

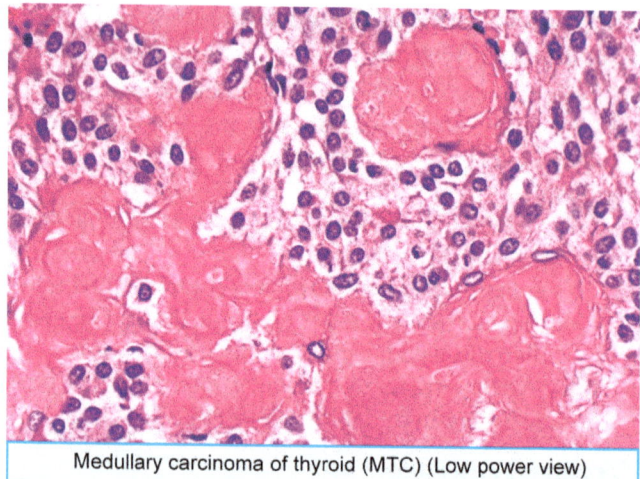

Medullary carcinoma of thyroid (MTC) (Low power view)

FIG. 18: Histopathological features of MTC: Nuclei with neuro-endocrine features (round nuclei with salt-and-pepper chromatin), +/–amyloid deposits (fluffy appearing acellular eosinophilic material), and +/–C-cell hyperplasia.
Courtesy: Professor Masud Parvez.

approximately to 30% if based on focal positron emission tomography (PET) scan.

Management of such a lesion requires five-step process:
1. Risk stratification for malignancy
2. Ultrasound-guided FNA of lesion with suspicious for malignancy
3. Surgical treatment for FNAC positive for malignancy
4. Nonsurgical treatment for FNAC negative for malignancy
5. Follow-up of benign and no suspicious incidentaloma

1. Risk stratification for malignancy is done on total score with size of the lesion. They are: (i) Benign—score 0 with nodule size <2.5 cm; (ii) Not suspicious—score up to 2 with nodule size <2.5 cm; (iii) Mildly suspicious—score 3 with nodule size >2.5 cm; (iv) Moderately suspicious—score 4-6 with nodule size >1.5 cm, and (v) Highly suspicious—score >7 with nodule size >1.0 cm **(Tables 15 and 16)**.
2. Ultrasound-guided FNA of lesion is to be done on cases with suspicious for malignancy risk—high, moderate, and mild suspicious.
3. Surgical treatment to be given to all cases with FNAC positive for malignancy.
4. Nonsurgical ablation techniques (percutaneous ethanol injection therapy, interstitial laser photocoagulation, or radiofrequency ablation) may be given to in cases negative for malignancy.

5. Persons with follow-up of benign and no suspicious risk can be discharged from medical care or kept in follow-up ultrasonogram evaluation protocol to see any increase in size and/or score at an interval of 6 months to 1 year.

FURTHER READINGS

1. Anatomy and Physiology by ©2017 Rice University. Textbook content produced by OpenStax. [online] Available from https://openstax.org/ [Last accessed September, 2023].
2. Standring S (Ed). Gray's Anatomy: The Anatomical Basis of Clinical Practice, 41st edition. [online] Available from https://www.amazon.com/Garys-Anatomy-Henry-Gray/dp/B00DXO9JRA) [Last accessed September, 2023].
3. Barrett K, Barman S, Yuan J, Brooks H (Eds). Ganong's Review of Medical Physiology, 26th edition. [online] Available from https://www.amazon.com/Ganongs-Review-Medical-Physiology-Twenty/dp/1260122409 [Last accessed September, 2023].
4. Melmed S, Koenig R, Rosen C, Auchus R, Goldfine A. Williams Textbook of Endocrinology, 14th edition. [online] Available from (https://www.elsevier.com/books/williams-textbook-of-endocrinology/bresnahan/978-0-323-55596-8 [Last accessed August, 2023].
5. Gardner D, Shoback D (Eds). Greenspan's Basic and Clinical Endocrinology, 10th edition. McGraw Hill; 2017. [online] Available from https://www.amazon.com/Greenspans-Basic-Clinical-Endocrinology-Tenth/dp/1259589285 [Last accessed September, 2023].
6. Ahmed T, Mahtab H, Tofail T (Eds). (2021). Thyroid Function Status by Paired Test. Lambart Academic Publication. [online] Available from https://www.amazon.com/THYROID-FUNCTION-STATUS-PAIRED-TEST/dp/6203580619 [Last accessed September, 2023].
7. Ahmed T, Mahtab H, Tofail T, Morshed AHG, Khan SA. (2021). Use of Paired Test in Management of Thyroid Disorders. [online] Available from https://www.longdom.org/open-access-pdfs/use-of-paired-test-in-management-of-thyroid-disorders.pdf [Last accessed September, 2023].
8. Tessler FN, Middleton WD, Grant EG, Hoang JK, Berland LL, Teefey SA, et al. ACR Thyroid Imaging, Reporting and Data System (TI-RADS): White Paper of the ACR TI-RADS Committee. J Am Coll Radiol. 2017;14(5):587-95.
9. Pacini F, Castagna MG, Brilli L, Pentheroudakis G. Thyroid cancer: ESMO Clinical Practice Guidelines for diagnosis, treatment and follow-up. Ann Oncol. 2019;30:1856-83.
10. Russ G, Bonnema SJ, Erdogan MF, Durante C, Ngu R, Leenhardt L. European Thyroid Association guidelines for ultrasound malignancy risk stratification of thyroid nodules in adults: The EU-TIRADS. Eur Thyroid J. 2017;6:225-37.

CHAPTER 4

Disorders of Parathyroid Gland

- ❑ Introduction to parathyroid gland
  - ➢ Anatomy of parathyroid gland
  - ➢ Parathyroid vascular anatomy
  - ➢ Parathyroid development
  - ➢ Physiology of parathyroid glands
- ❑ Parathyroid disorders
  - ➢ Hypoparathyroidism
  - ➢ Hyperparathyroidism
- ❑ Rickets, osteomalacia, and osteoporosis
  - ➢ Rickets and osteomalacia
  - ➢ Osteoporosis
- ❑ Incidentalomas of parathyroid

This chapter is about parathyroid gland, which begins with an introduction to applied anatomy and physiology. It covers hypoparathyroidism states, hyperparathyroidism, nonparathyroid hypercalcemia and rickets, osteomalacia, and osteoporosis. This chapter consists of 10 Figures, 4 Flowcharts, 12 Tables, and 5 Boxes to illustrate its text. This chapter ends with how to deal with incidentalomas of parathyroid.

INTRODUCTION TO PARATHYROID GLAND

■ Anatomy of Parathyroid Gland

There are four parathyroid glands in two pairs—superior and inferior. Normally they lie at the posterior aspect of the thyroid gland. The superior pair of *glands is usually located in the posterolateral side of the superior pole of the thyroid gland at the level of cricothyroid cartilage junction. They are at 1 cm above the intersection of the inferior thyroid artery and the recurrent laryngeal nerve. The position of inferior pair is usually variable—they may lie near the lower thyroid pole*. The shape of the gland is like a bean and weight is about 20–40 mg. The glands are encapsulated, and their surface is smooth. So, they can be differentiated from the thyroid gland or lymph nodes that have a more lobular surface or more pitted in appearance, respectively. There are three types of cells in a parathyroid gland. Of which chief cells and fat cells are constant and placed within thin fibrous capsules dividing the gland into lobules. The third type of cell is oxyphil cells, which appear at about puberty. The parathyroid glands appear light brown to tan. This color depends on their fat content, vascularity, and amount of oxyphil cells. Each parathyroid gland has a distinct hilar vessel, which is hallmark to differentiate from fatty tissue.

- *Chief cells* are of 6–8 µm size, polygonal shape with centrally placed round nuclei. They contain granules of parathyroid hormone (PTH). Cytoplasm is basophilic and most of them have intracellular fat. They are sensitive to changes in ionized calcium in serum.
- *Oxyphil cells* are larger than chief cells (12 µm). They do not contain secretory granules. Cytoplasm is acidophilic due to mitochondria. They appear at puberty as single cells, then pairs, and then nodules at the age of 40 years **(Figs. 1A and B)**.

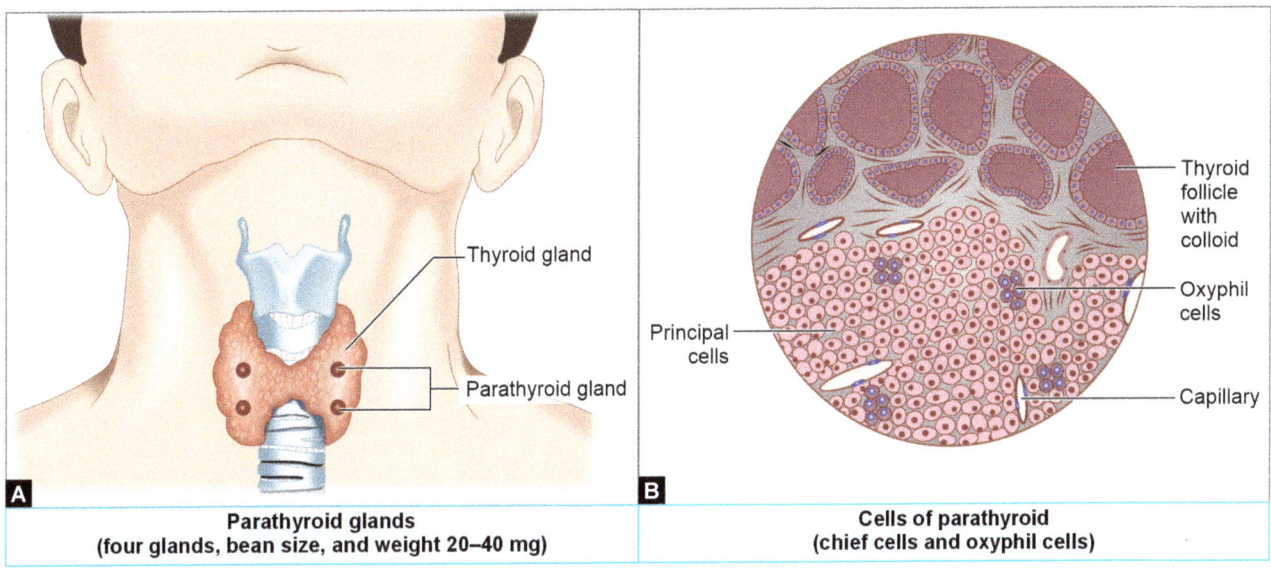

FIGS. 1A AND B: Anatomy and histology of parathyroid glands.

Parathyroid Vascular Anatomy

The inferior thyroid artery, from the thyrocervical trunk, supplies the inferior parathyroid gland. In approximately 1/10th of patients, the inferior thyroid artery is absent in one side (most commonly on the left side). The inferior parathyroid gland in that situation is supplied by a branch from the superior thyroid artery. In case a parathyroid is in the mediastinum, the inferior parathyroid glands descend into the anterior mediastinum. It may also be supplied by a thymic branch of the internal thoracic artery or even a direct branch of the aortic arch.

The inferior thyroid artery or an anastomotic branch between the inferior thyroid and the superior thyroid artery usually supplies the superior parathyroid gland. In about 20–45% of cases, the superior parathyroid glands receive significant vascularity from the superior thyroid artery.

Parathyroid Development

From the endoderm of the third and fourth pharyngeal pouches, the parathyroid glands develop. From the third, pharyngeal pouches give inferior pair, and the fourth pharyngeal pouches give superior pair. The inferior parathyroids are derived from the dorsal part of pharyngeal pouch, and the thymus arises from the ventral part of pharyngeal pouch. Usually, the inferior parathyroid glands become localized near the inferior poles of the thyroid, but thymus migrates toward the mediastinum.

From the fourth pharyngeal pouch, the superior parathyroid glands and the ultimobranchial bodies are derived. They migrate together, get detach from the pharyngeal wall, and fuse with the posterior aspect of the main body of the thyroid. These cells differentiate into the parafollicular cells (C cells) that secrete calcitonin. The superior parathyroid glands migrate in the inferior glands and remain in contact with the posterior part of the middle third of the thyroid lobes **(Figs. 2A and B)**.

Anatomic anomalies of the parathyroid gland may occur. The most common is the ectopic—the superior parathyroid commonly goes to tracheoesophageal groves, retroesophageal area, or posterior mediastinum, and those of inferior parathyroids to within thymus, anterior mediastinum, or thyroid. There may be supernumerary parathyroid glands also **(Fig. 3)**.

Physiology of Parathyroid Glands

The four parathyroid glands produce PTH. PTH helps to maintain calcium homeostasis in the body. Target tissues of PTH are renal tubule and bones. They have indirect action on gut epithelium via the activation of vitamin D.

Calcium and Phosphate Homeostasis

- Maintenance of normal serum calcium levels involves the regulation of the flux of calcium between the intestinal tract, kidneys, and bone.
- Calcium itself, PTH, and 1,25-dihydroxyvitamin D3 all play a role in calcium regulation.
- 1,25-dihydroxyvitamin D3 facilitates intestinal calcium absorption, whilst both 1,25-dihydroxyvitamin D3 and PTH stimulate calcium release from bone.
- PTH also stimulates the conversion of 25-hydroxyvitamin D3 to 1,25-dihydroxyvitamin D3 enabling distal renal tubular calcium reabsorption.

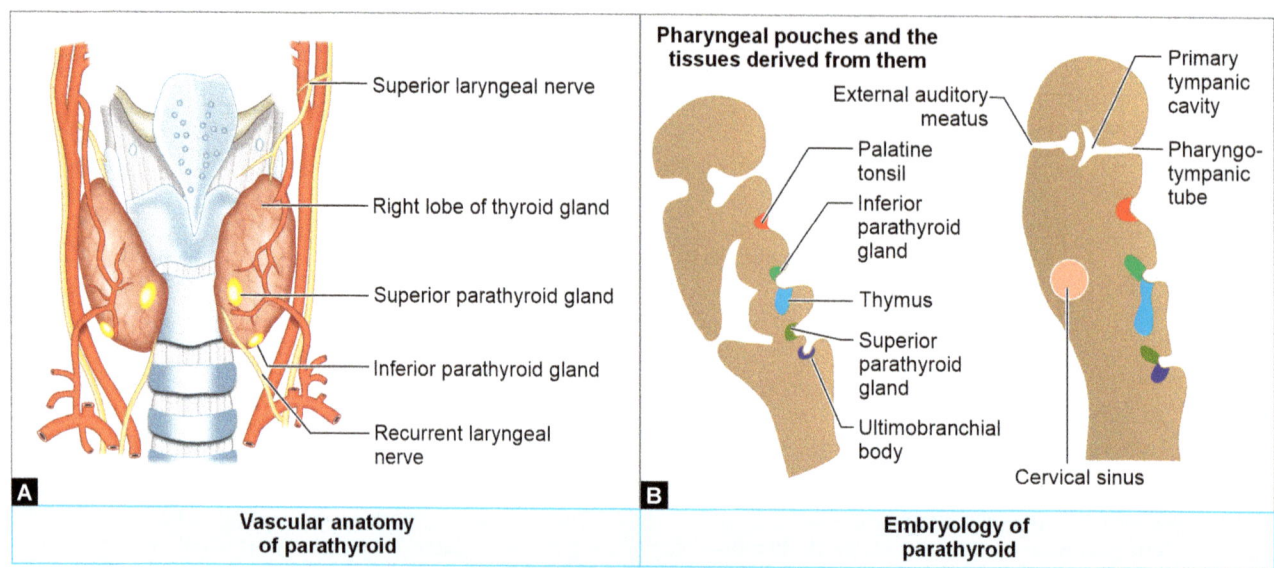

FIGS. 2A AND B: Vascular and developmental anatomy of parathyroid glands.

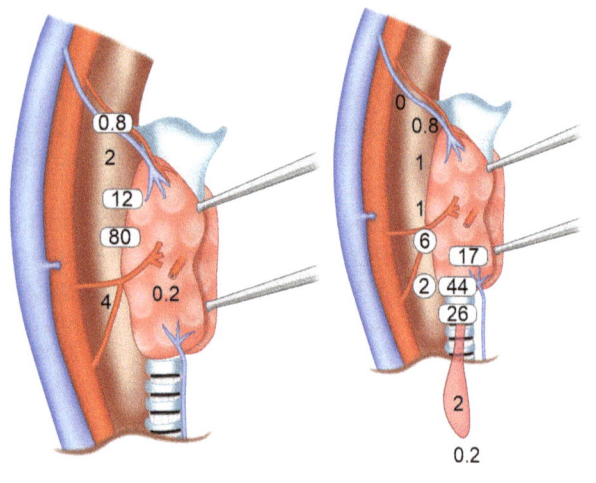

Ectopic positions of parathyroid glands

FIG. 3: Superior parathyroid goes to tracheoesophageal groves, retroesophageal area, or posterior mediastinum, and inferior parathyroid to within thymus, anterior mediastinum, or thyroid.

- High concentrations of serum calcium inhibit PTH secretion while low concentrations stimulate it.
- Phosphate reabsorption from the kidney is reduced by PTH. Thus, if PTH levels are low, serum phosphate will rise (more will be reabsorbed) **(Fig. 4)**.

PARATHYROID DISORDERS

Parathyroid disorders can either be hypofunctioning (hypoparathyroidism) or hyperfunctioning (hyperparathyroidism). Each of them is subdivided into

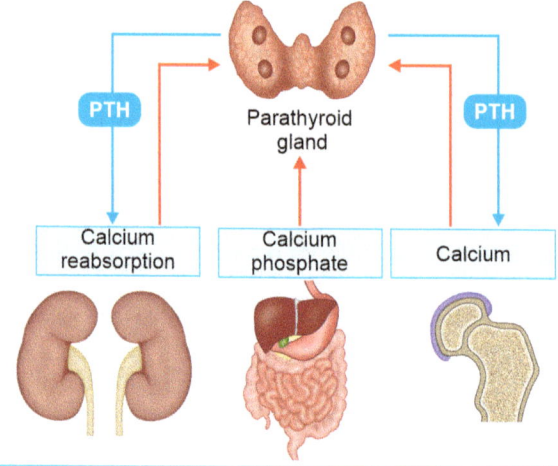

Calcium and phosphate homeostasis by PTH

FIG. 4: (1) Maintenance of normal serum calcium levels involves the regulation of the flux of calcium between the intestinal tract, kidneys, and bone. (2) Calcium, parathyroid hormone (PTH), and 1,25-dihydroxyvitamin D3 play a vital role in calcium regulation. (3) 1,25-dihydroxyvitamin D3 facilitates intestinal calcium absorption, whilst both 1,25-dihydroxyvitamin D3 and PTH stimulate calcium release from bone. (4) PTH also stimulates the conversion of 25-hydroxyvitamin D3 to 1,25-dihydroxyvitamin D3 enabling distal renal tubular calcium reabsorption. (5) High concentrations of serum calcium inhibit PTH secretion, while low concentrations stimulate it. (6) Phosphate reabsorption from the kidney is reduced by PTH. Thus, if PTH levels are low, serum phosphate will rise (more will be reabsorbed).

three subtypes—Hypoparathyroidism into hypoparathyroidism, pseudohypoparathyroidism (PHP), and pseudopseudohypoparathyroidism (PPHP).

CHAPTER 4: Disorders of Parathyroid Gland

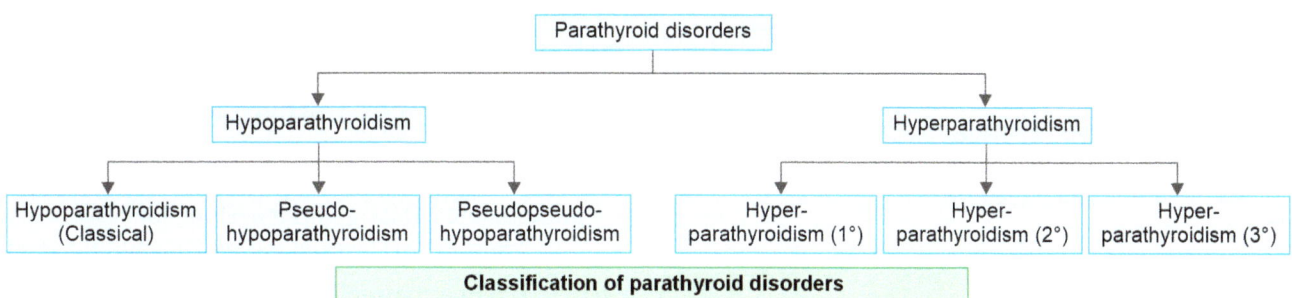

FLOWCHART 1: Parathyroid disorders can be either hypoparathyroidism or hyperparathyroidism. Each of them is subdivided into three subtypes.

Basic abnormality in classical hypoparathyroidism is hypocalcemia due to low secretion of parathormone, in PHP is hypocalcemia due to resistance parathormone action, and in PPHP there is no hypocalcemia and parathormone secretion is normal, but there are physical stigmata common with PHP.

Hyperparathyroidism is categorized into primary hyperparathyroidism, secondary hyperparathyroidism, and tertiary hyperparathyroidism. Basic abnormality in primary hyperparathyroidism is hypercalcemia due to high secretion of parathormone, in secondary hyperparathyroidism there is high secretion of parathormone due to low serum calcium level, and in tertiary hyperparathyroidism, there is high secretion of parathormone and high serum calcium level due to prolong period of secondary hyperparathyroidism **(Flowchart 1)**.

Hypoparathyroidism

Hypoparathyroidism is a clinical syndrome resulting from parathormone deficiency/inactivity. It is characterized by clinical (neuromuscular hyperactivity and others) and biochemical features (hypocalcemia and hyperphosphatemia), and hypocalcemia is considered as the hallmark.

Causes of hypoparathyroidism include:
- Surgery such as (1) thyroid surgery, (2) parathyroid surgery, or (3) neck surgery
- Idiopathic/autoimmune such as (1) early-onset genetic syndrome such as DiGeorge's syndrome or (2) multiple endocrine deficiency-Addison disease-candidiasis (MEDAC) syndrome
- *Functional (hypomagnesemia)*: These hypoparathyroid patients have very low serum megnesium level and improve dramatically on magnesium salt supplement **(Table 1 and Fig. 5)**.

Grading of the severity of hypoparathyroidism is done and shown in **Table 2**.

TABLE 1: The cause list of hypoparathyroidism.

Group	Disease
Surgical	- Thyroid surgery - Parathyroid surgery - Neck surgery
Autoimmune	- Early-onset genetic syndrome such as DiGeorge's syndrome - Multiple endocrine deficiency-Addison disease-candidiasis (MEDAC) syndrome
Functional	Functional (hypomagnesemia) hypoparathyroidism

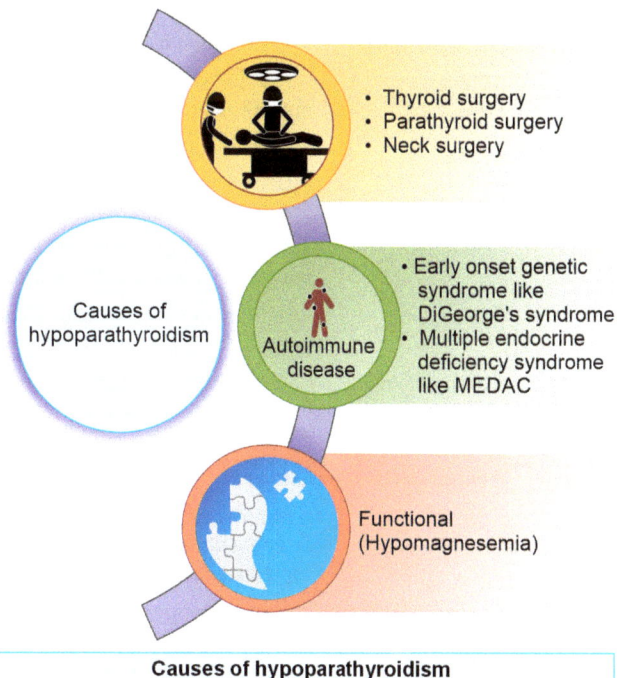

FIG. 5: There are three types of causes: (1) surgical, (2) autoimmune, (3) and functional.
(MEDAC: multiple endocrine deficiency-Addison disease-candidiasis)

Clinical Features of Hypoparathyroidism

Clinical features of hypoparathyroidism depend on the severity and chronicity of hypocalcemia. Features belong to two different types **(Table 3)**.
1. Neuromuscular hyperactivity
2. Nonneuromuscular features

TABLE 2:	Grading of severity of hypoparathyroidism.
Grade	Serum calcium level
1	Normal
2	Spontaneous inconstant hypocalcemia
3	<8.5 and up to 7.5 mg/dL
4	<7.5 and up to 6.5 mg/dL
5	<6.5 mg/dL

According to Parfitt hypoparathyroidism grading system.

Some features of hypoparathyroidism are given in **Figures 6A and B**.

Diagnosis of Hypoparathyroidism

A two-step diagnostic test include:
- *Step 1*: Documentation of hypocalcemia and hyperphosphatemia (along with renal function test).
- *Step 2*: Serum PTH level (along with magnesium level).

Step 1: Documentation of hypocalcemia and hyperphosphatemia (in absence of impaired renal function) is *virtually diagnostic* of hypoparathyroidism. In cases of relative phosphate-depleted state, such as low dietary intake or nonabsorption due to binding with drugs, (such as aluminum hydroxide gel) serum phosphate may not rise with hypocalcemia of hypoparathyroidism. In that case, nonparathyroid disorders producing hypocalcemia (such as rickets, osteomalacia, malabsorption syndrome, pancreatitis, etc.) should be excluded.

TABLE 3:	Clinical features of hypoparathyroidism.	
Types	Features of hypoparathyroidism	
Type 1	*Features of neuromuscular hyperactivity of hypoparathyroidism*	
1	Paresthesia	Numbness and tingling around mouth and fingertips
2	Tetany	Attack of tetany usually begins with paresthesia. Commonly occurs in the muscles of face and extremities. Signs of latent tetany such as *Chvostek's sign and Trousseau's sign* are positive in pretetanic stage, so they are used as follow-up tool for patient on calcium replacement and after thyroid surgery
3	Hyperventilation	May arise from fear of tetany and can lead to hypocapnia and alkalosis
4	Adrenergic symptoms	Tachycardia, sweating, and pallor in the face, and extremities are seen due to increased secretion of epinephrine
5	Convulsion	Younger patients are more prone to develop convulsion. It may be of two forms: 1. Generalized tetany followed by prolonged tonic spasm and typical epileptic sizers (grand mal, Jacksonian, focal, or petite mal) 2. They have typical electroencephalographic changes Both the forms respond to correction of hypocalcemia
6	Papilledema	Rare findings in hypoparathyroidism mostly present in association with convulsion and mimic brain tumors
7	Extrapyramidal signs	Chronically hypocalcemia may present with an extrapyramidal neurological syndrome such as Parkinsonism. They are sensitive to dystonic side effects of phenothiazine drugs. Calcification of basal ganglia is seen on X-ray of some cases
Type 2	*Nonneuromuscular features*	
1	Cataract	A common sequela of hypoparathyroidism is the formation of a confluent opacity in the posterior segment of the lens called *posterior lenticular cataract*. The change can be halted or even reverted to some extent on adequate treatment of hypocalcemia
2	Cardiac manifestation	Refractory congestive cardiac failure (CCF); resistance to digitalis therapy *Electrocardiogram (ECG) changes*: Prolongation of Q-T interval. Eucalcemia reverses all the cardiac manifestations
3	Dental manifestation	Childhood hypoparathyroidism is associated with: • Abnormal enamel formation • Dental eruption, delayed or absent • Defective dental root, short or blunted root

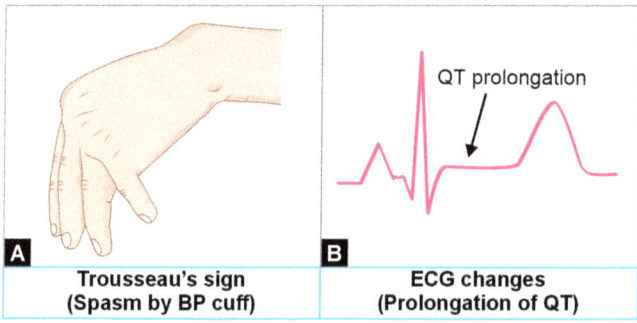

FIGS. 6A AND B: Some features of hypoparathyroidism.
(BP: blood pressure; ECG: electrocardiogram)

> **BOX 2: Calcium preparations used for the treatment of hypoparathyroidism.**
>
> - Calcium gluconate
> - Calcium lactate
> - Calcium chloride
> - Calcium carbonate
>
> Gluconate and lactate contain relatively small amount of elemental calcium, so large number of tablets are required. Chloride contains large amount of calcium, but tends to cause gastric irritation. Carbonate is preferred preparation, but it may tend to produce alkalosis.

> **BOX 1: Indications for search of hypoparathyroidism (hypocalcemia and hyperphosphatemia).**
>
> - Person underwent neck surgery (yearly)
> - Person suspected of MEDAC (multiple endocrine deficiency-Addison disease-candidiasis) syndrome (yearly)
> - Delay in dental development
> - Convulsive disorders (any form)
> - Basal ganglia calcification, skin candidiasis, and cataract

TABLE 4: Vitamin D preparations used in hypoparathyroidism.

Vitamin D preparation	Daily dose range
Vitamin D2 (ergocalciferol/ergosterol)	25,000–50,000 units
Dihydrotachysterol	0.2–1 mg
Calcifediol	25–200 µg
Calcitriol (1,25-dihydroxyvitamin D3)	0.25–5 µg

Satisfactory maintenance dose of calcium supplement and vitamin D for an individual is to be ascertained biochemical eucalcemia. Regular reexamination at an interval of 6 months to 1 year is to be done to detect complications of hypercalciuria and vitamin D toxicity.

Step 2: Serum PTH and magnesium level.
- An almost undetectable level of parathormone in cases of hypocalcemia and hyperphosphatemia *confirms the diagnosis* of hypoparathyroidism.
- All cases of hypoparathyroidism need to be checked for serum magnesium level. Hypomagnesemia is then dialogistic of functional hypoparathyroidism. A high level of PTH excludes hypoparathyroidism and may be due to (1) PHP, (2) vitamin D deficiency state, (3) secondary hyperparathyroidism, etc.

Indications for search of hypoparathyroidism are given in **Box 1**.

Treatment of Hypoparathyroidism

The aim of treatment is to restore serum calcium level by using calcium and vitamin D/synthetic analog therapy and maintain within physiological range. There is no practical scope for PTH therapy.

- *Maintenance therapy*:
  - Diet supplement: Diet should contain high calcium and low phosphate.
  - Calcium supplement: Calcium supplement to be made so that total calcium (diet + supplement) is >1 g/day for below 40 years of age and approximately 2 g/day for above 40 years of age population **(Box 2)**.
- *Vitamin D therapy*: Vitamin D preparations that are used in hypoparathyroidism are shown in **Table 4**.
- *Emergency therapy/measure of tetany*: Tetany due to hypoparathyroidism is a medical emergency. Aim of treatment is to prevent convulsion and stridor.
  - Intravenous (IV) calcium supplement: After assuring the airway, 10% calcium gluconate sodium 10–20 mL is given IV slowly, until symptoms subside or serum calcium is above 7 mg/dL.
  - Oral calcium: It should be started simultaneously with IV preparations such as:
    – Calcium gluconate 6 g three times daily or
    – Calcium lactate 5 g three times daily.
    – If serum calcium level falls below 7 g/dL after 6 hours, enforce IV therapy again.

Pseudohypoparathyroidism and Pseudopseudohypoparathyroidism

Pseudohypoparathyroidism

A familial syndrome resulting from resistance to PTH caused by mutation of *GNAS1* or *STX16* gene is characterized by:
- Hypocalcemia with other features of hypoparathyroidism
- Raised serum PTH level

- Developmental abnormalities, mostly marked on skeleton

Developmental abnormalities of pseudohypoparathyroidism:
- Short stature
- Mild obesity with round face
- Short metatarsal/metacarpal bones (usually fourth)
- Delayed dentation, defective enamel, or absence of teeth
- Bony exostosis, ectopic calcification, coxa vara/coxa valga, bowing of radius, tibia, and fibula.
- Mental retardation and hyperthyroidism may coexist. Some features of PHP are given in **Figures 7A and B**.

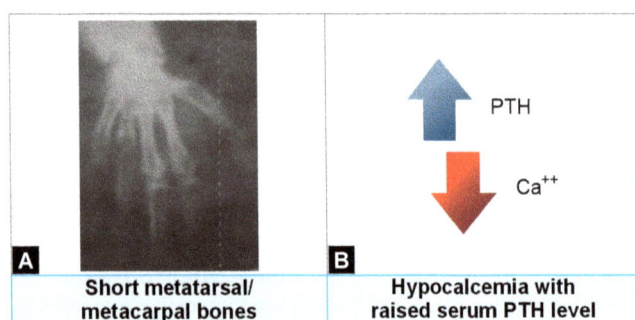

FIGS. 7A AND B: Features of pseudohypoparathyroidism.
(PTH: parathyroid hormone)

Pseudopseudohypoparathyroidism

Definition: Rare familial disorder, presents with developmental features of PHP, but serum calcium, phosphate, and PTH levels are normal.

Treatment of Pseudohypoparathyroidism and Pseudopseudohypoparathyroidism

- Treatment of PHP is same as hypoparathyroidism.
- No specific treatment of PPHP is required.

Comparison between three forms of hypoparathyroidism is given in **Table 5**.

Stepwise diagnostic approach to PHP and PPHP see in **Table 6**.

Decision-making investigation steps (DMIS) of a case suspected for primary hypoparathyroidism are given in **Table 7**.

Hyperparathyroidism

Hyperparathyroidism is a clinical syndrome resulting from excess parathormone.

This is characterized by:
1. Classical features of hypercalcemia, nephrolithiasis, and osteitis fibrosa cystica.

   Present trend of using serum calcium as a routine biochemical test, most cases are identified as (1) asymptomatic cases or (2) with nonspecific features such as excessive weakness.

TABLE 5: Comparison between three forms of hypoparathyroidism.

Condition	Appearance	PTH	Calcitriol	Calcium	Phosphates
Hypoparathyroidism	Normal	Low	Low	Low	High
Pseudohypoparathyroidism	Skeletal defects	High	Low	Low	High
Pseudopseudohypoparathyroidism	Skeletal defects	Normal	Normal	Normal	Normal

(PTH: parathyroid hormone)

TABLE 6: Diagnostic approach to pseudohypoparathyroidism and pseudopseudohypoparathyroidism.

Step	Check for	Finding	Conclusion/Diagnosis
1	Developmental abnormalities	Absent	Excluded
		Present	Go to step 2
2	Serum calcium, phosphate, and PTH levels	Calcium low but phosphate and PTH high	PHP
		Calcium, phosphate, and PTH normal	PPHP
		Calcium low, phosphate normal/low, and PTH normal/high	Check for vitamin D-related disorders

(PHP: pseudohypoparathyroidism; PPHP: pseudopseudohypoparathyroidism; PTH: parathyroid hormone)

TABLE 7: Decision-making investigation steps of a case suspected for primary hypoparathyroidism.

Step	Investigation	Result	Action/Inference
Initial step	Assay of serum calcium	Normal/High	Primary hypoparathyroidism excluded
		Low	Go to step 2
Step 2	Assay of serum phosphate level	Normal	Go to step 4
		High	Go to step 3
Step 3	Assay of serum creatinine	Normal	Go to step 4
		High	Treat as CKD
Step 4	Assay of serum PTH	Normal/High	Review from the initial step/skeletal stigma of pseudohypoparathyroidism
		Low	Go to step 5
Step 5	Assay of serum magnesium	Normal	Confirm hypoparathyroidism—treat and go to step 6
		Low	Confirm functional hypoparathyroidism—treat and go to step 7
Step 6	Monitor with serum calcium	Normal	Continue management by Ca^{++} and vitamin D
		Low/High	Adjust treatment
Step 7	Monitoring of serum calcium and magnesium	Normal	Continue management of Mg with/without Ca^{++} and vitamin D
		Low/High	Adjust treatments

(CKD: chronic kidney disease; PTH: parathyroid hormone)

BOX 3: Clinical features of primary hyperparathyroidism.

- *Central nervous system features of hypercalcemia*:
  - Impaired mentation
  - Recent memory loss
  - Emotional lability
  - Depression
  - Anosmia
  - Somnolence
  - Coma
- *Neuromuscular features*:
  - Proximal muscle weakness
  - Hypoactive deep tendon reflexes
  - Pain and vibration sensation loss
  - Abnormal tongue movements (resembling fascination)
  - Lingual atrophy
  - Ataxic gait
  - Abnormally strong (hard) fingers
- *Rheumatological feature*: Joint pain from gout, pseudogout, calcific tendinitis, and chondrocalcinosis
- *Dermatological features*: Pruritus due to metastatic calcification of skin
- *Gastrointestinal features*: Anorexia, nausea, vomiting, dyspepsia, and constipation
- *Renal features*: Polyuria, nocturia, renal colic, and intermittent passage of stone with urine
- *Other features*:
  - Palpable or visible parathyroid nodule in the thyroid (rare)
  - Conjunctivitis (due to calcium phosphate crystal)
  - Band keratopathy
  - Bony deformity and tenderness
  - Peptic ulcer disease

Classification of hyperparathyroidism with its causes is as follows:
- Primary hyperparathyroidism due to adenoma of single parathyroid gland (most common), hyperplasia of multiple parathyroid glands, and carcinoma of parathyroid gland(s) rare
- Secondary hyperparathyroidism due to hyperparathormonemia in response to chronic hypoalcemia as in chronic renal failure
- Tertiary hyperparathyroidism due to development of classical hyperparathyroidism (primary) in a secondary hyperparathyroidism case

Clinical Features of Primary Hyperparathyroidism

Box 3 shows the clinical features of primary hyperparathyroidism.

Radiological Features of Primary Hyperparathyroidism

Box 4 shows the radiological features of primary hyperparathyroidism.

Management of Primary Hyperparathyroidism

Management of primary hyperparathyroidism starts with documentation of its biochemical hallmark hypercalcemia. If hypercalcemia is coupled with high PTH, it ascertains primary hyperparathyroidism. The third step of management is to localize the source of high PTH by imaging [(sonography, ^{99m}Tc-sestamibi scintigraphy, magnetic resonance imaging (MRI), or computed

BOX 4: Radiological features of primary hyperparathyroidism.

- *In bone*:
  - Osteitis fibrosa cystica (subperiosteal bone resorption) best seen in fingers
  - Pepper pot appearance of skull film
  - Generalized osteopenia
  - Bone cyst (brown tumor)
  - Erosion of distal phalangeal tufts
  - Erosion of distal end of clavicles
- *In soft tissue*:
  - Nephrocalcinosis
  - Stone formation in kidney, gallbladder, pancreas, etc.

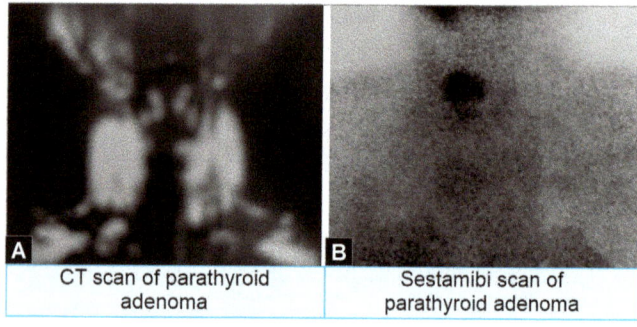

FIGS. 8A AND B: Parathyroid adenomas image in computed tomography (CT) and sestamibi scan.

Step	Action	Remarks
1	Documentation of hypercalcemia: • Total serum calcium (in fasting free-flowing venous blood) • Serum albumin (to do calculation by correction factor)*	Biochemical hallmark
2	Documentation of high PTH level	Automated sandwich-type immunoassay preferred
3	Localization of parathyroid lesion(s)	Sonography, ^{99m}Tc-sestamibi scan, MRI, and CT
4	Treatment of hypercalcemia	See management of hypercalcemia
5	Surgery	See table of extent of parathyroidectomy
6	Postsurgical management (including hungry bone syndrome)	See postoperative care of parathyroid surgery in primary hyperparathyroidism

TABLE 8: Steps of management of primary hyperparathyroidism.

*Calculated serum calcium (mg/dL) = Measured calcium (mg/dL) − (serum albumin in g/dL − 4).

(CT: computed tomography; MRI: magnetic resonance imaging; PTH: parathyroid hormone)

tomography (CT)]. The definite modality treatment of choice is surgery, and medical management of pre- and postoperative control of serum calcium is done. **Table 8** summarizes the management steps.

^{99m}Tc-sestamibi scan and CT scan of parathyroid adenoma are shown in **Figures 8A and B**.

Treatment of Hypercalcemia of Hyperparathyroidism (Preoperative)

- *Rehydration*: In general, patient becomes dehydrated due to anorexia, nausea, vomiting, and polyuria. All these result in significant volume depletion. Initial step of therapy is rehydration by using about 3–4 L of normal saline infusion over 24–48 hours.
- *Removal of calcium from blood*: Loop diuretic (20–80 mg/day) is used with the saline infusion to enhance renal clearance of calcium.
- *Reduction of calcium entry from bone*: Several agents are used such as calcitonin, plicamycin, gallium nitrate, and bisphosphonates.
  - Calcitonin, a peptide hormone, inhibits osteoclast. 4–8 units/kg body weight is given subcutaneously, intramuscular or IV. It can reduce calcium within 2–4 hours, and generally efficacy is lost in 1–8 days.
  - Plicamycin, a cytotoxic antibiotic, inhibits osteoclast. 15–25 µg/kg IV can bring down calcium to target within 24–72 hours. The agent is quite toxic to liver, kidney, and bone marrow.
  - Gallium nitrate binds to bone mineral and inhibits bone resorption. Continuous infusion at a rate of 200 mg/m^2/day can normalize serum calcium after 5–8 days. The age is somewhat nephrotoxic and should be used cautiously in dehydrated patient.
  - Bisphosphonates such as chlodronate and pamidronate are in use in acute or severe hypercalcemia. Chlodronate 300–600 mg or pamidronate 3–60 mg is infused over 2–4 hours. Serum calcium gradually falls to normal in 2–5 days and remains normal for several weeks. Once weekly dose is repeated until defiant surgical treatment is performed.
  - Reduction of calcium entry from gut: Glucocorticoid antagonized the action of vitamin,

TABLE 9: Extent of parathyroidectomy.	
Gland(s) involved	Surgical procedure
One	• Removal of the affected gland • Identify all other and suture tagging
Two/Three	• Removal of all but half of healthy gland • Suture tagging of preserved half of the normal gland
All four	• Removal of all but 35–50 g of one gland • Suture tagging of preserved portion of the gland

1,25-dihydroxyvitamin D, in intestine. So, it is useful in hypercalcemia of granulomatous and lymphomatous disorders also.

- *Parathyroid surgery in primary hyperparathyroidism*: Surgery is ideal for all cases. It is considered important when person is younger if bony change occurs or active nephrolithiasis is present. Localization of parathyroid lesion(s), if failed by noninvasive imaging, may require thyroid arteriography or selective venous catheterization for PTH assay. Extent of parathyroidectomy depends on the number of gland(s) involved **(Table 9)**.

Postoperative Care of Parathyroid Surgery in Primary Hyperparathyroidism

In postoperative period, serum calcium level usually goes to hypocalcemia within 24 hours. It can be mild to moderate, which is amenable to oral supplement of calcium with or without vitamin D. If there is bony change and preoperatively management of hypercalcemia is not satisfactory, patient can develop hungry bone syndrome (HBS) and requires specific management (see *Hungry Bone Syndrome*). Other complications during postoperative period are bone pain, metabolic acidosis, pancreatitis, etc.

Nonparathyroidal Causes of Hypercalcemia

Box 5 shows the lists of nonparathyroidal causes of hypercalcemia.

Williams syndrome: Williams syndrome or Williams–Beuren syndrome (WBS) is a rare genetic disorder characterized by (1) hypercalcemia, (2) supravalvular aortic stenosis, (3) short stature, (4) mental defect, and (5) Elfin-like facies. The typical facial features are high forehead, medial broadening of the eyebrows, periorbital fullness, depressed nasal bridge, malar hypoplasia, thick lips, and long nasolabial philtrum. WBS is caused by a 1–2-Mb microdeletion in 7q11.23, a region that contains 28 genes. Approximately 90% of WBS patients have a 1.55 Mb microdeletion and 8% have a 1.84 Mb microdeletion **(Fig. 9)**.

BOX 5: Nonparathyroidal causes of hypercalcemia.

- *Malignancy*:
  - Metastatic
  - Nonmetastatic
  - Multiple myeloma
- *Lymphoproliferative disorders*:
  - β-cell lymphoma
  - Hodgkin's disease
  - Lymphoid granuloma
- Hyperthyroidism
- Vitamin D intoxication
- *Immobilization*:
  - Paget's disease
  - Children
- Idiopathic infantile hypercalcemia (IIH)
- Vitamin A intoxication
- Williams syndrome
- Total parental nutrition (TPN)
- Thiazide
- *Granulomatous disorders*:
  - Tuberculosis
  - Silicosis
  - Candidiasis
  - Leprosy
- Familial hypocalciuric hypercalcemia (FHH)

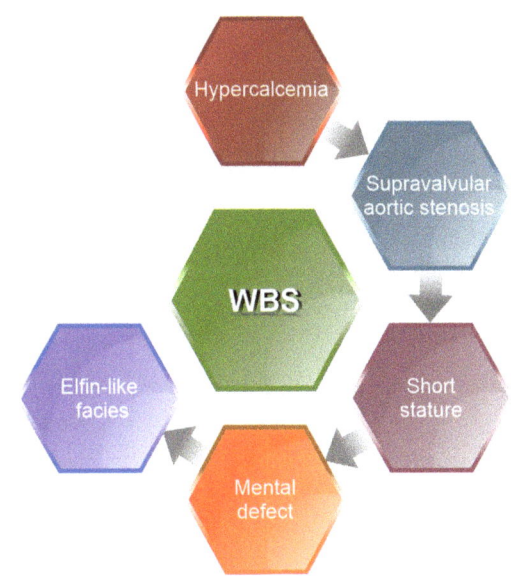

FIG. 9: Williams–Beuren syndrome (WBS) characterized by (1) hypercalcemia, (2) short stature, (3) supravalvular aortic stenosis, (4) mental defect, and (5) elfin-like facies.

Familial hypocalciuric hypercalcemia (FHH): It is an inherited disorder. In most cases, there are inactivating mutations of the gene for the calcium-sensing receptor of the parathyroid glands and in the thick ascending limb of the loop of Henle. FHH is characterized by:
- Onset of hypercalcemia before 10 years of age
- Serum PTH level high
- 1,25-dihydroxyvitamin D level normal
- Magnesium high
- Urinary clearance to calcium and magnesium low

People with FHH usually do not have any symptoms and are often diagnosed by chance during routine blood tests **(Fig. 10 and Table 10)**.

Hungry Bone Syndrome

It develops during postoperative period of parathyroidectomy in persons with primary hyperparathyroidism and preoperative high bone turnover having bone changes such as osteitis fibrosa cystica or brown tumor. It is characterized by (1) the rapid, profound, and prolonged hypocalcemia and (2) with hypophosphatemia and hypomagnesemia. The severe hypocalcemia is due to increased influx of calcium into bone after the sudden removal of the effect of high circulating levels of PTH on osteoclastic resorption.
- Treatment is aimed at replenishing the severe calcium deficit by using high doses of calcium, supplemented by high doses of active metabolites of vitamin D.

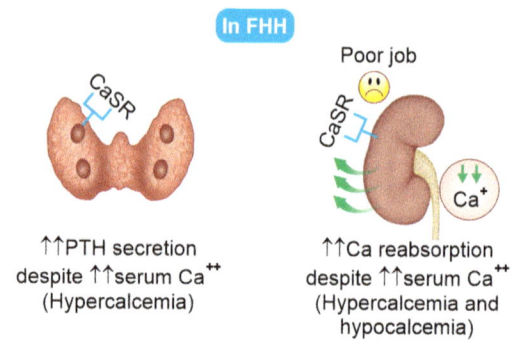

FIG. 10: Familial hypocalciuric hypercalcemia (FHH) is characterized by: (1) Onset of hypercalcemia before 10 years of age, (2) serum parathyroid hormone (PTH) level high, (3) 1,25-dihydroxyvitamin D level normal, (4) magnesium high, and (5) urinary clearance to calcium and magnesium low.

TABLE 10: Decision-making investigation steps (DMIS) of a case suspected of primary hyperparathyroidism.

Step	Investigations	Finding	Action/inference
Initial step	Assay of serum calcium	Normal	Primary hyperparathyroidism excluded
		High	Go to step 2
Step 2	Assay of PTH level	Normal	Go to step 4
		High	Go to step 3 (confirm primary hyperparathyroidism)
Step 3	Localization of parathyroid lesion(s) by imaging*	Normal	Go to step 4
		Localized	Go to step 5
Step 4	Assay of PTH-like peptide	High	Check for malignancy (steps 6 and 8)
		Not High	Go to step 6
Step 5	Primary hyperparathyroidism due to adenoma/carcinoma	Adenoma/carcinoma(s)	Management by surgery
Step 6	Assay of serum vitamin 1,25-dihydroxyvitamin D3 level	High	Check for granulomatous lymphoproliferative disorders
		Not High	Go to step 7
Step 7	Assay for FT_4 and TSH	Hyperthyroidism	Treat hyperthyroidism
		Normal	Go to step 8
Step 8	Serum/urine for protein electrophoresis	Myeloma	Treat myeloma
		Normal	Go to step 9
Step 9	Urinary calcium clearance	Low	Consider hypocaloric hypercalcemia (?FHH)
		Normal/high	Review whole data

*Parathyroid imaging—sonography, ^{99m}Tc-sestamibi scintigraphy, MRI, or CT. Steps can be interchanged according to clinical judgment.
(FT_4: free thyroxine; PTH: parathyroid hormone; TSH: thyroid-stimulating hormone)

- Adequate correction of magnesium deficiency and normalization of bone turnover is required for resolution of the hypocalcemia, which may last for a number of months after successful surgery.
- Prevention can be made by preoperative treatment with bisphosphonates.

RICKETS, OSTEOMALACIA, AND OSTEOPOROSIS

Rickets and Osteomalacia

Rickets and osteomalacia are clinical syndromes resulting from deficiency of vitamin D, producing rickets in childhood and osteomalacia in adults (Table 11).

Features of rickets and osteomalacia are given in Table 12.

Biochemical Features of Rickets and Osteomalacia

- Serum calcium and phosphate low or at lower normal range
- Serum alkaline phosphate high
- Vitamin D level in blood low

Radiological Features of Rickets and Osteomalacia

- *In children*:
  - Widen epiphyseal bone
  - Metaphysis is expanded and irregular.

- *In adult*:
  - Development of pseudofratcure or looser's zones (translucent zones passing through the cortex)
  - Subperiosteal erosions (Flowchart 2)

Treatment and Prevention of Rickets and Osteoporosis

Vitamin D supplement:
- For infants, vitamin D drops 400 IU/day
- For older children, vitamin D tablets 500 mg 2–3 tablets daily for treatment and one tablet daily for prevention. Simple vitamin D deficiency should not be treated with potent vitamin D metabolites.

Other Forms of Rickets and Osteoporosis

- Renal osteodystrophy
- Vitamin D-dependent rickets
- Vitamin D-resistant rickets

Renal Osteodystrophy

Renal osteodystrophy is the term used to describe the different patterns of the skeletal abnormalities that occur in patients with chronic kidney disease.

Clinically, it is characterized by profound muscle weakness and bone pain.

TABLE 11: Causes of rickets and osteomalacia.

Group	Cause
Malabsorption due to	- Crohn's disease - Small bowel resection - Chronic pancreatic insufficiency - Cystic fibrosis - Primary biliary cirrhosis
No exposure to sunlight	
Dietary deficiency	
Hypoparathyroidism	

TABLE 12: Features of rickets and osteomalacia.

Neonate	Growing children	Adult
- Failure to thrive - Fits for hypocalcemia - Small for height - Increased perinatal mortality - Radiological changes and multiple fractures	- Bone pain (mostly knee joint) - Knocked knee - Bow legs - Delayed dentation - Swollen and tender wrist - Short stature - Chostochondral junction prominent (rachitic rosary) - Indented ribs at attachment with diaphragm (Harrison's sulcus)	- Diffuse bone pain (rib, back, and pelvis) - Proximal muscle weakness waddling gait - Pseudo fracture—pelvis and neck of femur

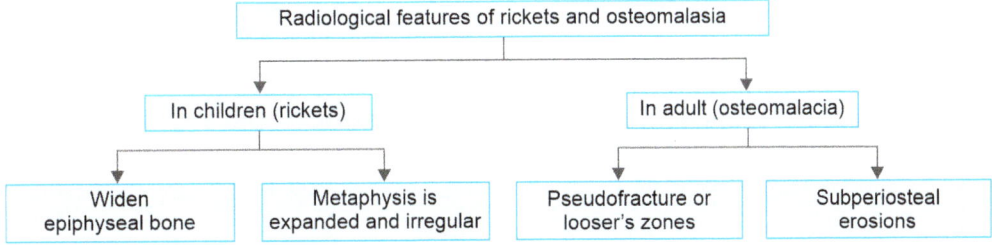

FLOWCHART 2: Radiological features of rickets and osteomalacia.

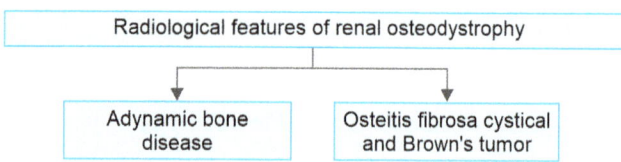

FLOWCHART 3: Radiological features of renal osteodystrophy.

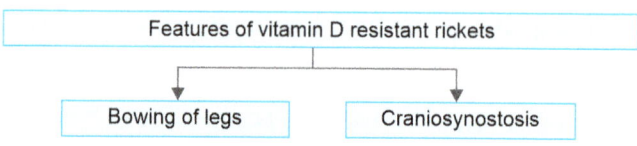

FLOWCHART 4: Features of vitamin D-resistant rickets.

The skeletal abnormalities are usually of two different forms:
1. Osteitis fibrosa, characterized by high bone turnover, increased osteoclastic and osteoblastic activity, and high levels of circulating PTH.
2. Adynamic bone disease is characterized by low bone turnover and low levels of circulating PTH **(Flowchart 3)**.

Decreased serum levels of calcitriol—1,25-dihydroxyvitamin D3, serum ionized calcium and elevated phosphorus, reduced numbers of vitamin D receptors and calcium sensors in the parathyroid gland, and skeletal resistance to the calcemic action of PTH play a major role in the development of renal osteodystrophy.

Renal replacement therapy plays a practical role in the treatment and prevention of renal osteodystrophy although calcitriol has some role in the treatment of bony changes.

Vitamin D-dependent Rickets

Vitamin D-dependent rickets are a group of genetic disorders (autosomal recessive) characterized by early-onset rickets due to:
- Inability to maintain adequate concentrations of active forms of vitamin D or
- A failure to respond fully to activated vitamin D in small/usual dose
- But response to large dose of vitamin D (>50,000 units/day)
- And patients have a lifelong "dependency" on administration of high dose of vitamin D replacement.

The term "vitamin D-dependent rickets" describes a group of genetic disorders that are characterized by early-onset rickets due to the inability to maintain adequate concentrations of active forms of vitamin D or a failure to respond fully to activated vitamin D.

Vitamin D-resistant Rickets or Hypophosphatemic Rickets

It is a disorder in which the bones become painfully soft and bend easily due to low levels of phosphate in the blood.

Symptoms usually begin in early childhood and can range in severity. Severe forms may cause bowing of the legs and other bone deformities; bone pain; joint pain; poor bone growth; and short stature. In some affected babies, the space between the skull bones closes too soon (craniosynostosis).

Treatment consists of the oral administration of large doses of vitamin D. Careful observation of patients during vitamin D therapy to prevent overdosage and hypercalcemia is of crucial importance. Surgical correction of the bony deformities is rarely necessary **(Flowchart 4)**.

Osteoporosis

Osteoporosis refers to decreased bone strength to cause to increased chance of fracture. It is due to low bone mass and microarchitectural disruption. Nowadays, the mostly accepted definition of osteoporosis is on the basis of bone mass density (BMD) using DXA (dual-energy X-ray absorptiometry) scan. The definition of osteoporosis is based on BMD score that compares BMD of a young adult reference population (T-score). Diagnosis of by T-score is as follows: (1) Osteoporosis = T-score < −2.5 SD (standard deviation); (2) Osteopenia = T-score between −1.1 and −2.4 SD; and (3) Normal = T-score > −1 SD.

Postmenopausal women with osteoporosis have bone loss related to estrogen deficiency and/or age. Initial history for risk factors for fracture, physical examination, and basic laboratory tests may reveal clues to potentially reversible causes of osteoporosis.

A low BMD Z-scores (age-matched comparison) may require further evaluation for secondary causes of osteoporosis. Early diagnosis and fracture risk are important because of the availability of therapies that can slow or even reverse the progression of osteoporosis. The clinical manifestations, diagnosis, and evaluation of osteoporosis in postmenopausal women will be reviewed here. The evaluation of osteoporosis in premenopausal women and men and the treatment of osteoporosis are reviewed separately.

Therapeutic of Osteoporosis

For practical aspect, it will be discussed on the basis of sex.

Osteoporosis in Female

Postmenopausal women with high risk of fractures are treated with some pharmacological agents. They are:
- Bisphosphonates
- Human monoclonal antibody—denosumab
- Parathyroid hormone-related protein (PTHrP) analog or
- Selective estrogen receptor modulators (SERMs)

Bisphosphonates

These molecules are recommended as the first choice to reduce fracture risk. Available bisphosphonates are alendronate, risedronate, zoledronic acid, and ibandronate. Ibandronate is less effective in reducing nonvertebral or hip fracture risk compared to rest of the three.

After 3-5 years of initiation of bisphosphonates, reassessment of fracture risk should be done. If the risk of fractures remains high, treatment should be continued, but if the risk of fractures becomes low to moderate, they may go to a "bisphosphonate holiday" for up to 5 years depending on BMD and clinical circumstances of the individual patient.

Doses of bisphosphonates:
- Alendronate can be taken in daily or weekly doses.
- Risedronate is in daily, weekly, and twice monthly doses.
- Ibandronate is once a month or as an IV injection administered once every 3 months.
- Zoledronic acid is an IV injection administered once yearly.

Oral bisphosphonates are given in empty stomach and with a full glass of water in the morning. Person should remain in an upright position and refrain from eating or drinking for at least 30 minutes.

Side effects of oral bisphosphonates are gastrointestinal problems including difficulty swallowing, inflammation of the esophagus, and gastric ulcer. Side effects of IV bisphosphonates include flu-like symptoms, fever, pain in muscles or joints, and headache. These side effects can occur initially for 2-3 days. Rare there are reports of osteonecrosis of the jaw and of visual disturbances in people taking oral and IV bisphosphonates.

Human Monoclonal Antibody: Denosumab

It is used to initial treatment for the prevention of osteoporosis as an alternative of bisphosphonate. It is given 60 mg subcutaneously once in every 6 months. Bone remodeling is the primary mode of action of this drug. Duration of action is 6 months. So, unlike bisphosphonate, a drug holiday or treatment interruption is not recommended with denosumab. Reassessment for fracture risk after 5-10 years and those remain at high risk of fractures should either continue denosumab or be treated with other osteoporosis therapies.

Parathyroid Hormone-related Protein Analog

Teriparatide and Abaloparatide are parathyroid hormone-related protein (PTHrP) analog available for use. They are indicated in women with osteoporosis at very high risk of fracture. Their mode of action is stimulation of new bone formation in the spine and the hip. Side effects of PTHrP include nausea, dizziness, and leg cramps. After initial treatment for up to 2 years, treatment should be switched to other agents.

Selective Estrogen Receptor Modulators

To reduce the risk of vertebral fractures, SERMs, raloxifene or bazedoxifene, are used. Patient characteristics for whom are (1) with a high risk of breast cancer, (2) with a risk of deep vein thrombosis, and (3) for whom bisphosphonates or denosumab are not appropriate. They act by preventing bone loss in the spine, hip, and total body. Side effects are uncommon with raloxifene, occasionally there may be hot flashes and blood clots in the veins.

Hormone Replacement Therapy (HRT) and Tibolone

In women, surgical menopause (with hysterectomy) can be on HRT using estrogen only [called estrogen replacement therapy (ERT)] to prevent all types of fractures. In postmenopausal women with osteoporosis at high risk of fracture and with the patient characteristics, HRT with tibolone can prevent vertebral and nonvertebral fractures.

Calcitonin and Teriparatide

Nasal spray calcitonin may be prescribed in postmenopausal women at high risk of fracture with osteoporosis. It is given to women who cannot tolerate other drugs such as raloxifene, bisphosphonates, estrogen, denosumab, tibolone, abaloparatide, or teriparatide. Calcitonin inhibits bone resorption resulting in increased bone mass.

Teriparatide is an injectable synthetic form of human PTH. This helps in new bone formation and therefore can be used even after fracture, and it also prevents the risk of fracture by improving bone mineral density. It is not recommended for >2 years.

Calcium and Vitamin D

Calcium and vitamin D should be used as an adjunct to osteoporosis therapies for postmenopausal women with low BMD and at high risk of fractures with osteoporosis.

Monitoring of osteoporosis: During the treatment of osteoporosis, BMD of the spine and hip should be on every 1-3 years. Monitoring of bone turnover markers (serum C-terminal cross-linking telopeptide for antiresorptive therapy or procollagen type N-terminal propeptide for bone anabolic therapy) is used to identify poor response or nonadherence to therapy.

Osteoporosis in Male

Males above 70 years are prone to osteoporosis.

Younger men (aged 50-69) should be tested if additional risk factors are present.

The risk factors of osteoporosis in male include:
- Diseases/conditions such as delayed puberty and hypogonadism, hyperparathyroidism, hyperthyroidism, or chronic obstructive pulmonary disease
- Drugs such as glucocorticoids or gonadotropin-releasing hormone (GnRH) agonists
- Alcohol abuse or smoking
- Other causes of secondary osteoporosis

For diagnosis of osteoporosis in men, tests used are—DXA of the spine and hip for osteoporosis or by a fracture risk calculator—*FRAX* (Fracture Risk Assessment Tool).

A complete history and physical examination for men is to be evaluated for osteoporosis and consideration for pharmacological therapy. Laboratory investigation should include serum calcium, phosphate, creatinine (with estimated glomerular filtration rate), alkaline phosphatase, liver function test, 1,25-dihydroxyvitamin D, total testosterone, and complete blood count.

Treatment is indicated:
- Men with a hip or vertebral fracture without any major trauma
- Men without a spine or hip fracture but BMD of the spine, femoral neck, and/or total hip is 2.5 SD or more below the mean of normal young white males
- FRAX calculator shows 10-year risk of hip fracture ≥3%
- Receiving long-term glucocorticoid therapy in pharmacological doses (e.g., prednisone or equivalent >7.5 mg/day) and/or androgen deprivation therapy (ADT) for prostate cancer.

Drugs used in male osteoporosis treatment are alendronate, risedronate, zoledronic acid, and teriparatide. Denosumab is used for men receiving ADT.

Other measures for osteoporosis prevention in male:
- *Calcium and vitamin D*: Daily consumption of 1,000-1,200 mg calcium from diet and/or with calcium supplements for men with or at risk for osteoporosis should be maintained.
- Men should receive vitamin D supplement if found low vitamin D levels [<30 ng/mL (75 nmol/L)] to achieve the blood level least 30 ng/mL (75 nmol/L).
- Weight-bearing activities for 30–40 min/session, three to four sessions per week should be done by men at risk of osteoporosis.
- Men at risk of osteoporosis should restrict or quit consumption of alcohol intake and smoking.

INCIDENTALOMAS OF PARATHYROID

Parathyroid incidentaloma was first reported in 1967 by discovering of parathyroid tumors during surgical exploration of neck by Allie et al. With the use of high-resolution ultrasonogram, parathyroid incidentaloma may be revealed prior to surgery. The incidence of these lesions is rare during thyroid surgery and varies between 0.2 and 4.5%.

Management of such a lesion requires a five-step process:
1. Clinical evaluation
2. Biochemical screening for hyperfunction of the lesion
3. Imaging study of the lesion
4. Surgical treatment for lesion
5. Follow-up of nonfunctional incidentaloma

1. *Clinical evaluation of*:
    i. Nonspecific symptoms, such as weakness, easy fatigability, weight loss, and epigastric distress
    ii. Symptoms referable to kidney
    iii. Symptoms referable to the skeleton system such as bone pain, pathological fractures, and deformities
2. Biochemical screening either measures serum calcium and intact PTH levels before every thyroidectomy or in patients found to have enlarged parathyroid.
3. *Imaging study*:
    i. *Sestamibi scan*: The sestamibi scintiscan in cases identified by ultrasonogram can show expected good sensitivity, but can miss almost half of parathyroid incidentalomas because of low sensitivity of sestamibi scanning in small lesions.
    ii. *Routine frozen sections*: Frozen sections cannot always differentiate normal from abnormal lesions. Its main function is to determine if the removed specimen is parathyroid tissue.
    iii. *Immunostaining*: Enlarged and hyperfunctioning gland takes immunostaining, so it can be used to detect hyperfunctioning parathyroid. But some authors documented in overt PH there was no biochemically hyperfunctioning. Thus, gross enlargement of parathyroid could be the first step toward hyperparathyroidism before biochemical disturbances develop.
    iv. *Fine-needle aspiration biopsy-parathyroid hormone (FNAB-PTH)*: Routine cytology with fine-needle aspiration has limited diagnostic value. The at present combination of FNAB with PTH assay on the needle washout after preparation of cytological specimens is used as a reliable method in investigation of parathyroid incidentaloma.

4. *Surgical treatment*:
    i. The management of parathyroid incidentaloma if biochemically proven to HP with or without clinical features of hyperfunction is—surgical removal of the enlarged gland(s) after identification of all the glands during operation.
    ii. Parathyroid incidentaloma if biochemically normal—it is recommended for a neck exploration to look for all four parathyroid glands for abnormally enlarged gland(s) and to remove all grossly enlarged parathyroid glands as long as at least one normal parathyroid gland remains. The glandular enlargement is considered as the prestage of biochemically abnormality in the natural process of development of parathyroid adenoma.
    iii. Postoperative biochemical follow-up should include serum calcium and intact PTH (iPTH) level. Both are either normal or transiently low in cases of cure of the condition.
5. *Follow-up*: Follow-up of nonfunctional parathyroid incidentaloma should include serum calcium and iPTH level at least once after 6 months.

FURTHER READINGS

1. Anatomy and Physiology by ©2017 Rice University. Textbook content produced by OpenStax. [online] Available from https://openstax.org/ [Last accessed September, 2023].
2. Standring S (Ed). Gray's Anatomy: The Anatomical Basis of Clinical Practice, 41st edition. [online] Available from https://www.amazon.com/Garys-Anatomy-Henry-Gray/dp/B00DXO9JRA) [Last accessed September, 2023].
3. Barrett K, Barman S, Yuan J, Brooks H (Eds). Ganong's Review of Medical Physiology, 26th edition. [online] Available from https://www.amazon.com/Ganongs-Review-Medical-Physiology-Twenty/dp/1260122409 [Last accessed September, 2023].
4. Melmed S, Koenig R, Rosen C, Auchus R, Goldfine A. Williams Textbook of Endocrinology, 14th edition. [online] Available from (https://www.elsevier.com/books/williams-textbook-of-endocrinology/bresnahan/978-0-323-55596-8) [Last accessed August, 2023].
5. Gardner D, Shoback D (Eds). Greenspan's Basic and Clinical Endocrinology, 10th edition. McGraw Hill; 2017. [online] Available from https://www.amazon.com/Greenspans-Basic-Clinical-Endocrinology-Tenth/dp/1259589285 [Last accessed September, 2023].
6. Katz AD, Kong LB. Incidental preclinical hyperparathyroidism identified during thyroid operations. Am Surg. 1992;58(12): 747-9.
7. Frasoldati A, Pesenti M, Toschi E, Azzarito C, Zini M, Valcavi R. Detection and diagnosis of parathyroid incidentalomas during thyroid sonography. J Clin Ultrasound. 1999;27(9):492-8.
8. Consensus Development Conference Panel NIH conference. Diagnosis and management of asymptomatic primary hyperparathyroidism: Consensus Development Conference statement. Ann Intern Med. 1991;114(7):593-7.

CHAPTER 5

Disorders of Adrenal Gland

- ❏ Introduction to the adrenal glands
  - ➢ Anatomy of adrenal glands
  - ➢ Physiology of adrenal glands
- ❏ Diseases of adrenal glands
  - ➢ Hypercortisolemia
  - ➢ Cushing's syndrome
  - ➢ Hyperaldosteronism
- ➢ Adrenal (adrenocortical) insufficiency
- ➢ Congenital adrenal hyperplasia
- ❏ Pheochromocytoma
  - ➢ Identification and treatment
  - ➢ Diagnosis of pheochromocytoma
- ❏ Adrenal incidentaloma

This chapter is about Adrenal Gland, which begins with an introduction to applied anatomy and physiology. It covers hyperfunctional states and hypofunctional states, adrenal cortex, congenital adrenal hyperplasia, and adrenal medullary disorder—pheochromocytoma. This chapter consists of 22 Figures, 8 Flowcharts, 18 Tables, and 1 Box to illustrate its text. This chapter ends with how to deal with Adrenal Incidentalomas.

INTRODUCTION TO THE ADRENAL GLANDS

(Anatomy and applied Embryology; Physiology)

■ Anatomy of Adrenal Glands

Two adrenal glands are retroperitoneum structures lie on the upper ends of the two kidneys. The right adrenal gland is pyramidal and the left one is crescentic in shape. The maximum width of right adrenal gland is 6.1 mm and that of the left adrenal gland is 7.9 mm. Glands are yellowish small and they weight about 4–5 g.

The glands have rich blood supply. Each receives three adrenal arteries arising from (1) inferior phrenic artery, (2) renal artery, and (3) abdominal aorta.

Venous drainage: The right gland flows directly into the inferior vena cava and the left gland into the left renal vein. Lymphatics drain to the aortic lymph nodes **(Fig. 1)**.

There are two distinct parts of each adrenal gland, one lie inside the other: (1) the outer one is adrenal cortex and (2) the inner one is adrenal medulla. The adrenal cortex is divided into three zones. From exterior to interior the zones are named as (1) zona glomerulosa, (2) zona fasciculata, and (3) zona reticularis **(Fig. 2)**.

The adrenal glands are better visualized by computed tomography (CT) scan than other modalities. After contrast administration their density reaches to approximately 50–60 Hounsfield units (HU) and seen as inverted V and coma shape in right and left sides respectively.

Embryology: The adrenal cortex and medulla are mesodermal and ectodermal in origin respectively. From the mesoderm of the posterior abdominal wall at 6th week of gestation the adrenal cortex starts developing. The fetal cortex is a predominant structure during entire fetal life, it starts steroid secretion very early. At 4th month of gestation its size is four times of the kidney but at birth it is one-third of the size of the kidney. In fetal life, only a small proportion of the gland consists zona glomerulosa and fasciculata but there is no zona reticularis. After birth, the fetal cortex starts rapid regression and disappears almost

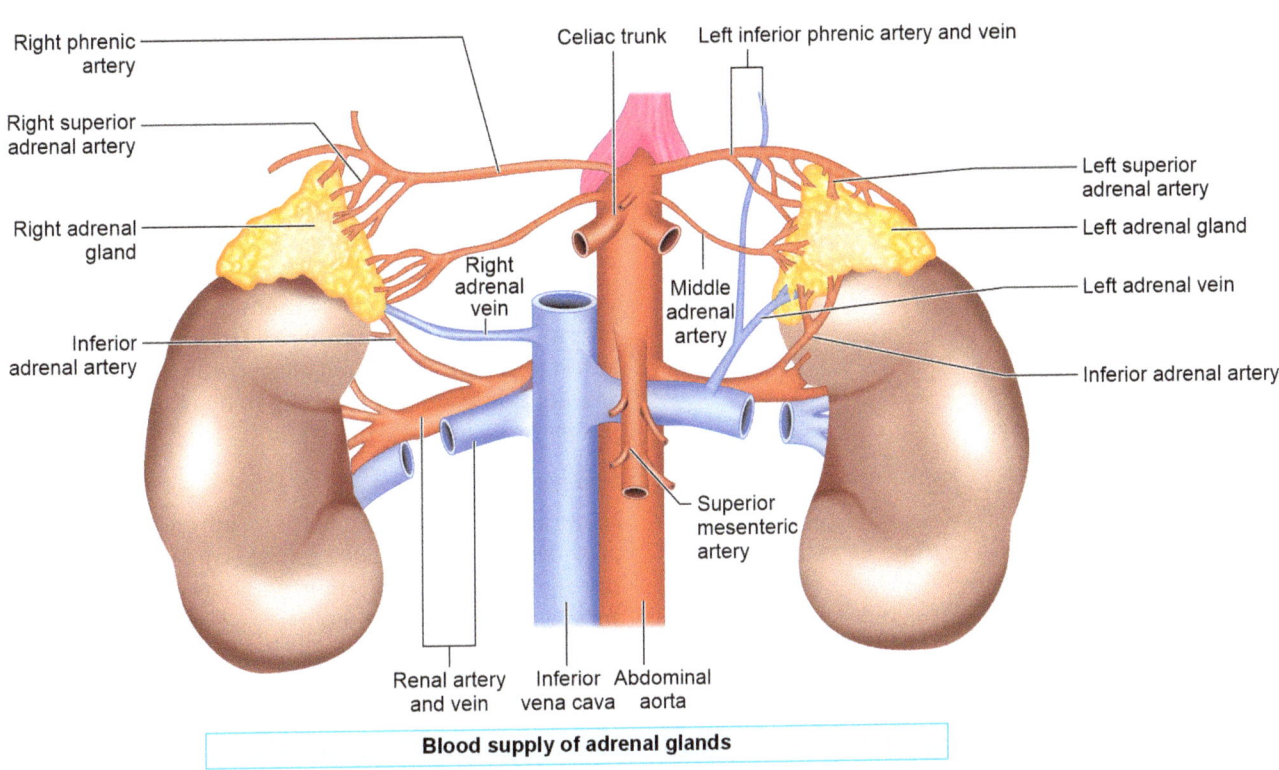

Blood supply of adrenal glands

FIG. 1: The arterial supply comes from three sources—adrenal arteries arising from (1) inferior phrenic artery, (2) renal artery, and (3) abdominal aorta. Venous drainage flows directly to two veins (1) on right side into the inferior vena cava and (2) on left side into the left renal vein.

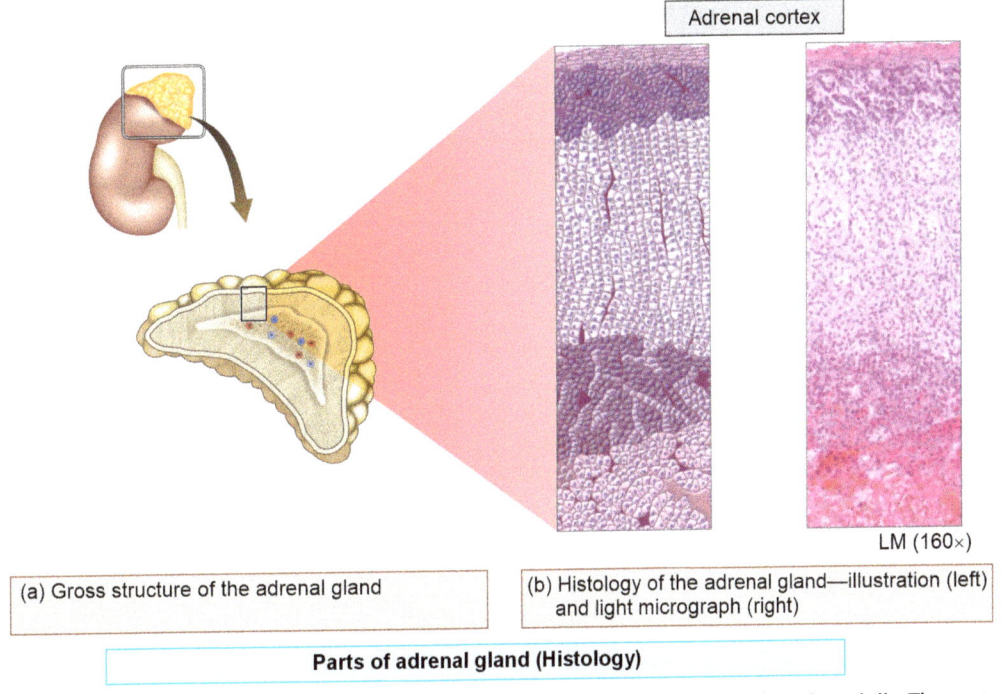

(a) Gross structure of the adrenal gland

(b) Histology of the adrenal gland—illustration (left) and light micrograph (right)

Parts of adrenal gland (Histology)

FIG. 2: There are two distinct parts of each adrenal gland: (1) the adrenal cortex and (2) the adrenal medulla. The cortex is divided into three zones. From exterior to interior the zones are: (1) zona glomerulosa, (2) zona fasciculata, and (3) zona reticularis.

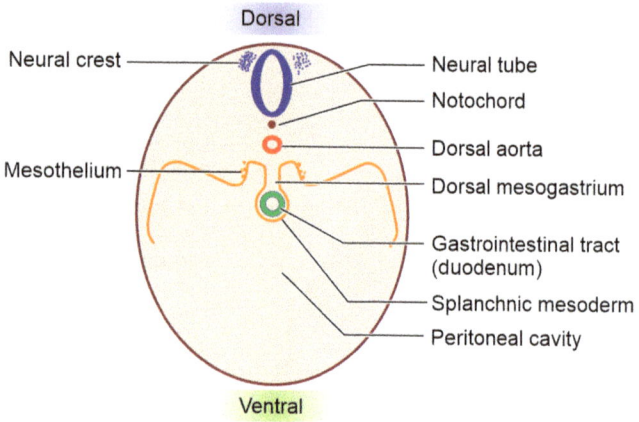

Adrenal gland development

FIG. 3: Adrenal cortex starts developing from mesoderm at 6 weeks and soon begins steroid secretion. Cortex is predominant in entire fetal life; at 4 months it is four times of kidney and at birth it is one-third. Zona glomerulosa and fasciculata make up only a small proportion but zona reticularis is absent. After birth, the fetal cortex rapidly regression and disappears by age of 1 year. The permanent adult-type adrenal cortex is fully developed by age of 4–5 years. The adrenal medullas arise from neural crest cells that migrate to the medial aspect of the developing cortex. The cells have neuron-like morphology. Two cell types (1) secrete epinephrine and norepinephrine.

completely by age of 1 year. The permanent adult-type adrenal cortex is fully developed by 4–5 years of age.

The adrenal medullas develop from neural crest cells. Neural crest cells migrate to the medial aspect of the growing adrenal cortex. The cells of the medulla have neuron-like morphology. There are two cell types (1) secrete epinephrine (adrenaline) 80% and norepinephrine (noradrenaline) 20% respectively **(Fig. 3)**.

Birth Anomalies

Some anatomic anomalies of the adrenal gland may occur. Anomalies are usually associated with renal anomalies. Examples are (1) agenesis of an adrenal gland can be associated with agenesis of the kidney of same side and (2) fused adrenal glands (the two glands join across the midline posterior to the aorta) usually associated with a fused horseshoe kidney.

■ Physiology of Adrenal Glands

Physiology of Adrenal Cortex

Three types of steroid hormones are synthesized and secreted from the adrenal cortex. Hormones are more or less zone specific:
1. The zona glomerulosa secretes mineralocorticoids (the most important of which is aldosterone)
2. The zona fasciculata secretes mostly glucocorticoids (predominantly cortisol)
3. The zona reticularis secretes adrenal androgen [mainly dehydroepiandrosterone (DHEA)] and a small quantity of androgens also released from the zona fasciculata

About half of aldosterone is bound to protein in the blood. Most of cortisol (approximately 90%) binds to cortisol-binding globulin or transcortin. The liver is the site of degradation of all adrenocortical steroids. The degraded products are conjugated mostly to glucuronides or rest to sulfates. Excretion of approximately 75% of these degradation products form the body is in urine and the rest in the stool by means of bile.

Mineralocorticoids

Mineralocorticoid activities of adrenal steroids are provided by aldosterone, deoxycorticosterone, corticosterone, and cortisol. About 90% of mineralocorticoid activity is due to aldosterone, its concentration in the blood changes with posture and also has diurnal variation—in supine position concentration ranges from 2 to 16 ng/dL and in upright position 5 to 41 ng/dL. Its daily secretory rate is generally 150–250 µg.

Site of action of aldosterone is at the renal tubular epithelial cells of the collecting and distal tubules. It promotes sodium reabsorption and potassium excretion. Sodium is reabsorption is coupled with passive water flow in extracellular fluid. This leads to an increase in the extracellular fluid volume with little or no change in the plasma sodium concentration. The elevated extracellular fluid volumes can rise blood pressure. This high pressure helps to minimize further increases in extracellular fluid volume by causing a pressure diuresis. This phenomenon is called aldosterone escape.

In state of aldosterone lack, the kidney will lose excessive amounts of sodium and water, leading to severe dehydration. In imbalances (1) with high in aldosterone will lead to hypokalemia and muscle weakness and (2) with low in aldosterone will lead to hyperkalemia with cardiac toxicity.

Mild metabolic alkalosis may develop with aldosterone excess because there will be loss hydrogen also.

In addition to the renal tubules, other sites of aldosterone action include the sweat glands, salivary glands, and intestine, especially the colon. So, clinical manifestations of deficiency or excess of this hormone can be seen in these organ dysfunctions.

Factors affecting aldosterone secretion include the renin-angiotensin system, changes in the plasma potassium and sodium concentration, adrenocorticotropic hormone (ACTH), etc. The renin-angiotensin system and plasma potassium concentration are the most important factors.

- The renin-angiotensin system—(1) any decreased blood flow to the kidney, due to hypovolemia, hypotension, or renal artery stenosis, the juxtaglomerular apparatus to releases and enzyme called renin; (2) renin activates angiotensinogen to release a peptide hormone called angiotensin I; (3) in the lung, angiotensin-converting enzyme (ACE) converts angiotensin I to angiotensin II which is a more potent vasoconstrictor and stimulator of aldosterone release from the adrenal cortex.
- Concentration of potassium—increases in the plasma potassium concentration stimulate the release of aldosterone to encourage potassium excretion by the kidney.
- Concentration of sodium—decreases in sodium concentration stimulate aldosterone release.
- *Adrenocorticotropic hormone secretion*: It primarily causes release of glucocorticoids by the adrenal also stimulates aldosterone release to a lesser extent.

Glucocorticoids

Zona fasciculata of adrenal cortex is the site of glucocorticoid hormone production. Most (approximately 95%) of glucocorticoid activity is from the cortisol hormone. Corticosterone, a glucocorticoid less potent than cortisol is also secreted by this zone of cortex. In blood averages concentration of cortisol is 12 µg/dL and average daily secretory is 5-20 mg.

Adrenocorticotropic hormone secretion of the anterior pituitary gland stimulates cortisol secretion. ACTH secretion is again controlled by corticotropin-releasing hormone (CRH) of the hypothalamus. Normally, CRH, ACTH, and cortisol secretory rates show a circadian rhythm, with peak(s) in the early morning and a nadir in the evening. Various stresses can also stimulate ACTH secretion and thereby also increase cortisol secretion. Blood cortisol level has a negative feedback effect on the anterior pituitary and the hypothalamus that helps to regulate plasma cortisol concentrations **(Figs. 4 and 5)**.

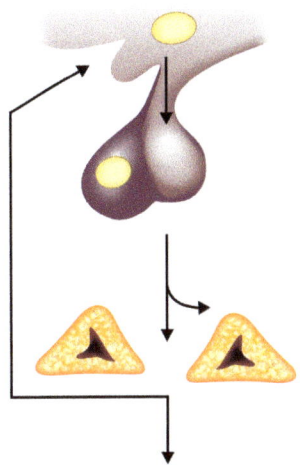

Normal relation between pituitary and adrenals

FIG. 4: Cortisol release is almost entirely controlled by the secretion of adrenocorticotropic hormone (ACTH) by the anterior pituitary gland and their negative feedback.

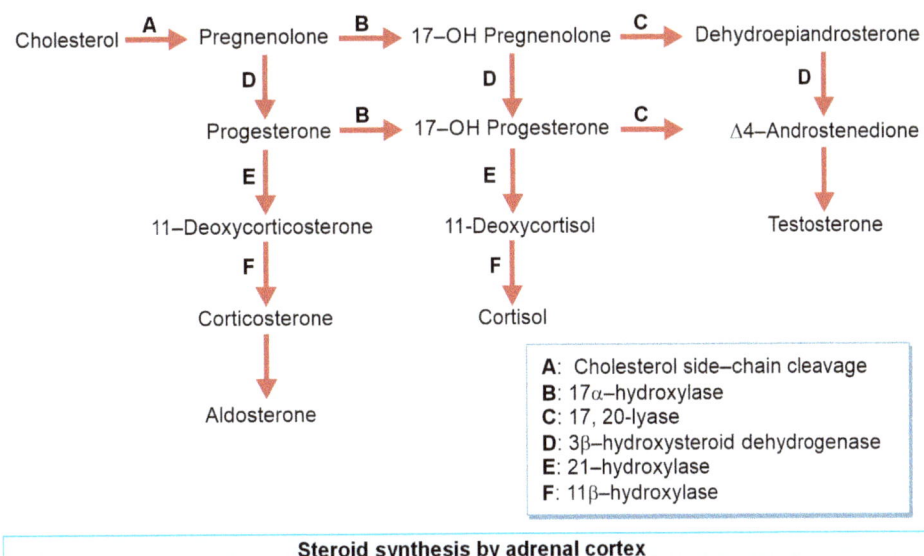

Steroid synthesis by adrenal cortex

FIG. 5: Adrenal cortex secretes three types of steroid hormones: (1) Zona glomerulosa secretes mineralocorticoids—aldosterone. (2) Zona fasciculata and zona reticularis secretes—glucocorticoids—predominantly cortisols. (3) Adrenal androgens are predominantly secreted by the zona reticularis, with small quantities released from the zona fasciculata.

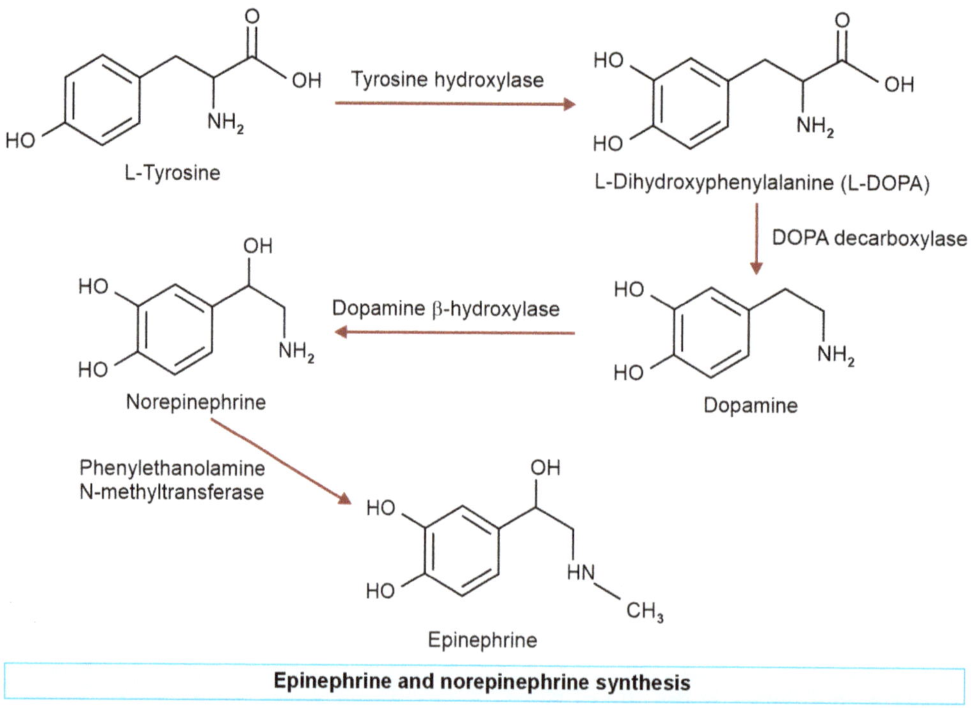

Epinephrine and norepinephrine synthesis

FIG. 6: Epinephrine (80%) and norepinephrine (20%), with minimal amounts of dopamine, are secreted into the bloodstream due to direct stimulation by acetylcholine release from sympathetic nerves.

Cortisol has many effects on different system/organs of the body; some of them are as follows:
- *In the liver*: Cortisol stimulates gluconeogenesis by stimulating the involved enzymes and mobilizing necessary substrates—amino acids from muscle and free fatty acids from adipose tissue. Cortisol also decreases glucose use by extrahepatic cells in the body. So, the overall result is increase in blood glucose and increased glycogen stores in the liver.
- *In body (except in the liver)*: Cortisol decreases protein stores by inhibiting protein synthesis and stimulating catabolism of muscle protein.
- *Anti-inflammatory effects*: It blocks the early stages of inflammation by stabilizing lysosomal membranes, preventing excessive release of proteolytic enzymes, decreasing capillary permeability and consequently edema and decreasing chemotaxis of leukocytes. It also induces rapid resolution of inflammation that is already in progress.
- *In blood*: Cortisol decreases eosinophil and lymphocyte counts in the blood which affects immunity adversely.

Adrenal androgens

The adrenal cortex secretes several male and female sex hormones. Male sex hormones include DHEA, dehydroepiandrosterone sulfate (DHEAS), androstenedione, and 11-hydroxyandrostenedione. Female sex hormones are progesterone and estrogen—these are small in amount. Most of the androgens are converted to testosterone extra-adrenally. All these hormones have weak effects, but they play an important role in early development of the male sex organs in childhood and induction of pubarche of women. ACTH of pituitary stimulates androgen release by the adrenal.

Adrenal medulla

Adrenal medullary glands lie within the adrenal cortex gland but they are different in structure and function. They are of neural crest origin and secrete mainly epinephrine (80%) and norepinephrine (20%) and a minimal amount of dopamine. They are secreted into the bloodstream due to direct stimulation by acetylcholine release from sympathetic nerves. The adrenal medulla cell receives preganglionic sympathetic nerve fibers of the sympathetic chains and splanchnic nerves which pass from the intermediolateral horn cells of the spinal cord. The hormones cause increase in cardiac output and vascular resistance **(Fig. 6)**.

DISEASES OF ADRENAL GLANDS

Adrenal disorders present with hormonal disturbances. Diseases of adrenal cortex are described as hyperfunctioning states of mineralocorticoid aldosterone (hyperaldosteronism) and glucocorticoid—cortisol

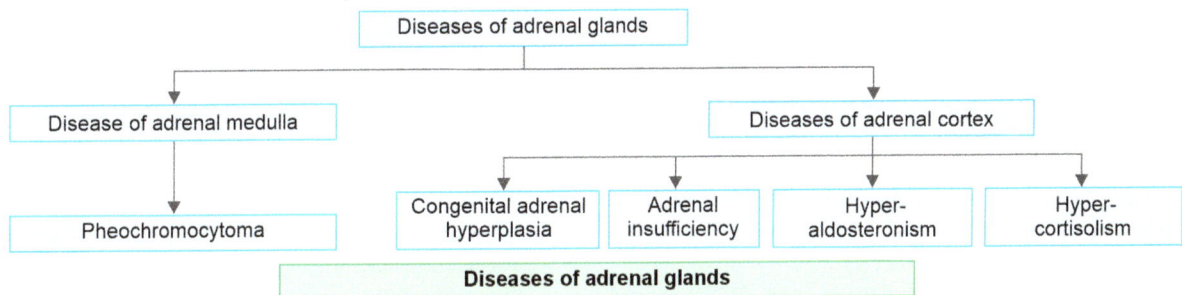

FLOWCHART 1: (A) Diseases of adrenal cortex are described as (1) Hyperfunctioning states (hyperaldosteronism) and hypercortisolism, (2) Deficiency of cortisol with or without aldosterone (adrenal insufficiency), and (3) Production of abnormal steroid (CAH) and (B) Disease of adrenal medulla—pheochromocytoma.

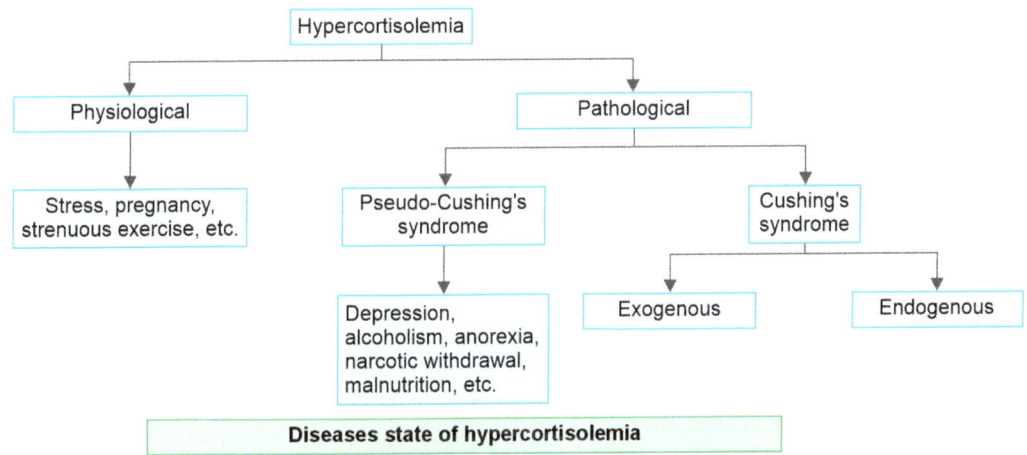

FLOWCHART 2: Hypercortisolemia may be either a physiological response or a pathological state: (1) Pathological hypercortisolemias are Cushing's syndrome or pseudo-Cushing's syndrome and (2) Physiological hypercortisolemias are due to stress, pregnancy, strenuous exercise, etc.

(hypercortisolism), deficiency of cortisol with or without aldosterone (adrenal insufficiency), and production of abnormal steroid [congenital adrenal hyperplasia (CAH)]. Disease of adrenal medulla is excess productions of catecholamine—pheochromocytoma.

Diseases of adrenal cortex are:
1. Hypercortisolism (excess cortisol)
2. Hyperaldosteronism (excess aldosterone)
3. Adrenal insufficiency (diminish cortisol with or without diminish aldosterone)
4. Congenital adrenal hyperplasia (abnormal steroid genesis)

Disease of adrenal medulla: Pheochromocytoma (excess catecholamine) **(Flowchart 1)**.

■ Hypercortisolemia

A state of hypercortisolemia may be either a physiological response or a pathological state due to a wide range of

TABLE 1: Class and causes of Cushing's syndrome.

Class (~%)	Causes (~ % within class)
Adrenocorticotropic hormone (ACTH) dependent (85%)	Pituitary ACTH-producing lesions (Cushing's disease ~80%)
	Ectopic ACTH-producing tumors (ectopic ACTH syndrome ~20%)
ACTH independent (15%)	Adrenal adenoma (~30%)
	Adrenal carcinoma (~70%)

causes which may be either physiological or pathological. Physiological causes include stress, pregnancy, or chronic strenuous exercise. Pathological cause includes Cushing's syndrome—endogenous or exogenous (mostly iatrogenic), psychiatric conditions, such as depression, alcoholism, anorexia, narcotic withdrawal and malnutrition **(Table 1)** of which we will study Cushing's syndrome in brief **(Flowchart 2)**.

Cushing's Syndrome

Cushing's syndrome can be defined as symptoms and signs of associated with prolong exposure to inappropriately high plasma cortisol (hypercortisolism).

Classification of hypercortisolism is initially done as endogenous or exogenous according to the source of cortisol and then endogenous class is further on the basis of ACTH dependency **(Flowchart 3)**.

Causes of Cushing's syndrome are (1) Adrenal adenoma or carcinoma, (2) Pituitary ACTH-producing lesions, and (3) Ectopic ACTH-producing tumors **(Table 1)**.

Clinical Presentation of Cushing's Syndrome (For All Age Group)

- Obesity (trunkal; mild-to-moderate)
- Thin skin, easy bruising, and purple skin striae
- Moon face, plethora, acne, and hirsutism **(Figs. 7A to F)**.

With the relative early detections (as in routine health checkup), the time-old list of presenting symptoms and

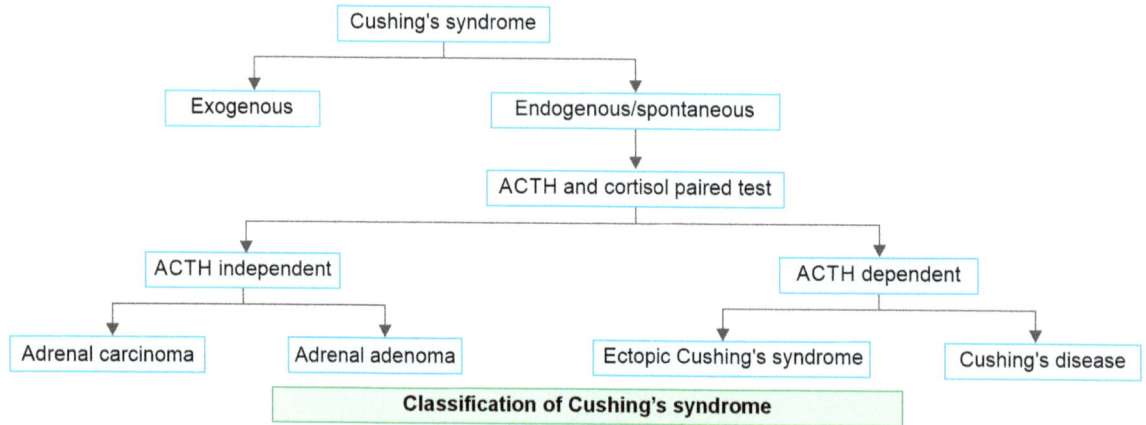

FLOWCHART 3: Spontaneous Cushing's syndrome is either adrenocorticotropic hormone (ACTH)-dependent or ACTH-independent. ACTH level is very high in ectopic Cushing's syndrome.

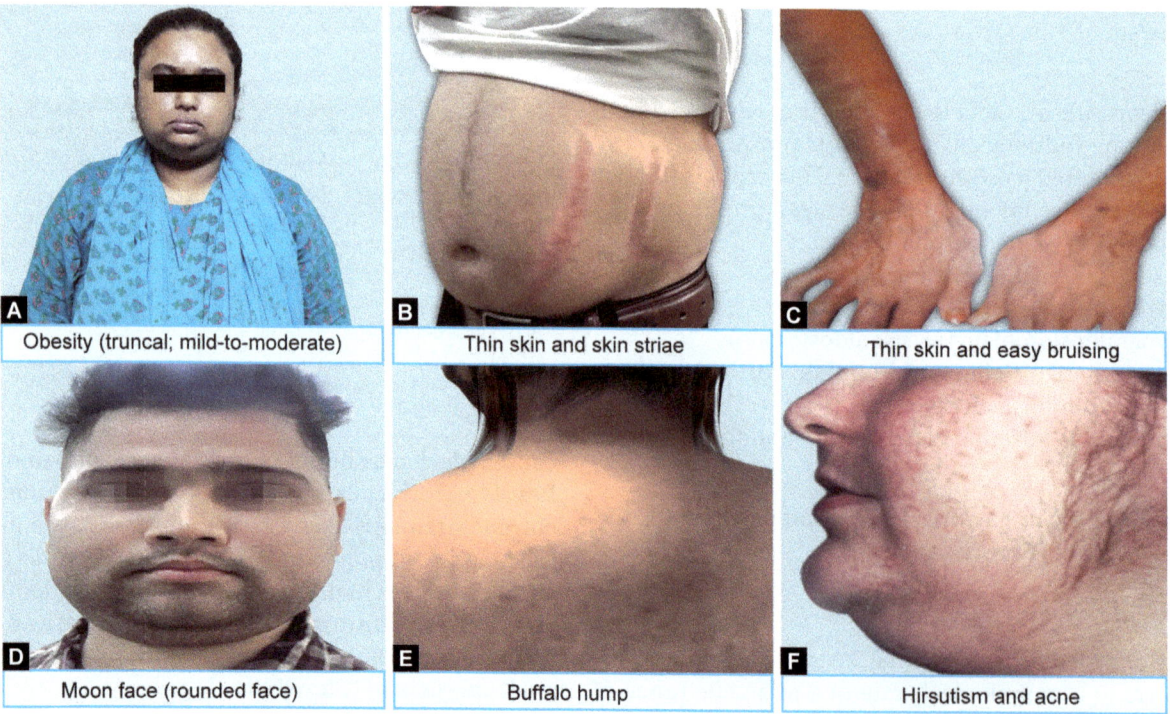

FIGS. 7A TO F: Presentation of Cushing's syndrome.

signs has changed nowadays. The other common features are as follows:
- Thin skin texture
- High blood sugar and pressure
- Menstrual irregularity and infertility
- Depression, emotional instability, and sleep disorders
- Undue fatigability
- Osteoporosis, etc.

Clinical Presentation of Cushing's Syndrome (For Children Age up to 18 Years)
- Growth arrest
- Rapid weight gain (obesity)
- Avascular necrosis of hip
- Fatigue/weakness
- Pubertal arrest
- Easy bruising and purple skin striae
- Moon face, plethora, acne, and hirsutism
- Hyperpigmentation
- Hypokalemic alkalosis

Tumors causing ectopic ACTH syndrome **(Table 2)**.
Useful clinical hints to etiology of Cushing's syndrome:
- *Virilization*: Adrenal carcinoma
- *Sings of aldosterone excess (hypertension and hypokalemic alkalosis)*: Ectopic ACTH
- *Severe hyperpigmentation*: Ectopic ACTH

TABLE 2: List of tumors causing ectopic adrenocorticotropic hormone (ACTH) syndrome.

Location	Tumors	Percentage
Within thorax (65%)	Oat cell carcinoma	50%
	Thymic carcinoid	10%
	Bronchial carcinoid	5%
Within abdomen and pelvis (23%)	Pancreatic islet cell tumors	10%
	Pheochromocytoma	5%
	Ovarian tumor	2%
	Prostatic carcinoma	<2%
	Cervical carcinoma	<2%
	Gastric carcinoma	<2%
	Gallbladder carcinoma	<2%
Neck and head region (7%)	Medullary carcinoma of thyroid	5%
	Parathyroid carcinoma	<2%
	Parotid carcinoma	<2%
Uncertain location (5%)		

Diagnosis of Cushing's Syndrome
Diagnosis as well as treatment of Cushing's syndrome is still representing a challenge for endocrinologist. Correct interpretations of data of diagnostic tools involving other disciplines like imaging, neurosurgery, etc. in step-by-step fashion have made remarkable progress in this regards.

There are three steps of evaluation for and management (1) Step 1: To establish spontaneous hypercortisolemia, (2) Step 2: To establish ACTH dependency of hypercortisolemia—paired ACTH and cortisol test, and (3) Step 3: Imaging study (±biochemical study) to ascertain etiology for therapeutic action.

Step 1: To establish spontaneous hypercortisolemia:
- Indicated for all cases either with clinically suspected for Cushing's syndrome after exclusion of exogenous intake of steroid (by history) or for an incidentaloma of at adrenal/pituitary.
- Biochemical test(s) for hypercortisolemia examples:
  o *Urinary free cortisol (UFC)*: UFC is measured a value more than the upper limit of normal range is considered positive of Cushing's syndrome and there may be 20-25% false negative report. Most of pseudo-Cushing's syndrome cases can be excluded by this test. But, it is not effective in detection of adrenal insufficiency.
  o *Late-night salivary cortisol*: It is a sensitive diagnostic test for Cushing's syndrome. Elevated cortisol between 11:00 PM and midnight appears to have a sensitivity of 93-100%. Normal range of <3.0-4.0 nmol/L or 0.10-0.15 µg/dL. Normal levels exclude the diagnosis of Cushing's syndrome due to an ACTH-secreting tumor; but there may be false negative for some patients with Cushing's syndrome due to an adrenal tumor.
  o *Low dose overnight dexamethasone suppression test (LODST)*: 1 mg of dexamethasone is orally given at 11 PM and cortisol is measured from next morning at 9 AM sample of blood, a value >50 mg/dL is considered positive for Cushing's syndrome. 40 out of a series of 154 cases were detected as identified as Cushing's syndrome by using LODST in our institute BIRDEM **(Fig. 8)**.

Step 2: To establish ACTH dependency of hypercortisolemia.

A simple paired ACTH and cortisol test result can provide valuable information for next step (step 3) action(s)—(1) very low or undetectable ACTH (say <10 pg/mL) with hypercortisolemia lesion(s) at adrenals,

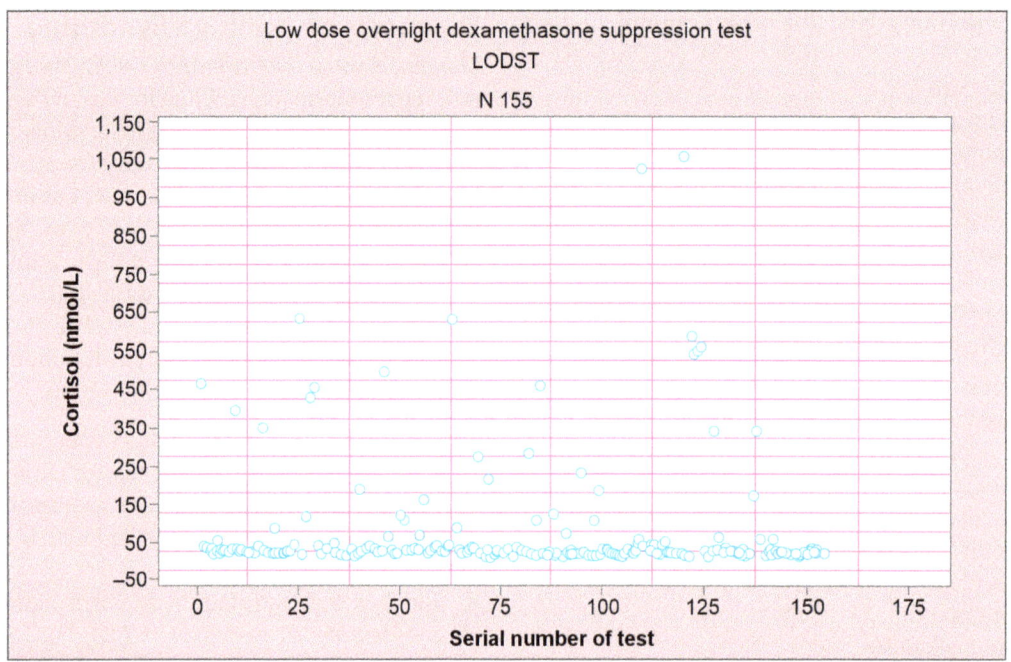

FIG. 8: 1 mg of dexamethasone is orally given at 11 PM and cortisol is measured from next morning at 9 AM sample of blood, a value >50 mg/dL is considered positive for Cushing's syndrome (CS). 40 out of a series of 154 cases were detected as identified as CS by using LODST in our institute BIRDEM.

Source: Ahmed T, Mahtab H, Tofail T, Morshed AHG, Rahman FB, Khan SA. Current status of low dose overnight dexamethasone supression test (LODST). J Obes Diabetes. 2020;4:5-8.

(2) very high ACTH (say >20 pg/mL) with hypercortisolemia lesion is likely to be ectopic ACTH syndrome, and (3) above normal or high normal ACTH (say 10–20 pg/mL) with hypercortisolemia lesion might be due to Cushing's disease (CD).

Step 3: Imaging study (+biochemical study) depending on paired ACTH and cortisol test result **(Figs. 9 to 11 and Flowchart 4)**.
- For ACTH independent cases of adrenal imaging
- Pituitary and adrenal imaging for ACTH-dependent cases
- Bilateral inferior petrosal sinus sampling combine ovine-sequence CRH stimulation test for cases of hypercortisolemia with microadenoma or negative image of pituitary region
- For cases with very high ACTH search for source of ectopic ACTH syndrome cases

Iodocholesterol scan can be used to:
- Differentiate between ACTH-dependent hypercortisolemia (bilateral high uptake—either for CD or ectopic ACTH syndrome) from ACTH-independent macronodular adrenal (unilateral adenoma/carcinoma) causing Cushing's syndrome
- Establish remnant hyperplasia after bilateral adrenalectomy
- Identify ectopic adrenal tissue

Treatment of Cushing's Syndrome

- *Surgeries for Cushing's syndrome are as follows*:
  - Unilateral adrenalectomy for unilateral adenoma or carcinoma
  - Bilateral adrenalectomy for bilateral macronodular hyperplasia, adenoma, or carcinoma
  - Surgery of primary tumor with metastasis if feasible in carcinoma.
- *Drug therapies for Cushing's syndrome are as follows*:
  - Use of mitotane, metyrapone, aminoglutethimide, trilostane, ketoconazole, or RU486 to control hypercortisolism.
  - Use of mitotane at very high dose (12 g/day) for carcinoma hypercortisolism; partial response is seen in 15–20% cases.
  - Use of Cytoxan, adriamycin, 5 Flurouracil, methotrexate (MTX), suramin, and gossypol as chemotherapy of carcinoma.

Treatment Options of Cushing's Disease

Treatment options are as follows:
- Transsphenoidal (microscopic or endoscopic) surgery or hemiphysectomy is the first line of treatment for CD by one school of thought. In events of failure resurgery or second-line options like radiotherapy (including Gamma Knife radiosurgery) or medical therapy or bilateral adrenalectomy can be tried.

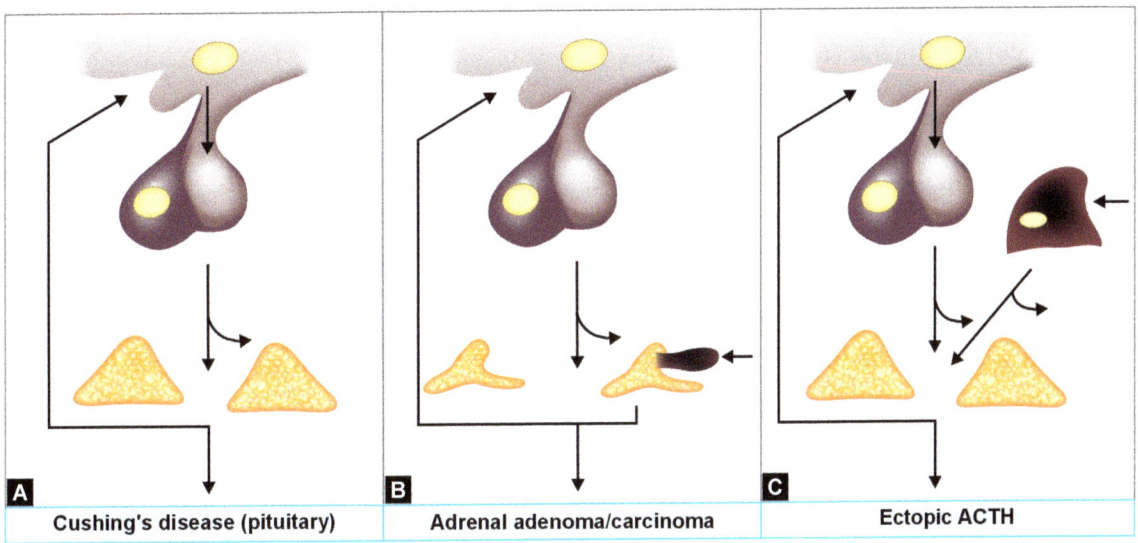

FIGS. 9A TO C: Different site of pathology in spontaneous hypercortisolemia.
(ACTH: adrenocorticotropic hormone)

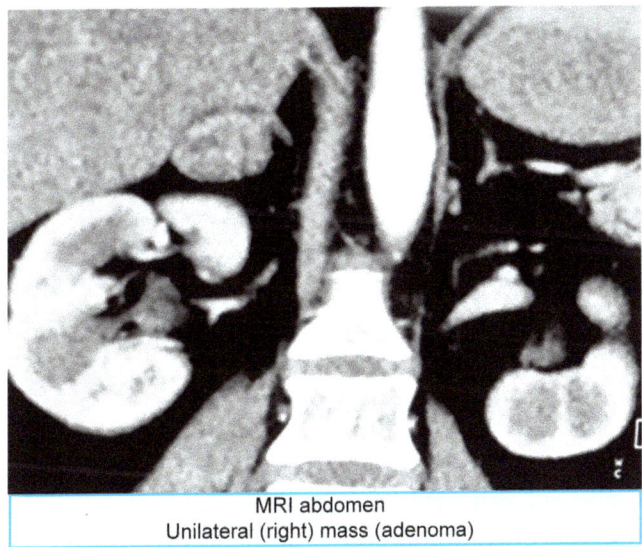

FIG. 10: Magnetic resonance imaging (MRI) of adrenal adenoma.

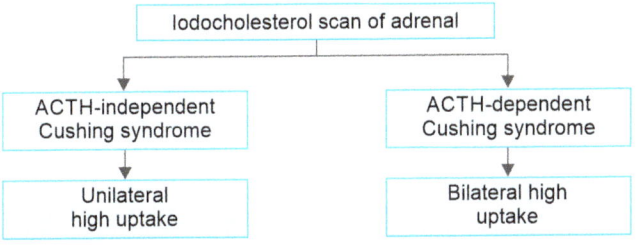

FLOWCHART 4: Iodocholesterol scan of adrenal— adrenocorticotropic hormone (ACTH)-dependent versus independent Cushing syndrome.

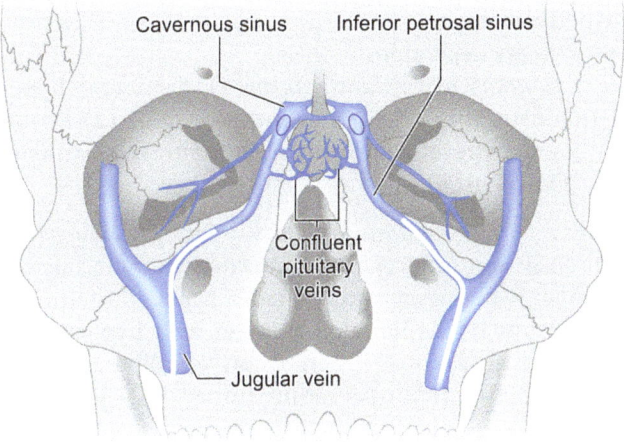

Bilateral simultaneous inferior petrosal sinus sampling (BIPSS)

FIG. 11: BIPSS with corticotropin-releasing hormone (CRH) stimulation provides the "gold standard" in the differential diagnosis of Cushing's syndrome (CS). An IPS:P ratio ≥2.0 in basal samples conclusive of Cushing's disease (CD). And a peak IPS:P ratio ≥3.0 after CRH injection identified CD. In CD patients difference of ≥1.4-fold between concentrations in two sinuses ascertain location of microadenoma.

- Gamma Knife or stereotactic radiosurgery may become the future first line of treatment for CD.
- Pituitary external irradiation with mitotane. Total 5,000 rad in 100–200 rads fractions over 5–6 weeks (full effects may take years together). Mitotane is gradually tapered as irradiation takes effects.

- Medical therapy with ketoconazole (usual dose of 0.4–1.2 g/day), mitotane (usual dose of 1–4 g/day), metyrapone (usual dose of 1–4 g/day), aminoglutethimide (usual dose of 0.5–2 g/day), trilostane (usual dose of 0.2–1 g/day). Relapse is common after withdrawal of the drug.
- Bilateral adrenalectomy is in practice in case of nonavailability of other options or intolerance to medical therapy. But it requires lifelong steroid replacement therapy, risk to develop Nelson's syndrome in 10–15% of cases due to high ACTH level and may recur due to remnant hyperplasia.

■ Hyperaldosteronism

Hyperaldosteronism is characterized by salt retention, hypokalemia, and metabolic alkalosis with or without hypertension.

Hyperaldosteronism is initially classified as primary or secondary; the secondary hyperaldosteronism is further subclassified into secondary hyperaldosteronism with hypertension or secondary hyperaldosteronism without hypertension.
- Primary hyperaldosteronism
- *Secondary hyperaldosteronism*: (1) Secondary hyperaldosteronism with hypertension and (2) Secondary hyperaldosteronism without hypertension **(Flowchart 5)**.

Causes of hyperaldosteronism: (1) Primary hyperaldosteronism due to adrenal adenoma or carcinoma, bilateral nodular hyperplasia, and idiopathic hyperaldosteronism. (2) Secondary hyperaldosteronism with hypertension due to renovascular hypertension, accelerated hypertension, and renin-secreting tumor. (3) Secondary hyperaldosteronism without hypertension due to sodium wasting nephropathy, renal tubular acidosis (RTA), pseudohypoaldosteronism, Bartter's syndrome, and diuretic/laxative abuse **(Fig. 12)**.

Table 3 summarizes a list of hyperaldosteronism.

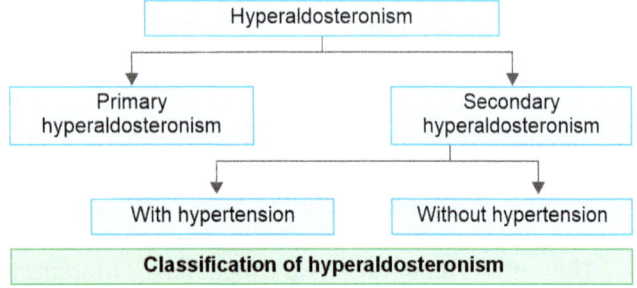

FLOWCHART 5: Hyperaldosteronism is initially classified as primary or secondary; the secondary hyperaldosteronism is further subclassified into two: with or without hypertension.

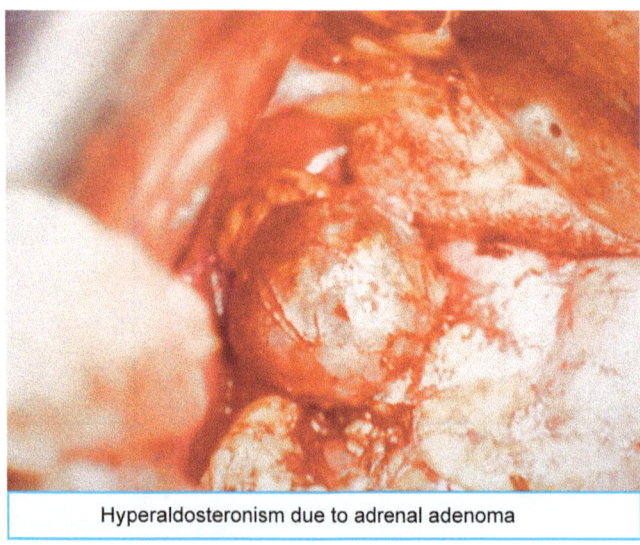

Hyperaldosteronism due to adrenal adenoma

FIG. 12: A large adenoma-secreting aldosterone.

TABLE 3: List of hyperaldosteronism.

Class/subclass	Causes
Primary hyperaldosteronism	• Adrenal adenoma or carcinoma • Bilateral nodular hyperplasia • Idiopathic hyperaldosteronism
Secondary hyperaldosteronism with hypertension	• Renovascular hypertension • Accelerated hypertension • Rennin-secreting tumor
Secondary hyperaldosteronism without hypertension	• Sodium wasting nephropathy • Renal tubular acidosis • Pseudohypoaldosteronism • Bartter's syndrome • Diuretic/laxative abuse

Primary Hyperaldosteronism
Clinical Presentation
- Patient seek medical attention for nonspecific complaints arise from hypokalemia:
  ○ Tiredness, loss of stamina, weakness, nocturia, and lassitude
  ○ Headache is a frequent incidental complaint.
- *When hypokalemia is severe with alkalosis*: Increased thirst, polyuria, and paresthesia may be present.
- Blood pressure ranges from borderline to severe hypertension:
  ○ Mean BP systolic 200 and diastolic 120 mm Hg
  ○ Malignant hypertension is rare (i.e., papilledema absent)
  ○ Clinical edema is also rare.
- Signs of subclinical tetany Trousseau's or Chvostek's sign may be present (indicating alkalosis).

Diagnosis of primary hyperaldosteronism made by documentation of hyperaldosteronism with suppressed plasma renin activity (PRA) and its cause is determined by localization of lesion by (1) CT scan, (2) adrenal venography, (3) I^{131} iodocholesterol scanning, or (4) aldosterone gradient by adrenal veins sampling with catheter **(Table 4)**.

Plasma Renin Activity Test

Plasma renin activity test estimate ability of renin to form angiotensin I from angiotensinogen in per unit of time (expressed as ng/mL/hour). Normal adult value is (0.5–4.0 ng/mL/hour with normal sodium intake and upright position). It is suppressed in (1) salt-retaining steroid therapy, (2) antidiuretic hormone (ADH) therapy, and (3) salt-sensitive essential hypertension—primary hyperaldosteronemia **(Fig. 13)**.

Decision-making investigation steps (DMIS) of primary hyperaldosteronism are shown in **Table 4**.

Treatment of Primary Hyperaldosteronism

- *For unilateral lesion*:
  Adrenalectomy: After preparing the patient with low sodium diet, potassium supplement and spironolactone. Spironolactone should be stopped a few days prior to surgery to avoid hyperkalemia. Cure rate is 50%, excellent reduction in hypertension in the rest.

- *For bilateral lesion (hyperplasia) or inoperable carcinoma*: Spironolactone and low sodium diet may control potassium wasting.

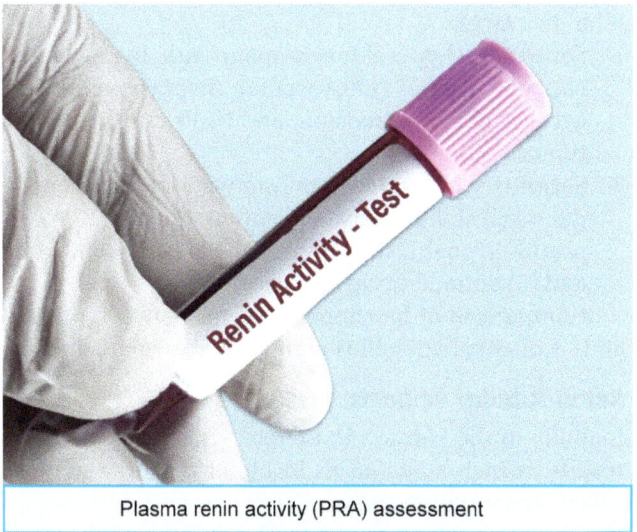

FIG. 13: Plasma renin activity (PRA) test estimate ability of renin to form angiotensin I from angiotensinogen in per unit of time (expressed as ng/mL/hour). It is low (suppressed) in primary hyperaldosteronism but not in secondary hyperaldosteronism.

TABLE 4: Decision-making investigation steps of primary hyperaldosteronism.

Step	Investigation	Result	Action/inference
Initial step	Serum electrolyte to document hypokalemia	Hypokalemia	Go to step 4
		Normokalemia but sodium intake low	Go to step 2
		Normokalemia but on diuretic therapy	Go to step 3
Step 2	Patient is given 1 g of NaCl, i.e., 1/5 teaspoon table salt with each meal for 4 days. Then serum electrolyte is repeated on 5th day	Hypokalemia	Go to step 4
		No hypokalemia	Exclude
Step 3	Discontinue diuretics for 3 weeks and then serum electrolyte is repeated	Hypokalemia	Go to step 4
		No hypokalemia	Exclude
Step 4	Plasma renin activity (PRA) assessment	PRA suppressed	Go to step 5
		PRA not suppressed	Exclude
Step 5	Assessment of aldosterone production by 24-hour urinary aldosterone excretion and or plasma aldosterone level* (both tests are preferred if patient is on high salt diet)	High	Go to step 6
		Not high	Exclude
Step 6	*Localization of lesion by*: • CT scan • Adrenal venography • I^{131} iodocholesterol scanning • Aldosterone gradient by adrenal veins sampling with catheter	Localization—Yes	Go to step 7
		Localization—No	Follow-up
Step 7	Adrenalectomy for unilateral lesion or medical therapy for bilateral and inoperable carcinomas		

*Normal excretion of aldosterone range 5–20 mg/24 hours and normal plasma aldosterone <10 mg/L. 10–20 for hyperplasia and >20 for adenoma or carcinoma.

Secondary Hyperaldosteronism

In secondary hyperaldosteronism, aldosterone hypersecretion is due to high renin production. So, it differs from primary hyperaldosteronism by absence of PRA suppression.

It has two forms:
1. Secondary hyperaldosteronism with hypertension caused by (i) renovascular hypertension, (ii) accelerated hypertension, and (iii) rennin-secreting tumor.
2. Secondary hyperaldosteronism without hypertension due to (i) sodium wasting nephropathy, (ii) RTA, (iii) pseudohypoaldosteronism, (4) Bartter's syndrome, and (5) diuretic/laxative abuse.

Comparison of biochemical events between primary and secondary hyperaldosteronism is shown in **Table 5**.

Renal Tubular Acidosis

Inability of the kidneys to excrete acids from the blood results in high acids levels in blood resulting acidosis called renal tubular acidosis (RTA).

There are many types of RTA. Of them, three are common/main types, namely type 1, 2, and 4 RTAs.

Type 1 RTA is due to defect at distal part of the renal tubules; type 2 RTA is due to defect at proximal part of the renal tubules cause; and type 4 RTA occurs when the tubules are unable to excrete enough potassium and as well as acid from the blood, its other name is hyperkalemic RTA.

Type 3 RTA was previously described as a rare type of RTA and now it is considered as a combination of type 1 and type 2 RTA.

Type 1 RTA is associated with autoimmune diseases such as Sjögren's syndrome and lupus. Other diseases and conditions related to type 1 RTA include (1) renal medullary cystic disease, (2) sickle cell anemia, (3) a hereditary form of deafness, (4) Ehlers–Danlos syndrome, and (5) recurrent urinary tract infections. Children with type 1 RTA grow more slowly. Adults with type 1 RTA develop progressive kidney disease and bone diseases. Both adults and children with type 1 RTA may develop renal stones formation.

Type 2 RTA is associated with Fanconi syndrome and viral hepatitis. In adults, with multiple myeloma, exposure to toxins—acute lead poisoning or chronic exposure to cadmium or certain drugs to treat human immunodeficiency virus (HIV), viral hepatitis, glaucoma, migraines, and seizures. Other diseases and conditions related to type 2 RTA include (1) cystinosis, (2) hereditary fructose intolerance, and (3) Wilson disease. Children with untreated type 2 RTA may grow slowly and remain short. There may be rickets and dental disease in both children and adults.

Type 4 RTA is associated with the renal transplant rejection. Due to hyperkalemia, people with type 4 RTA can have muscle weakness, heart disease, such as slow or irregular heartbeats and cardiac arrest **(Figs. 14A to C)**.

Treatment of RTA
- This is called alkali therapy. Drinking a solution of sodium bicarbonate or sodium citrate is given to all types of RTA to lower the acid level in blood. It can prevent kidney stones formation.

TABLE 5: Biochemical events primary versus secondary hyperaldosteronism.

Primary hyperaldosteronism	Secondary hyperaldosteronism
High aldosterone	High renin
High sodium retention	High angiotensinogen II
High potassium loss	High aldosterone
Low renin	High sodium retention
Low angiotensinogen II	High potassium loss

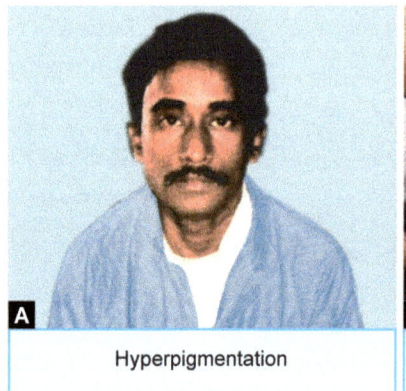
A: Hyperpigmentation

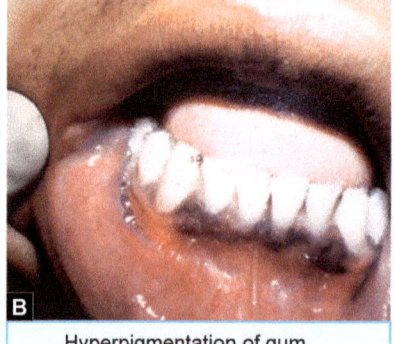
B: Hyperpigmentation of gum, mucosa, and tongue

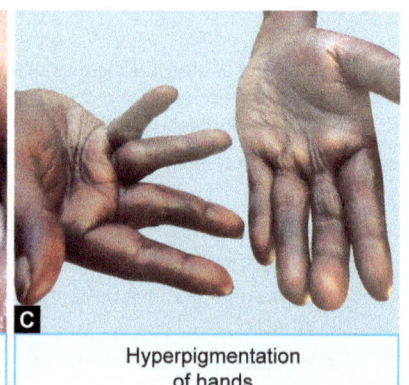
C: Hyperpigmentation of hands

FIGS. 14A TO C: Hyperpigmentation in chronic adrenal insufficiency.

TABLE 8: Replacement/maintenance therapy.

Glucocorticoid replacement (adult)	• Hydrocorticosterone 20–30 mg/day orally • Prednisolone 5–7.5 mg/day orally • Cortisone 25–35 mg/day orally
Glucocorticoid replacement (children)	Cortisone acetate or hydrocorticosterone phosphate 12–15 mg/m^2/day orally is preferred
	This is given in two divided doses in ratio of 2:1, one in the morning and at 4–5 PM respectively
Mineralocorticoid replacement	Fludrocortisone (9α-fludrocortisones) 50–300 μg/day orally if serum sodium is not maintained
Therapy during stress	
During minor stress	Dose of glucocorticoid is doubled in nausea, vomiting, fever >100°F, and minor surgery
During major stress (including major surgery)	Dose of glucocorticoid can be given as high as 10 times in oral, IM or IV routes. Mineralocorticoid replacement is not required at that time
Patient's education	
Identification and education	Education is mandatory. Every patient should have medical alert bracelets/steroid card and emergency kit

TABLE 9: Clinical presentation of secondary adrenocortical insufficiency.

Symptoms	Signs	Common biochemical features
Similar to that of primary adrenocortical insufficiency	Similar to that of primary adrenocortical insufficiency Except: • No hyperpigmentation • No vitiligo • No adrenal calcification	Similar to that of primary adrenocortical insufficiency Except: • No hyperkalemia
And	And	And
Headache and/or other central nervous system (CNS) symptoms (according to cause)	Other CNS signs (according to cause)	Other CNS findings (according to cause)

TABLE 10: Primary versus secondary adrenocortical insufficiency.

Test/tool	Procedure	Conclusions
Long ACTH stimulation test	1 mg of depot-ACTH$^{1-24}$ is given IM and plasma cortisol is measured at 1, 4, 8, and 24 hours after injection	Any value >550 nmol/L excludes primary adrenal insufficiency
Plasma ACTH measurement	Plasma ACTH is measured at basal state	• ACTH >250 pmol/mL is conclusive of primary adrenal insufficiency • A normal/low value is compatible with secondary adrenal insufficiency
oCRH stimulation test	1 μg/kg of body weight oCRH is given IV and plasma ACTH and cortisol is measured at 0, 30, 60, 90, and 120 minutes after injection	• Mark ACTH raise but no response to cortisol is conclusive of primary adrenal insufficiency • No ACTH raise and no or minimal response to cortisol is compatible of secondary adrenal insufficiency

(ACTH: adrenocorticotropic hormone; oCRH: ovine-corticotropin-releasing hormone)

Acute Adrenal Insufficiency or Adrenal Crisis

It is a medical emergency which can be either a de novo presentation of new case or acute deterioration in a known chronic adrenal insufficiency person.

The ominous sign of adrenal crisis is hypotension and circulatory collapse. Other features will be features of adrenal insufficiency (primary/secondary) and features of precipitating factors (stress factors or sudden stoppage of steroid).

Diagnosis and treatment of adrenal crisis

- Treatment should be start without waiting for diagnostic confirmation.
- If suspected collect blood for a paired ACTH and cortisol or rapid ACTH stimulation test and start treatment.

ABC of treatment of adrenal crisis is as follows **(Table 11)**:
A. Intravenous fluid to correct volume depletion, dehydration, and hypoglycemia.
B. *Glucocorticoid therapy*:
- Hydrocortisone phosphate 100 mg IV stat and 6 hourly
- Reduce the dose to 50 mg IV 6 hourly, if the patient becomes stable.
C. Identify the precipitating factor(s) and treat accordingly.

■ Congenital Adrenal Hyperplasia

Definition: Congenital adrenal hyperplasia is a family of autosomal recessive disorder of adrenal steroid production caused by deficient or defective enzyme action for cortisol biosynthesis.

Low cortisol production of CAH results in increase production of ACTH secretion. Excess ACTH stimulation results in hyperplasia of adrenal cortex. So, why the name is CAH?

Clinical Presentation

Its clinical presentation varies widely. It depends on the steroid profile changed by the defective enzyme.

The triad of clinical picture is as (1) deficiency of glucocorticoids, (2) imbalance of mineralocorticoids, and (3) excess androgens as shown in **Flowchart 7**.

Classification or type of CAH (on the basis of enzyme involved) is given in **Table 12**.

21-hydroxylase Deficiency Syndrome

The steroid synthesis defects are described in **Figures 15 and 16** and clinical features in **Table 13**.

There are three different clinical presentations of 21-hydroxylase deficiency **(Table 13)**.

11β-hydroxylase Deficiency Syndrome

The steroid synthesis defects are described in **Figure 17** and clinical features in **Table 14**.

TABLE 11: ABC of treatment of adrenal crisis.

A.	Fluid therapy	Intravenous fluid (DNS/NS) to correct volume depletion, dehydration, and hypoglycemia
B.	Glucocorticoid therapy	• Hydrocortisone phosphate 100 mg IV stat and 6 hourly (classically there will be marked improvement within 4 hours of first steroid injection) • Reduce the dose to 50 mg IV 6 hourly, if the patient becomes stable
C.	Precipitating factor(s)	Identify the precipitating factor(s) and treat accordingly

(DNS: dextrose normal saline; NS: normal saline)

TABLE 12: Classification of congenital adrenal hyperplasia (CAH).

Clinical class	Enzyme	Type
Simple non-salt wasting CAH	21-hydroxylase deficiency	Type I CAH
Severe classic salt wasting CAH	21-hydroxylase deficiency	Type II CAH
Mild nonclassic (late onset) CAH	21-hydroxylase deficiency	
	11β-hydroxylase deficiency	Type III CAH
	3β-hydroxylase deficiency	Type IV CAH
	17α-hydroxylase deficiency	Type V CAH
Lipoid adrenal hyperplasia	Cholesterol desmolase deficiency	Type VI CAH

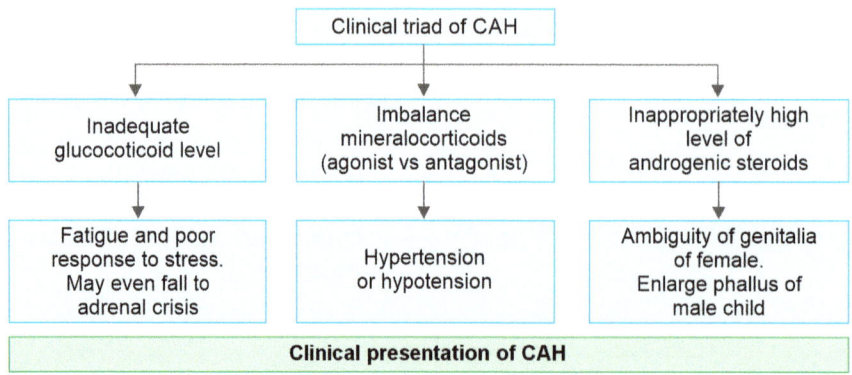

FLOWCHART 7: Clinical presentation of congenital adrenal hyperplasia (CAH) depends on degree of alteration in three types of steroid production.

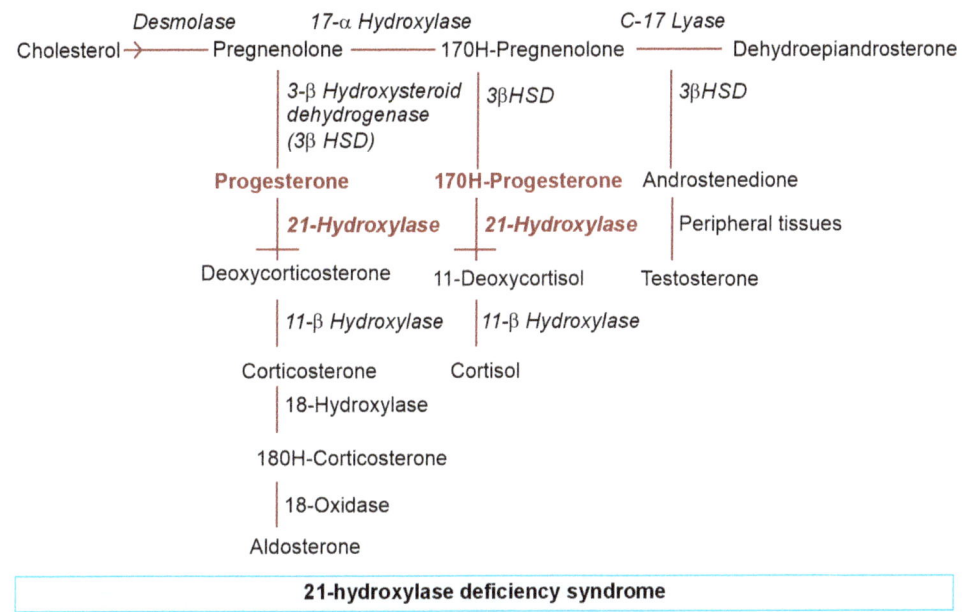

FIG. 15: 21-hydroxylase deficiency leads to deficiency of cortisol and aldosterone and excess androgens. Three clinical presentations (1) Simple non-salt wasting congenital adrenal hyperplasia (CAH) (type I); (2) Severe classic salt wasting CAH (type II), and (3) Mild nonclassic (late onset) CAH.

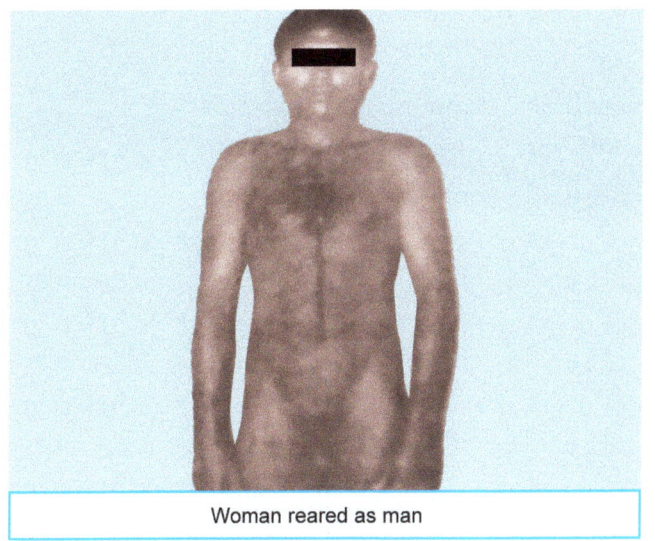

FIG. 16: An untreated adult female.

3β-hydroxysteroid Dehydrogenase Deficiency Syndrome

The steroid synthesis defects are described in **Figure 18** and clinical features in **Table 15**.

17α-hydroxylase/17,20-lyase Deficiency Syndrome

The steroid synthesis defects are described in **Figure 19** and clinical features in **Table 16**.

Cholesterol Desmolase Deficiency Syndrome

The steroid synthesis defects are described in **Figure 20** and clinical features in **Table 17**.

Treatment of CAH

Treatment of the virilizing CAHs involves hormone replacement therapy with glucocorticoids. The goal of treatment is suppression of excessive ACTH and adrenal androgen secretion without hypercortisolism. **Table 18** summarizes the treatment of CAH.

PHEOCHROMOCYTOMA

Pheochromocytoma is a catecholamine-producing tumor that typically produces labile hypertension and paroxysmal symptoms.
Common presentations are:
- *Sustained hypertension* difficult to control with usual drug and dose.
- *Hypertensive crisis*

Features	Simple non-salt wasting CAH (type I CAH)	Severe classic salt wasting CAH (type II CAH)	Mild nonclassic (late onset) CAH
Clinical features	• Ambiguous genitalia in female infants • Large erectile penis in male infants • Accelerated growth in childhood • Cliteromegaly with or without labial fusion (Prader type I or II) in female baby • Precocious puberty in male baby • Short final height due to early bone maturation	• Severe fluid and electrolyte loss due to diarrhea and vomiting within first week of life • Exaggerated features of simple non-salt wasting CAH • Features due adrenal insufficiency are dark complexion, postural hypotension, and poor tolerance to stress • Fond of taking large amount of table salt	• At birth normal external genitalia • Mild feature of androgen access around puberty, such as hirsutism in girls and oligospermia in boys • Symptom varies from asymptomatic to frank cases • Biochemical features are comparable with symptom score
Biochemical features	Serum 17-hydroxyprogesterone (17-OHP) high at basal and post-ACTH stimulation will be high	Serum 17-OHP high at basal and post-ACTH stimulation will be high	Serum 17-OHP high at basal and post-ACTH stimulation will be high
Neonatal screening	Hill prick blood spotted on filter paper on days 3–5 of life for high 17-OHP level.		

TABLE 13: Types of 21-hydroxylase deficiency syndrome [salt losing congenital adrenal hyperplasia (CAH)].

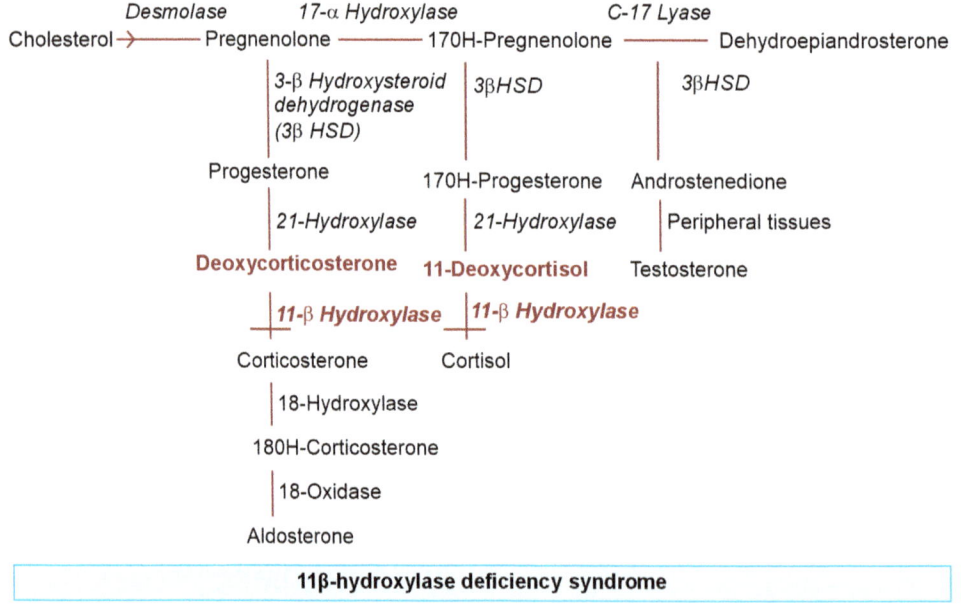

FIG. 17: 11β-hydroxylase deficiency leads to deficiency of cortisol and aldosterone and excess androgens. Two clinical presentations (1) classical congenital adrenal hyperplasia (CAH) (type III); (2) late onset/cryptic variant CAH.

TABLE 14: 11β-hydroxylase deficiency syndrome (hypertensive CAH) (type III CAH).

Clinical features	Biochemical features	Late onset/cryptic variant
• Severe hypertension • Sings of moderate virilization (cliteromegaly) in girls and precocious puberty in boys	• Low potassium, low plasma rennin activity, and there may be high sodium • Mineralocorticoid [desoxycorticosterone acetate (DOCA)] high • Androgens high	Present with hirsutism and primary amenorrhea in girls

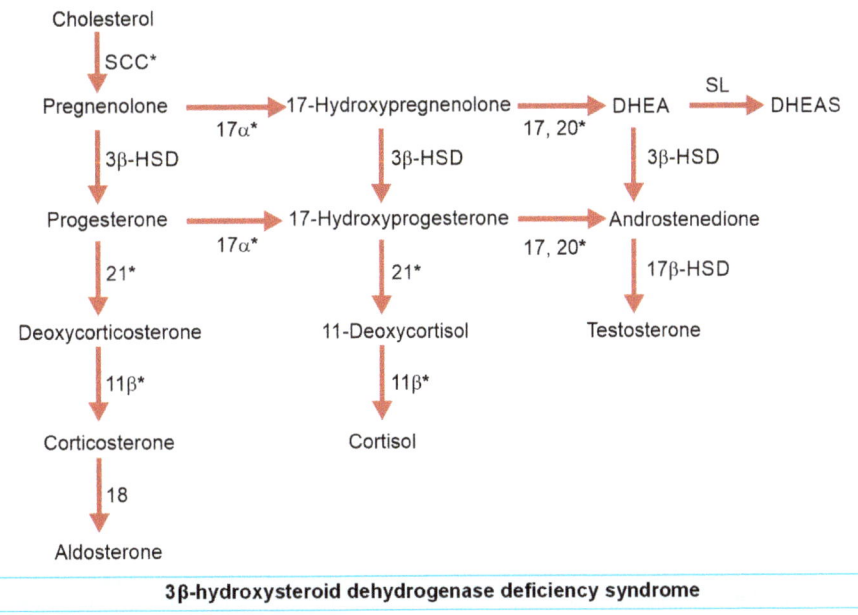

*Hydroxylase

FIG. 18: 3β-hydroxysteroid dehydrogenase deficiency (3β-HSD) leads to deficiency of cortisol, aldosterone, and testosterone but excess dehydroepiandrosterone (DHEA). Two clinical presentations (1) classical congenital adrenal hyperplasia (CAH) (type IV); (2) late onset/non-classical form.

TABLE 15: 3β-hydroxysteroid dehydrogenase deficiency syndrome (type IV CAH).		
Clinical features	**Biochemical features**	**Late onset/nonclassical form**
• Sings of androgens deficiency incomplete masculinization with hypospadias in boys but excess dehydroepiandrosterone (DHEA) clitoromegaly, and labial fusion in girls • Severe fluid and electrolyte loss due in infancy due to low aldosterone and cortisol • Frequent adrenal crisis	• Low adrenal and gonadal steroids • High DHEA	• Female present with hirsutism • Male with some degree of hypospadias

- Sign and symptoms of aortic dissection and myocardial infarction
- Paroxysmal episodes, suggestive of catecholamine release, their severity and clinical presentations are variable and generally include:
  ○ Frontal or occipital severe headache
  ○ Excessive sweating, palpitation, and apprehension for impending death along with chest and abdominal pain, nausea, and vomiting

The paroxysm last from few minutes to several hours, most episodes subside within 10 minutes.

Identification and Treatment

Such cases are important because of following characters:
- The hypertension is curable.
- The hypertensive paroxysms are sometimes lethal.
- The tumor itself may be malignant.
- Such cases can be a component of familial multiple endocrine neoplasia (MEN II and MEN III).

Findings suggestive of pheochromocytoma:
- *Clinical findings*:
  ○ Paroxysmal nature of attacks
  ○ Signs of adrenergic activity (1) tachycardia and (2) excessive sweating
  ○ Signs of hypermetabolism (1) raised body temperature and (2) weight loss
  ○ Orthostatic hypotension
  ○ Anxiety neurosis
  ○ Neurocutaneous manifestations (1) café-au-lait spots (>6), (2) neuromas of neurofibromas, (3) retinoblastoma, and (4) vertebral abnormalities.
- *Laboratory findings*:
  ○ Glucose intolerance
  ○ High hematocrit
- Family history of pheochromocytoma
- *Associated diseases*:
  ○ Hyperthyroidism
  ○ Medullary carcinoma of thyroid

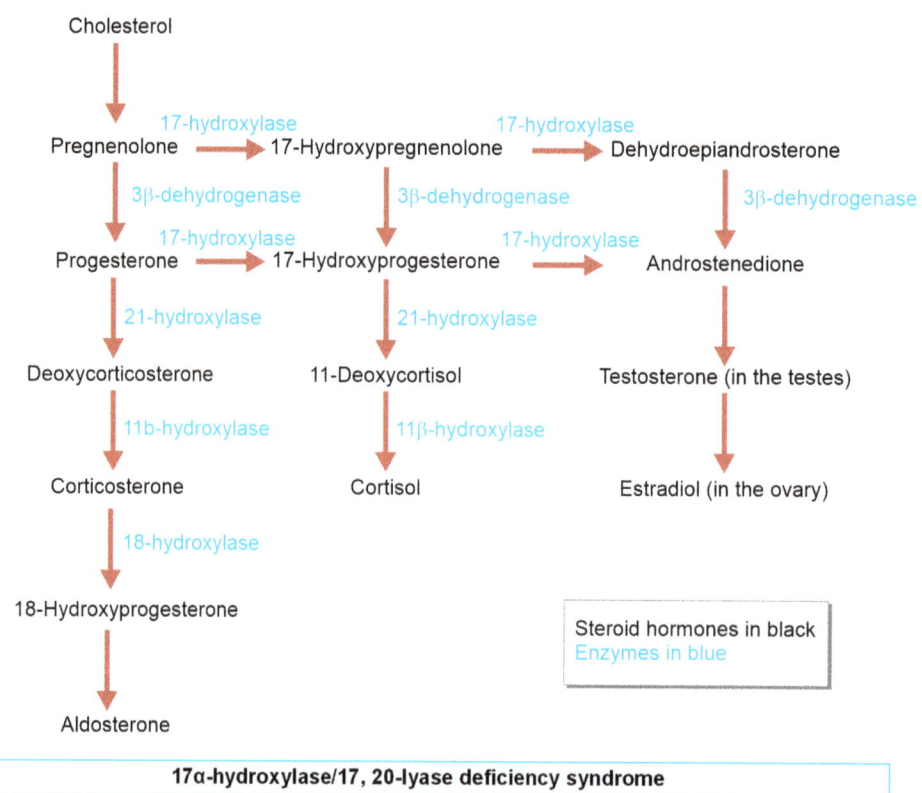

FIG. 19: 17α-hydroxylase/17,20-lyase deficiency syndrome leads to deficiency of gonadal steroids. One clinical presentation—congenital adrenal hyperplasia (CAH) type V.

TABLE 16: 17α-hydroxylase/17,20-lyase deficiency syndrome (type V CAH).		
Clinical features	**Biochemical features**	**Late onset/nonclassical form**
• At birth both boy and girl are with female phenotype • At puberty primary gonadal failure with enlarge breast and primary amenorrhea • Minimum or no adrenal crisis • Hypertension	• Low potassium, plasma rennin activity, and aldosterone • High FSH and LH	Absent
(CAH: congenital adrenal hyperplasia; FSH: follicle-stimulating hormone; LH: luteinizing hormone)		

- Islet cell tumor
- Neurofibromatosis

Diagnosis of Pheochromocytoma

There are two steps:
- *Step 1*: Biochemical confirmation of suspected case
- *Step 2*: Anatomical localization

Biochemical Confirmation of Suspected Case

- It is traditionally done by 24 hours urinary catecholamine by high-pressure liquid chromatography (HPLC).
- Substances are (1) dopamine (DA), (2) norepinephrine (NE), and (3) epinephrine.
- Metabolite measurement of 24 hours urinary vanillylmandelic acid (VMA) or total metanephrines is dine in most laboratories. Specific measurements of catecholamines are superior. In >90% cases of pheochromocytomas, catecholamines are more than twice of their upper limit of normal range. Most of the time, urinary catecholamine (especially norepinephrine) is elevated but occasionally they are normal if sampled when the person is normotensive or asymptomatic. Therefore, sample should be collected during a paroxysm.

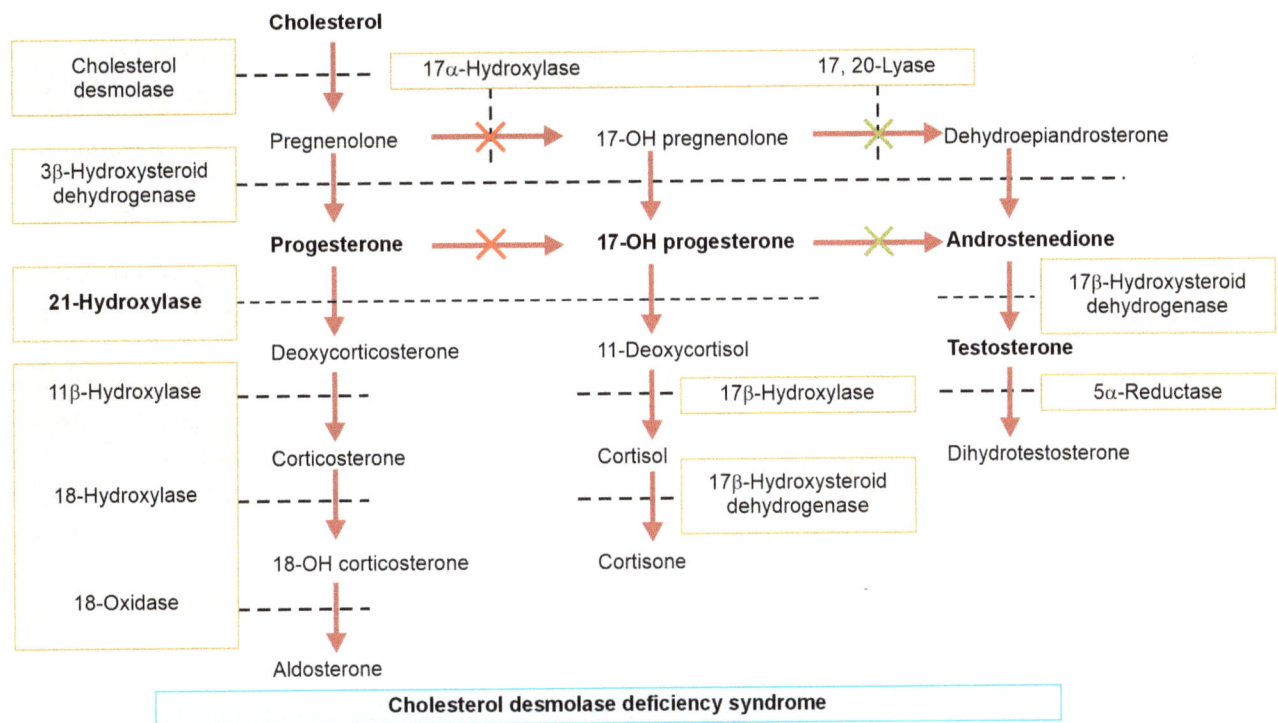

FIG. 20: Cholesterol desmolase deficiency syndrome leads to absolute deficiency of adrenal steroids. Phenotype female at birth. Usually die from adrenal crisis within first week of life (CAH type VI).

TABLE 17: Cholesterol desmolase deficiency syndrome (type VI CAH).		
Clinical features	**Biochemical features**	**Late onset/nonclassical form**
• Serious disorder • All steroid synthesis is blocked • Phenotype female at birth • Usually die from adrenal crisis within first week of life • With early recognition and treatment, they can survive	Absence of all type of steroid hormone in blood	Absent

TABLE 18: Treatment of CAH.		
Principle of treatment	**Glucocorticoid**	**Mineralocorticoid**
• In all forms of CAH glucocorticoid replacement with or without mineralocorticoid • It corrects all the metabolic disturbances, i.e., lower ACTH and androgens to normal; remission of hypertension, virilization, etc. improves	• In children, hydrocortisone is drug of choice (10–15 mg/day) • In adult, prednisolone or dexamethasone can be used. Dose is equivalent to 20 mg of hydrocortisone, i.e., 0.75 mg of dexamethasone or 7.5 mg of prednisolone in two divided doses in 2:1 ratio	Synthetic steroid 9α-fluorocortisone is used in salt wasting cases. Usual dose of 0.05–0.1 mg/day

(ACTH: adrenocorticotropic hormone; CAH: congenital adrenal hyperplasia)

Provocative Test

Pharmacological agents for provocation of attack, such as histamine, glucagon, or tyramine are not in use for their potential danger.

Adrenolytic (Phentolamine) Test

Intravenous bolus of phentolamine (up to 5 mg) is administered in a suspected individual after getting a stable blood pressure record. A fall in blood pressure start in 2–3 minutes and last approximately 10 minutes. The test is considered positive if fall in systolic is >35 mm Hg and >25 mm Hg in diastolic.

Anatomical Localization

Location of pheochromocytoma:
- Adrenal (90% is in adrenal medulla; 80% solitary, and 10% bilateral—most are having positive family history)
- Extra-adrenal (10%):
  - Cervical (2%)
  - Thoracic (10–20%)
  - Intra-abdominal (70–80%):
    - Upper abdominal (40%)
    - Organ of Zuckerkandl (30%)
    - Bladder (15%)

Localization procedures:
- *CT scan*: An adrenal pheochromocytoma with a diameter of >3 cm can be readily visualized with CT **(Fig. 21)**.
- It appears as a homogenous mass with a density >10 HU units on an unenhanced film and with contrast density is enhanced. Sometime hemorrhagic foci are see within the mass.
- *MRI*: Typical appearance of a pheochromocytoma in T1 image is slightly hypointense to the rest of the adrenal gland. But in T2 image, some are markedly hyperintense which called lightbulb sign **(Fig. 22)**.
- Iodobenzylguanidine scintigraphy (when CT/MRI fails to localize).
- Arteriography is also used in some specialized centers.

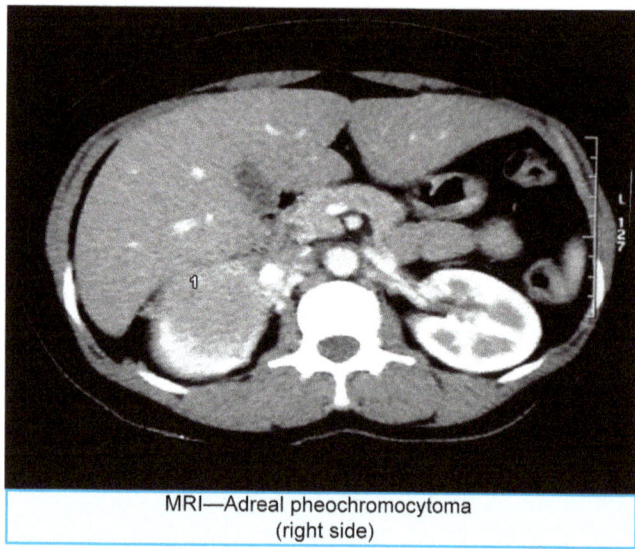

FIG. 22: A 26-year-old lady having hypodense mass in right adrenal in T2 image; some are markedly hyperintense, i.e., positive lightbulb sign.

Treatment of Pheochromocytoma

Surgical Excision

Preoperative treatment of hypertension with adequate dose of α-adrenergic antagonist (phenoxybenzamine) for adequate time to expand the contracted vascular volume.

Persistent hypertension in postoperative state may be due to:
- Missed pheochromocytoma
- Adrenomedullary hyperplasia
- Renal artery ligation
- Essential hypertension

All patients should undergo clinical as well as biochemical evaluation at least after 1 month of surgery.

ADRENAL INCIDENTALOMA

Adrenal incidentaloma is defined as a clinically unapparent adrenal lesion (≥1 cm in diameter) that is detected on imaging performed for indications other than adrenal disease evaluation. This definition excludes patients who are undergoing screening and surveillance because of hereditary syndromes or those with known extra-adrenal cancer who are undergoing imaging for staging or during follow-up after treatment. They are now identified more frequently than before because of widespread use of thoracic and abdominal imaging. All of them demand evaluation for hormonal activity and potentiality for malignancy.

Adrenal incidentaloma detected on imaging study may or may not be hormonally functional. A functional

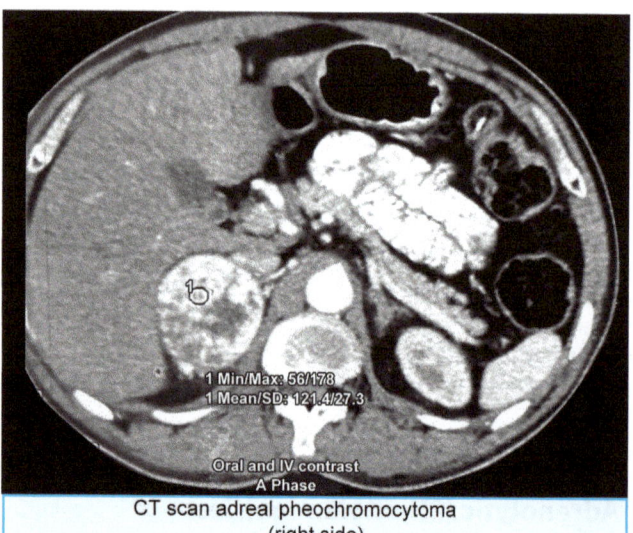

FIG. 21: A 50-year man with a fairly large dense mass showing enhancement after contrast and heterogenecity.

one may producing (1) cortisol (Cushing's syndrome), (2) aldosterone (primary hyperaldosteronism), or (3) pheochromocytoma. Large lesions (size >4 cm) are likely to be a malignant lesion.

Management of such a lesion requires to follow a six-step process:
1. Clinical evaluation for specific hormone excess
2. Biochemical screening study
3. Study of imaging features
4. Fine needle aspiration (FNAC) and/or surgery for cytological or histological study
5. Specific treatment
6. Follow-up of benign incidentaloma

Clinical evaluation of:
- Look for primary hyperaldosteronism in cases with resistant hypertension and hypokalemia (without papilledema and edema)
- Look for pheochromocytoma in episodic/sustain hypertension
- Look for Cushing's syndrome in cases with cushingoid features, glucose intolerance, hypertension, etc.

Biochemical screening study:
- For pheochromocytoma, either with plasma or urinary catecholamine measurements
- If negative in biochemical testing for pheochromocytoma, then for all patients should undergo biochemical testing for Cushing's syndrome and/or primary hyperaldosteronism.

Study of imaging features: A CT scan should be used to determine precontrast density, contrast washout along with its size and margins.
- A precontrast density is >10 HU; washout <50% are considered as a useful diagnostic information for suspecting malignant potentiality.
- Lesions with larger size (>4 cm) and/or irregular margin have more chance of malignancy.

Fine needle aspiration and/or surgery for cytological or histological study: For lesions with larger size (>4 cm) and/or irregular margin have more chance of malignancy **(Flowchart 8)**.

Treatment depending on functional status and histology of the lesion:
- For hormonally active adrenal incidentalomas are according to the surgical removal protocol of the disease/syndrome.
- For malignant adrenal incidentalomas are according to the oncology protocol.
- For hormonally inactive and nonmalignant adrenal incidentalomas follow-up protocol.

Follow-up:
- For masses that likely to be benign (<10 HU; washout >50%), small (<3 cm), and nonfunctioning, imaging, and biochemical reevaluation (pheochromocytoma and hypercortisolism only) can be advised to repeat after 1–2 year or more.
- For other indeterminate lesions, repeat evaluation for growth after 3–12 months is useful, and subsequent testing intervals will be based on the rate of growth.

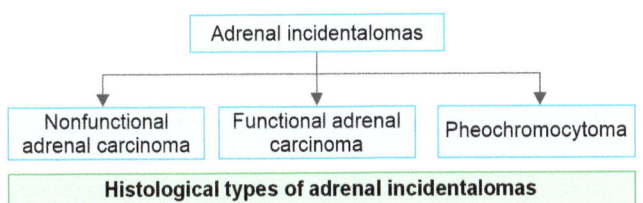

FLOWCHART 8: Histological types of adrenal incidentalomas fine needle aspiration (FNAC) material may of three types.

FURTHER READINGS

1. Betts JG, DeSaix P, Johnson E, Johnson JE, Korol O, Kruse D, et al. Anatomy and Physiology. Houston, Texas: OpenStax, Rice University; 2017.
2. Standring S. Gray's Anatomy: The Anatomical Basis of Clinical Practice, 41st edition. Philadelphia, PA, Elsevier; 2015.
3. Barrett KE, Barman SM, Yuan J, Brooks HL. Ganong's Review of Medical Physiology, 26th edition. New York: McGraw Hill-Medical; 2019.
4. Melmed S, Koenig R, Clifford JR, Richard J, Allison BG. Williams Textbook of Endocrinology, 14th edition. Philadelphia, PA, Elsevier; 2019.
5. Gardner DG, Shoback D. Greenspan's Basic and Clinical Endocrinology, 10th edition. New York: McGraw-Hill Education; 2018.
6. Coleman WB, Tsongalis GJ. Molecular Pathology, The Molecular Basis of Human Disease, 2nd edition. United Kingdom: Elsevier Inc; 2017.
7. Fassnacht M, Arlt W, Bancos I, Dralle H, Newell-Price J, Sahdev A, et al. Management of adrenal incidentalomas: European Society of Endocrinology Clinical Practice Guideline in collaboration with the European Network for the Study of Adrenal Tumors. Eur J Endocrinol. 2016;175(2):G1-G34.
8. Ahmed T, Mahtab H, Tofail T, Morshed AHG, Rahman FB, Khan SA. Current Status of Low Dose Overnight Dexamethasone Suppression Test (LODST). J Obes Diab. 2020;4:5-8.

CHAPTER 6

Diabetes Mellitus and Insulinoma

- ❑ Introduction to diabetes mellitus
  - ➢ Anatomical and physiological concept
  - ➢ Pathophysiology of diabetes
  - ➢ Insulin resistance and metabolic syndrome
- ❑ Definition, diagnosis, and classification of diabetes mellitus
  - ➢ Definition
  - ➢ Diagnosis
  - ➢ Classification of diabetes mellitus
- ❑ General principles in the management of diabetes mellitus
  - ➢ General treatment components of diabetes mellitus
  - ➢ Exercise and diabetes mellitus
  - ➢ Drug treatment of diabetes mellitus
- ❑ Insulinoma

This chapter is about Diabetes Mellitus and Insulinoma, which begins with an introduction to applied anatomy and physiology of beta cells. It covers diagnosis and treatment of diabetes, detection of acute complication of diabetes, and management of insulinoma. This chapter consists of 32 Figures, 17 Tables, and 10 Flowcharts to illustrate its text.

INTRODUCTION TO DIABETES MELLITUS

(Anatomical and Physiological Concept; Pathophysiological Concepts)

■ Anatomical and Physiological Concept

The pancreas is a retroperitoneal organ, which lays in the epigastric, left hypochondriac, and a portion of the umbilical abdominal regions. An adult pancreas weight averaged 91.8 g (range: 40.9–182 g). The size is up to 3 cm for the head, 2.5 cm for the neck and body, and 2 cm for the tail. Blood supply is from pancreaticoduodenal, splenic, gastroduodenal, and superior mesenteric arteries. Venous derange from head is by superior mesenteric branch of the hepatic portal vein. The rest is drain by pancreas to duodenal vein via splenic vein **(Fig. 1)**.

- The pancreas consists of exocrine (80%) and endocrine portions (2%); rest is formed by ducts, blood vessel, and connective tissue.
- Human pancreas contains 1–2 million islets of Langerhans. These are scattered throughout the pancreas, more plentiful in the tail.
- Each islet consists of at least four types of cells—A (alpha), B (beta), D (delta), and F (PP) cells.
- Beta cells account for 60–75% of cells of an islet; these are generally located in the center. They are surrounded by alpha cells, which make up about 20% of an islet **(Fig. 2)**.

The lymphatic drainage: The pancreas has a complex, intricate network of lymphatic vessels, and nodes responsible for the drainage of the head, neck, body, and tail of the pancreas.

CHAPTER 6: Diabetes Mellitus and Insulinoma

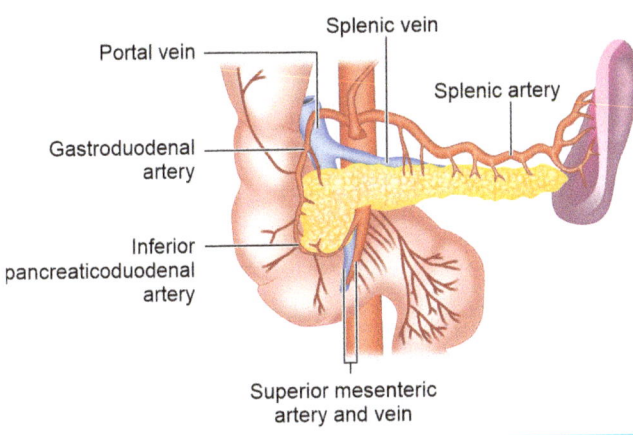

Anatomy of pancreas

FIG. 1: Pancreas is a retroperitoneal organ, weight averaged 91.8 g. The size is up to 3 cm for the head, 2.5 cm for the neck and body, and 2 cm for the tail. Blood supply is from pancreaticoduodenal, splenic, gastroduodenal, and superior mesenteric arteries. Venous derange from head is by superior mesenteric branch of the hepatic portal vein. The rest is drain by pancreatico-duodenal vein via splenic vein.

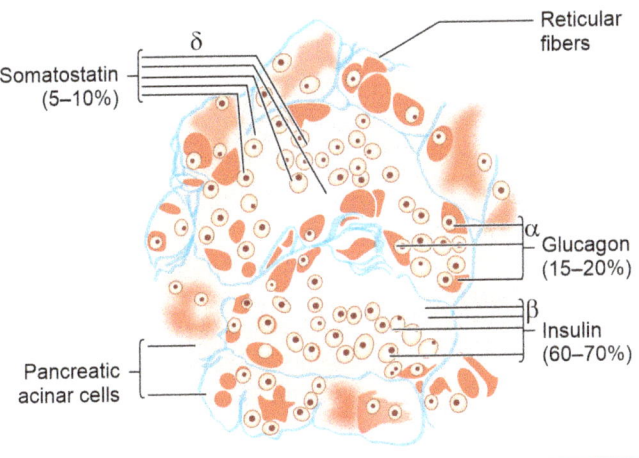

Human islets of Langerhans

FIG. 2: Pancreas contains 1–2 million islets of Langerhans. These are scattered throughout the pancreas, more plentiful in the tail. Each islet consists of at least four types of cells—A (alpha) B (beta), D (delta), and F (PP) cells. Beta cells account for 60–75% of cells of an islet; these are generally located in the center. They are surrounded by alpha cells, which make up about 20% of an islet.

Nerve supply: The pancreas receives parasympathetic nerve fibers from the posterior vagal trunk via its celiac branch. Sympathetic supply comes from T6–T10 via the thoracic splanchnic nerves and the celiac plexus.

Anatomic anomalies of the pancreas can be a fusion anomaly (pancreas divisum), migration anomaly (annular pancreas, ectopic pancreas), or duplication anomaly (number or form variation). Pancreas divisum is the most common congenital pancreatic ductal anatomic variant, occurring in approximately 4–14%.

Human Insulin Synthesis, Secretion, and Blood Profile

Human Insulin

Insulin is a hormone synthesized in the beta cells. It is first formed as preproinsulin in the rough endoplasmic reticulum. It is then cleaved immediately into proinsulin and transported to Golgi apparatus where packaging into secretory granules takes place. Then it is cleaved further into insulin and C peptide in equimolecular amounts. Insulin is composed of two peptides chains—A chain of 21 amino acids and B chain of 30 amino acids, connected by two disulfide bridges. Insulin has a circulatory half-life of 3–5 minutes. It is catabolized by the liver, kidney, and also placenta **(Fig. 3)**.

Insulin Synthesis in the Beta Cells (In Three Steps)

In the initial step, preproinsulin is formed in the rough endoplasmic reticulum. In next step, it is cleaved into proinsulin and transported to Golgi apparatus where packaging occurs to form secretory granules. The third or final step take place during insulin secretion where proinsulin is cleaved further into insulin and C peptide in equimolecular amounts **(Fig. 4)**.

Insulin Secretion

Blood glucose stimulates beta cell to secrete insulin, and so secretion of insulin of an individual is primarily regulated by his/her dietary events.

Events during the synthesis process are: (1) Blood glucose molecules enter into the beta cell through the glucose transporter-2 (GLUT2) of cell membrane. Glucose does not require insulin (this cell is an insulin-independent cell). (2) Within the cell adenosine triphosphate (ATP)/adenosine diphosphate (ADP) ratio goes up due to increased production of ATP from glycolysis. (3) ATP-sensitive potassium channels get blocked. (4) Membrane becomes depolarized. (5) Voltage-gated calcium channels get opened. (6) Entry of calcium within beta cell. (7) Insulin is released by exocytosis **(Fig. 5)**.

Insulin Secretion in Healthy Subjects

There is a continuous low-level secretion of insulin (approximately 1 unit/h) between meals and throughout night. It is called "*basal insulin*." So about 24 units of insulin is secreted as basal secretion. Following meals there is sharp rise, which is called "*prandial or bolus insulin*" release. The rate and amount of secretion are influenced by the amount and composition of meals.

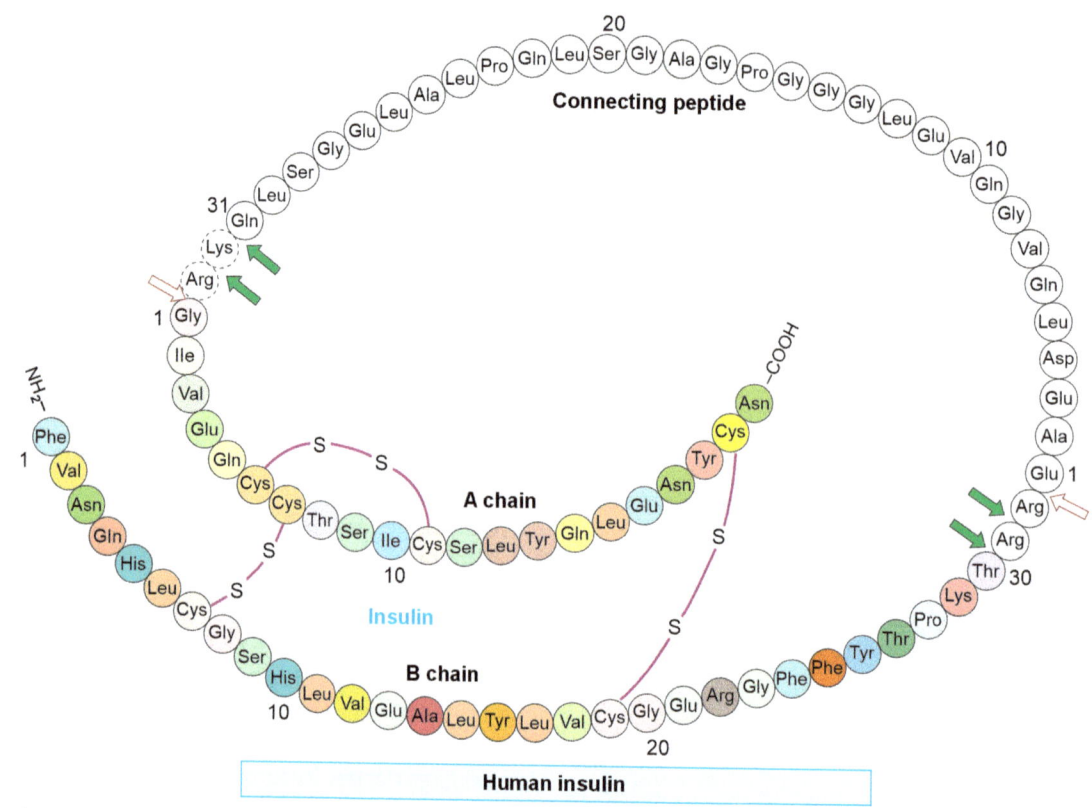

FIG. 3: Insulin is composed of two peptide chains—A chain of 21 amino acids and B chain of 30 amino acids, connected by two disulfide bridges. Molecular weight—5808 Daltons. Molecular formula: $C_{257}H_{383}N_{65}O_{77}S_6$.

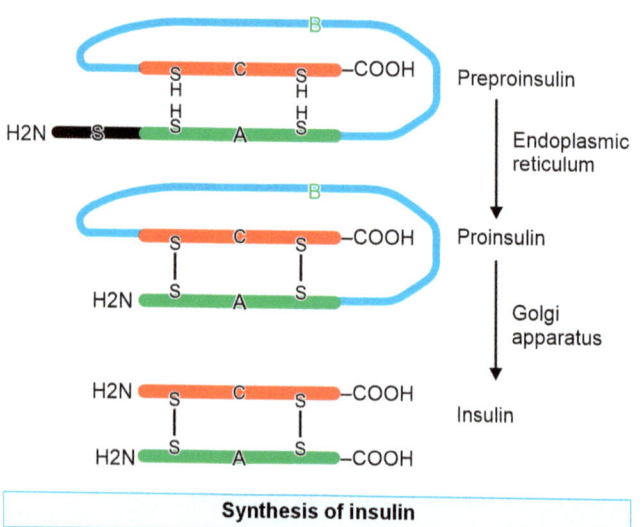

FIG. 4: Insulin is synthesized in three steps: Step 1—preproinsulin in rough endoplasmic reticulum. Step 2—cleavage to proinsulin and transported to Golgi apparatus to from secretory granules. Step 3—final cleavage to insulin and C-peptide during secretion.

On an average there is also another 24 units of insulin secretion per day as meal-related bolus. A *bolus release* shows two phases—*first phase* is sharp and transient rise lasting for <10 minutes; this is followed by *second phase* that is sustained and persists till the blood glucose goes back near to the basal state **(Fig. 6)**.

Glucose Homeostasis during Fasting State and after Intake of Food

In Fasting State

When there is no glucose supply to blood from the gut during night and between meals, our body mechanism is adjusted to ensure glucose supply to the vital tissues.

This adjustment takes place by the three processes—(1) insulin secretion goes down, (2) hepatic glucose output (HGU) increase, and (3) glucose uptake predominantly by insulin-independent cells (vital tissue brain and heart kidney).

Following an overnight fast, the majority (~75%) of glucose disposal occurs in insulin independent tissues.

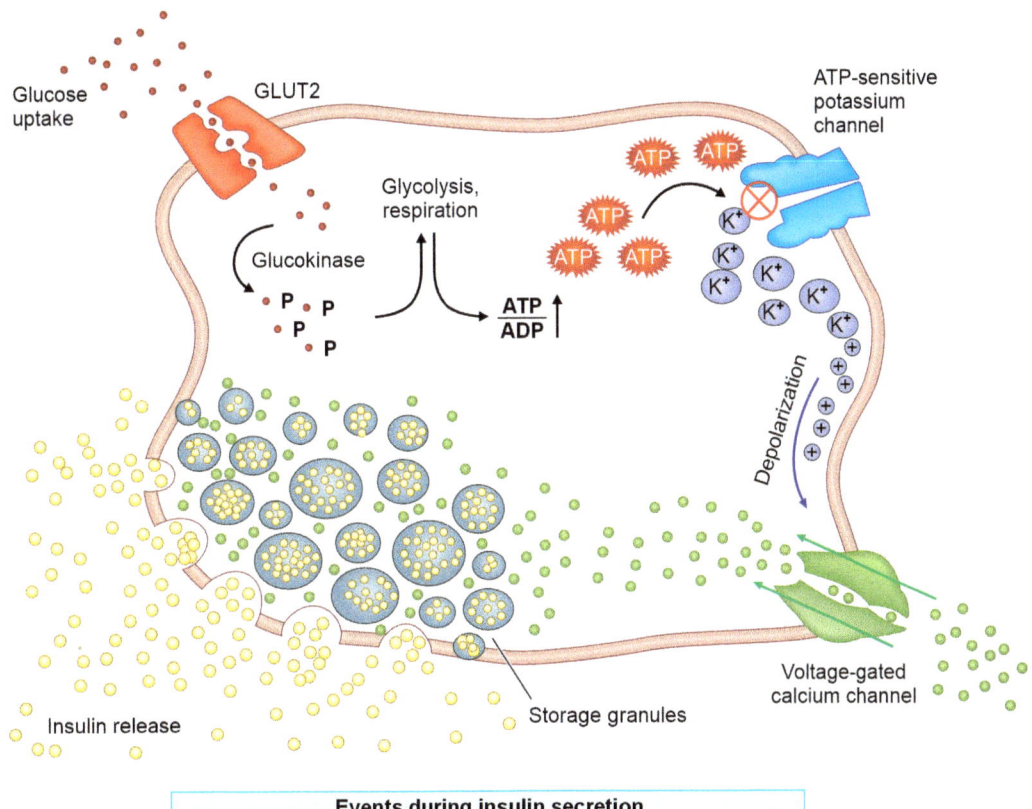

FIG. 5: Events are: Blood glucose molecules enter into beta cell through the glucose transporter-2 (GLUT2) of cell membrane. Within the cell adenosine triphosphate (ATP)/adenosine diphosphate (ADP) ratio goes up due to increased production of ATP from glycolysis. ATP-sensitive potassium channels get blocked. Membrane becomes depolarized. Voltage-gated calcium channels get opened. Entry of calcium within beta cell. Insulin is released by exocytosis.

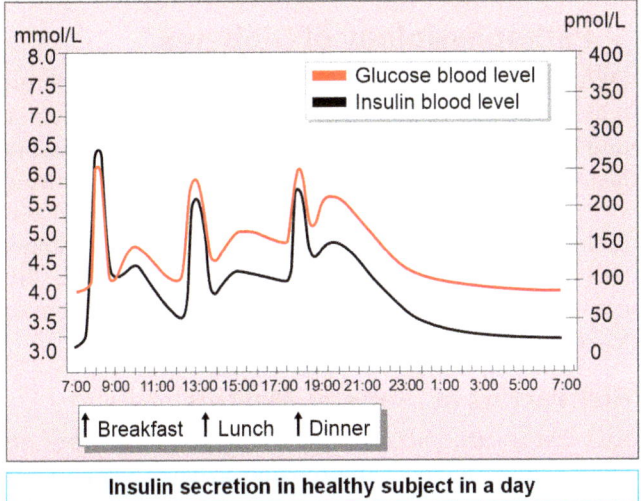

FIG. 6: There is a continuous low-level secretion of insulin (approximately 1 unit/h) between meals and throughout night. It is called *"basal insulin."* Following meals there is sharp rise, which is called *"prandial or bolus insulin"* release. The rate and amount of secretion are influenced by the amount and composition of meals.

Insulin-independent tissues, the brain and splanchnic organs, utilize ~50% and ~25%, respectively; insulin-dependent tissues, primarily in muscle, utilize only 25%.

Basal glucose utilization (~2 mg/kg/min) is precisely matched by glucose production by liver.

After Food Intake

Following ingestion of meal, when there is excess glucose supply to blood from the gut, our body mechanism is adjusted to ensure euglycemia by the following processes and effects:

Three adjustment processes occur: (1) Insulin secretion increase; (2) suppression of HGU, and (3) glucose uptake by insulin-dependent cells (muscle and fat).

There are two effects of hyperglycemia following meal: (1) Enhance muscle glucose uptake (mass effect) and (2) suppress HGU **(Fig. 7)**.

Our body cells/tissues can be divided in to two groups on the basis of their dependency on insulin for uptake of blood glucose: Insulin dependent and insulin independent. Gut epithelial cell, red blood cell, brain cell,

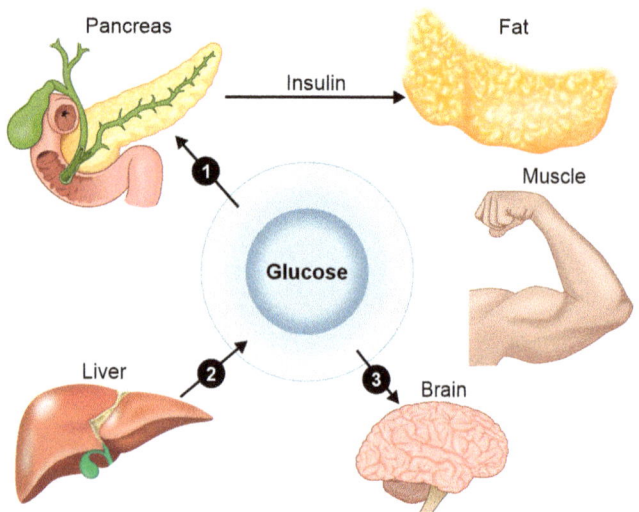

Feed-fast adjustment of insulin and glucose in healthy state

FIG. 7: *During fasting*: (1) Insulin secretion goes down; (2) Increased hepatic glucose output; (3) Glucose uptake by insulin-independent cells. *After feeding*: (1) Insulin secretion goes up; (2) Suppressed hepatic glucose output; (3) Glucose uptake by insulin-independent cells.

TABLE 1: Insulin action at tissue level.		
Liver	**Fats**	**Skeletal muscle**
• Increased protein synthesis • Increased lipid synthesis • Decreased glucose output (due to decreased gluconeogenesis, increased glycogen synthesis, and increased glycolysis)	• Increased glucose entry • Increased fatty acid synthesis • Increased triglyceride deposition • Activation of lipoprotein lipase • Inhibition of hormone-sensitive lipase	• Increased glucose entry • Increased glycogen synthesis • Increased protein synthesis • Decreased protein catabolism • Decreased release of gluconeogenic amino acids

In the fat tissue insulin: (1) Increased glucose entry, (2) increased fatty acid synthesis, (3) increased triglyceride deposition, (4) activation of lipoprotein lipase, and (5) inhibition of hormone-sensitive lipase.

In the skeletal muscle tissue insulin: (1) Increased glucose entry, (2) increased glycogen synthesis, (3) increased protein synthesis, (4) decreased protein catabolism, and (5) decreased release of gluconeogenic amino acids.
- Fats
- Increased glucose entry
- Increased fatty acid synthesis
- Increased triglyceride deposition
- Activation of lipoprotein lipase
- Inhibition of hormone-sensitive lipase **(Table 1)**.

Pathophysiology of Diabetes

Different pathophysiological mechanisms of different type of diabetes mellitus (DM) result in "Hyperglycemia" and it is the biochemical Hallmark of DM. Environmental factors trigger the diabetogenic process in a genetically susceptible individual. Impaired beta-cell function (insulin deficiency) and/or inefficient action [insulin resistance (IR)] are the central mechanisms of hyperglycemia. The complications in diabetic state are most likely secondary to hyperglycemia **(Table 2)**.

Risk Factors of Diabetes Mellitus

Risk factor varies according to the type of DM. They are either nonmodifiable or modifiable. In type 1 DM (T1DM), genetic factor is human leukocyte antigen (HLA) linked and environmental factors include immunological insult of beta cells by viruses, dietary factors such as cow milk, smoked and cured meat, coffee, and gluten, and stress. In type 2 DM (T2DM), genetic factor is polygenic. Aging

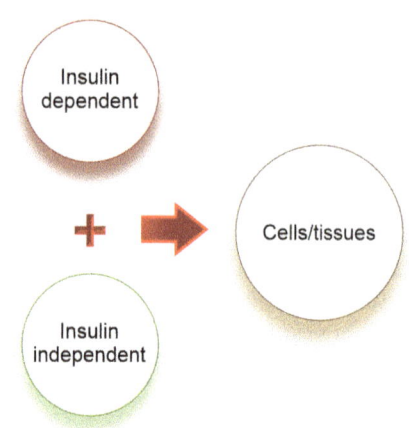

Insulin dependency for uptake of blood glucose

FIG. 8: Gut epithelial cell, red blood cell, brain cell, cell of nephrons, and pancreatic beta cell are insulin-independent cells.

cell of nephrons, and pancreatic beta cell are insulin-independent cells **(Fig. 8)**.

Insulin Action at Tissue Level

In the liver tissue insulin: (1) Increased protein synthesis, (2) increased lipid synthesis, and (3) decreased glucose output due to decreased gluconeogenesis, increased glycogen synthesis, and increased glycolysis.

TABLE 2: Pathophysiology of diabetes mellitus (DM).		
Biochemical hallmark of DM	**Diabetogenic process**	**Complications in DM**
Hyperglycemia, the biochemical Hallmark of diabetes mellitus, is the reflection of different physiopathological mechanisms, playing differently in different classes of diabetes	• Environmental factors trigger the diabetogenic process in a genetically susceptible individual • Impaired beta-cell functions (insulin deficiency) and/ or inefficient action (insulin resistance) are the central mechanisms of hyperglycemia	The complications in diabetic state are most likely secondary to hyperglycemia

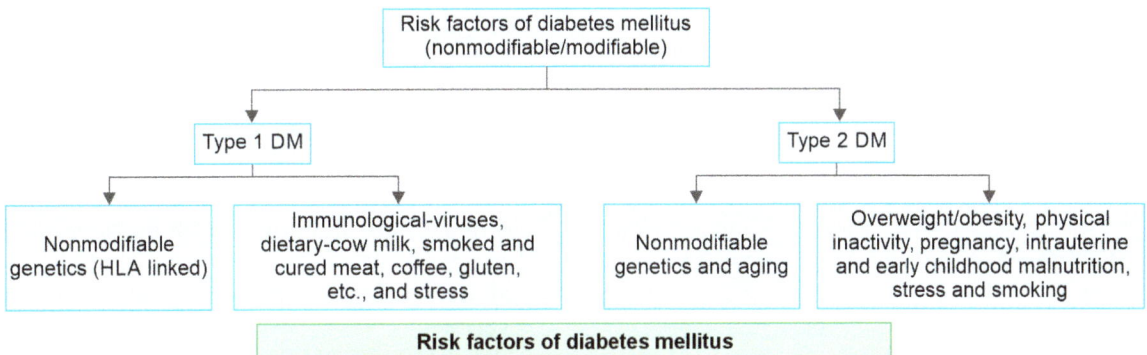

FLOWCHART 1: Risk factors for diabetes mellitus (DM) are either nonmodifiable or modifiable. So, there is scope of primary prevention approach through modifying them.
(HLA: human leukocyte antigen)

is a prominent factor and environmental factors include overweight/obesity, physical inactivity, pregnancy, intrauterine and early childhood malnutrition, stress, and smoking **(Flowchart 1)**.

Pathway to Development of Diabetes Mellitus

- Environmental factors trigger the diabetogenic process in a genetically susceptible individual.
- Impaired beta-cell function (insulin deficiency) and/ or inefficient action (IR) are the central mechanisms of hyperglycemia.
- The complications in diabetic state are most likely secondary to hyperglycemia **(Fig. 9)**.

Pathogenesis of Type 1 Diabetes Mellitus

- *Key defects*: Absolute insulin deficiency is the main defect.
- Hyperglycemia starts abruptly. If not treated with insulin, an acute complication like diabetic ketoacidosis (DKA) costs the life within a short period.
- *Insulin deficiency and "Honeymoon" phase*: The insulin deficiency is present at the time of clinical onset of the disease and throughout the entire course. Though some residual beta-cell function may be seen and transient periods of remission can occur producing the so-called "Honeymoon" phase of the disease.
- *Genetic and environmental factors*: The decrease in insulin secretory capacity is due to actual loss of

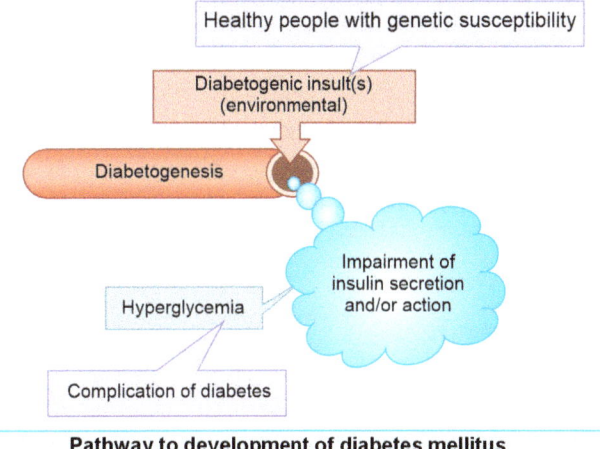

FIG. 9: Environmental factors trigger the diabetogenic process in a genetically susceptible individual. Impaired beta-cell function (insulin deficiency) and/or inefficient action (insulin resistance) are the central mechanisms of hyperglycemia. The complications in diabetic state are most likely secondary to hyperglycemia.

beta-cell mass. An immunological mechanism of beta-cell destruction is initiated and maintained by interplay of genetic and environmental factors.
- *Genetic influence*: The precise nature of the genetic influence in the pathogenesis of T1DM is still unclear. Monozygotic twins have a 20–50% concordance for T1DM. The risk for siblings of diabetic patients is

6-10%. The offspring of women with T1DM have a lower risk of disease (2.1%) than offspring of men with T1DM (6.1%).
- *HLA linkage*: HLA DR3 and DR4 are associated with three to fivefold increase in risk for T1DM. HLA B8 and B15 also show similar associations. Increasingly HLA B8/DR3 is associated with a persistence of islet cell antibodies (ICA), whereas HLA B15/DR 4 is associated with development of high titer of insulin autoantibodies (IAA) **(Figs. 10 and 11)**.

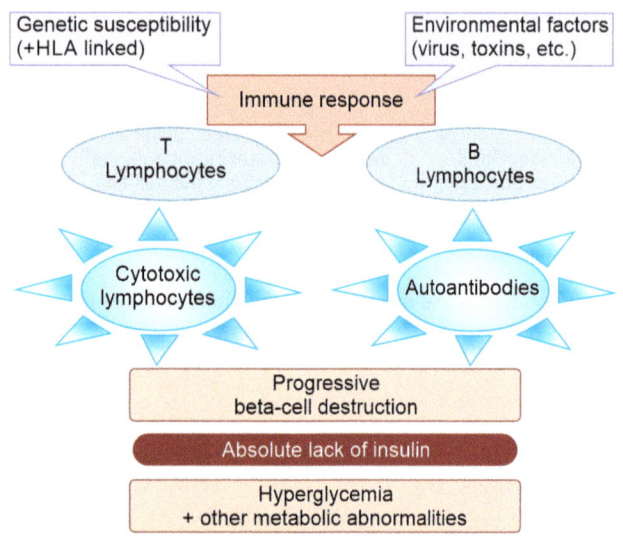

FIG. 10: Autoimmune destruction of beta-cell mass in genetically [human leukocyte antigen (HLA) linked)] susceptible person by environmental insults (virus, toxin, etc.).

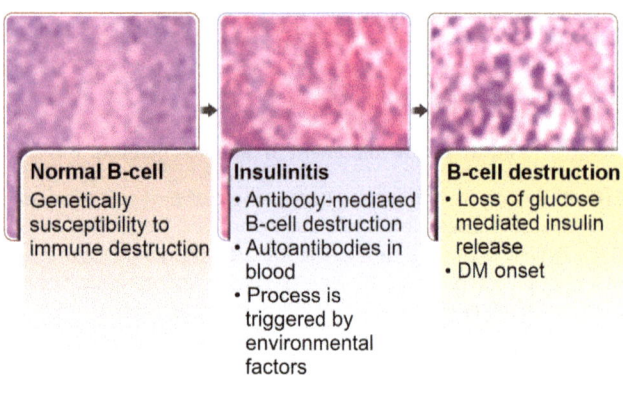

FIG. 11: Absolute lack of insulin occurs by loss of beta-cell mass by immunological process.

Pathogenesis of Type 2 Diabetes Mellitus
Key Points
- T2DM is heterogeneous disorder.
- Hyperglycemia is not only result of defective insulin action (sensitivity) but also contributed by progressive beta-cell destruction, leading to diminishing insulin release.
- The impact of the two defects—sensitivity and release of insulin—varies from person to person and in same person from time to time. One group of patients may exhibit severe impairment of insulin release and normal sensitivity. Another group of patients demonstrate exaggerated insulin release, mostly in the early phase of the disease.
- T2DM is polygenic disorder. The exact interaction of genetics and environment during its development is unclear.
- Monozygotic twins have a 60–90% concordance for T2DM.
- The risk for T2DM in siblings of diabetic patients is 10–33%. Connubial has more chance of T2DM than an offspring of single parent with diabetes.
- Off springs of women with T2DM have two to threefold greater risk of developing diabetes than do off springs of men with the disease.

Natural History of T2DM
- It starts by breakdown of healthy status of a genetically susceptible individual.
- Earliest abnormality is IR without any glucose intolerance.
- Glucose intolerance begins with the appearance of impaired fasting glucose (IFG) or impaired glucose tolerance (IGT).
- Ultimately, it reaches DM level with increasing glucose intolerance **(Flowchart 2 and Fig. 12)**.

Insulin Release in T2DM
- *Basal insulin secretion*:
  ○ In early stage, the basal insulin secretion is usually normal in nonobese and high in obese T2DM patients.
  ○ In late cases due to progressive failure of beta cells, the basal insulin secretion becomes low or low normal.
- *Postmeal insulin secretion*:
  ○ First phase is absent from very early stage (before the prediabetic stage).
  ○ Second phase may be high or normal in early stage but become low later **(Fig. 13)**.

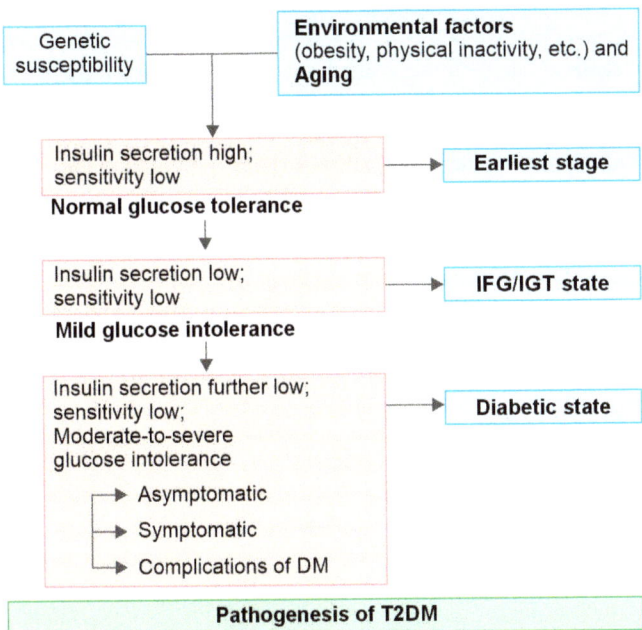

FLOWCHART 2: Two defects—sensitivity and release of insulin—varies from person to person and in same person from time to time. T2DM is a polygenic disorder. Monozygotic twins have a 60–90% concordance for T2DM.

(IFG: impaired fasting glucose; IGT: impaired glucose tolerance; T2DM: type 2 diabetes mellitus)

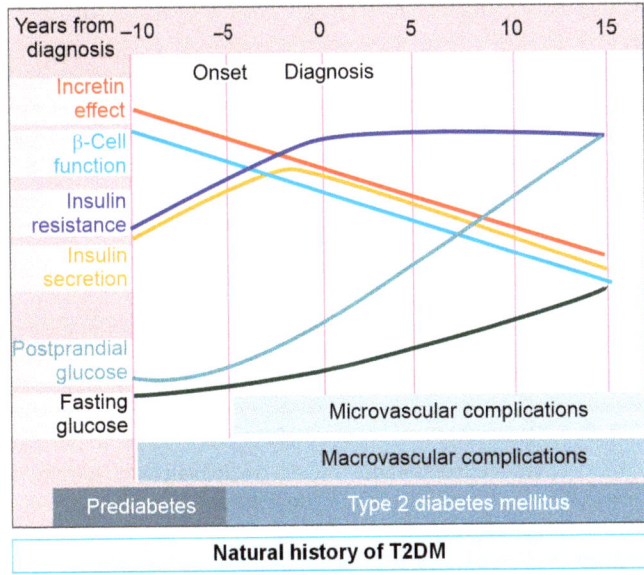

FIG. 12: T2DM starts by breakdown of healthy status of a genetically susceptible individual. Initially, there is insulin resistance without any glucose intolerance. Glucose intolerance begins with the appearance of IFG or IGT. Ultimately, it reaches DM level with increasing glucose intolerance.

(IFG: impaired fasting glucose; IGT: impaired glucose tolerance; T2DM: type 2 diabetes mellitus)

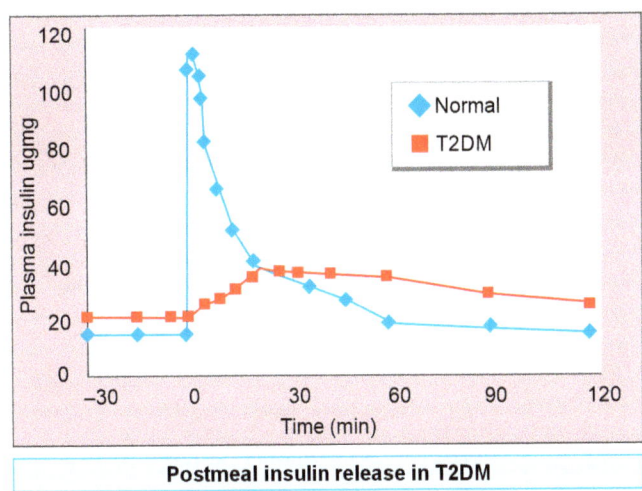

FIG. 13: First phase is absent from very early stage (before the prediabetic stage). Second phase may be high or normal in early stage but become low later.

(T2DM: type 2 diabetes mellitus)

Progressive Beta-cell Failure in Type 2 Diabetes Mellitus

It is a progressive disorder. Progressive beta-cell failure starts as a very early process of diabetogenesis of T2DM and is much advanced by the time hyperglycemia starts.

- As individuals progress from normal glucose tolerance to IFG state, there is a 50% decline in beta-cell mass, and
- A person in IGT state has already lost over 80% of their beta-cell function.

So, there is a significant loss of cell mass and function long before the onset of T2DM (**Fig. 14**).

Important Causes of Beta-cell Failure

- Advancing age
- Genetic factors
- Insulin resistance—causes beta-cell failure by continuous hypersecretion of insulin and amyloid polypeptide; direct—beta-cell impairment; and lipotoxicity.
- Glucotoxicity—chronically elevated glucose level impairs beta-cell function; it also plays role in hepatic and muscle IR.
- Lipotoxicity—elevated plasma free fatty acid (FFA) level and deposition of fat in the beta-cell impair insulin secretion.
- Glucagon-like peptide-1 (GLP-1) deficiency

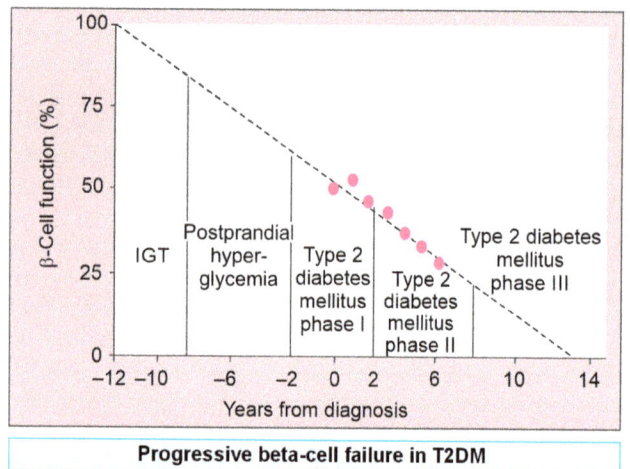

Progressive beta-cell failure in T2DM

FIG. 14: As individuals progress from normal glucose tolerance to IFG state, there is a 50% decline in beta-cell mass, and a person in IGT state has already lost over 80% of their beta-cell function. Apart from age and genetic factors, there are other factors for beta-cell failure.
(IFG: impaired fasting glucose; IGT: impaired glucose tolerance; T2DM: type 2 diabetes mellitus)

Insulin Resistance and Metabolic Syndrome

Insulin Resistance

Insulin Resistance and Type 2 Diabetes Mellitus
- Insulin resistance (IR) is also an early finding in T2DM, especially in obese and some nonobese patients.
- It may exist many years prior to the onset of diabetes.
- The molecular basis of the resistance seems to reside both at the receptor as well as postreceptor levels.

Evidences of Insulin Resistance
Observations that provide ample evidence to support this in T2DM are:
- Higher basal insulin level
- Low glucose–insulin ratio
- Decreased effect of exogenous insulin
- Glucose clamp with insulin infusion study, etc. **(Table 3)**

Insulin Resistance—Impact on Diabetogenesis
Figure 15 depicts the impact on diabetogenesis.

Metabolic Syndrome
Metabolic syndrome (MS) is associated with increased IR and plays key role in development of many noncommunicable diseases (NCDs) including T2DM.
- A waist circumference (WC) more than normal represents IR and regarded as the most important component of the syndrome.
- MS is diagnosed by three or more features of the five, namely (1) central obesity by weight circumference, (2) high blood pressure, (3) dyslipidemia [high triglyceride (TG) and low high-density lipoprotein (HDL) cholesterol], and (4) raised fasting blood glucose (FBG) **(Table 4)**.

TABLE 3: Insulin resistance (IR).

Liver	Fats	Skeletal muscle
The rate of basal HGP is increased by an increase in hepatic luconeogenesis. In addition, hepatic IR and other factors contribute to increased circulating glucagon level and enhanced hepatic sensitivity to glucagon, lipotoxicity, and glucotoxicity	IR causes—increased lipolysis, so high plasma FFA; chronically increased FFA stimulates gluconeogenesis, hepatic/muscle insulin resistance, and impaired insulin secretion	IR at muscle can account for over 85–90% of the impairment in total body glucose disposal in T2DM subjects. It results in a large increase in blood glucose

(FFA: free fatty acid; HGP: hepatic glucose production; T2DM: type 2 diabetes mellitus)

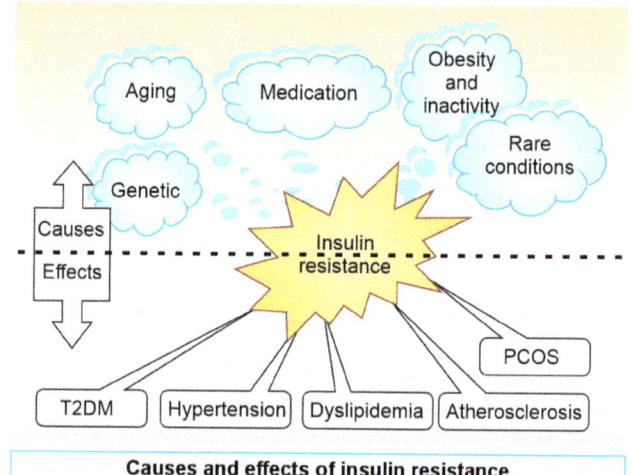

Causes and effects of insulin resistance

FIG. 15: (1) Causal agents: Genetic, aging, medication, obesity and inactivity, and rare conditions. (2) Effects: T2DM, hypertension, dyslipidemia, atherosclerosis, and PCOS.
(PCOS: polycystic ovary syndrome; T2DM: type 2 diabetes mellitus)

TABLE 4: Metabolic syndrome is the combination of three or more of the five features (IDF criteria number 1 plus any two from numbers 2 to 5).

Sl. No.	Parameter	Value
1.	Waist circumference	>90 cm (in male) and >80 cm (in female)
2.	Blood pressure	>130/85 mm Hg
3.	HDL cholesterol	<40 mg/dL (in male) and <50 mg/dL (in female)
4.	TG	>150 mg/dL
5.	Fasting blood glucose	>5.6 mmol/L

(HDL: high-density lipoprotein; IDF: International Diabetes Federation; TG: triglyceride)

DEFINITION, DIAGNOSIS, AND CLASSIFICATION OF DIABETES MELLITUS

Definition

Diabetes mellitus is a metabolic disorder characterized by raised blood glucose due to decreased cellular uptake of glucose by insulin sensitive cells as a result of insufficient insulin action or its availability. The blood glucose level of DM at fasting is >7.0 mmol/L and/or 120 minutes after a standard oral glucose drink is >11.1 mmol/L. An intermediate degree of glucose intolerance lies between normal and diabetic which is called *prediabetic* with two separate subtypes (1) abnormal fasting glucose (6–6.9 mmol/L)—called *IFG* or (2) abnormal blood glucose at 120 minute after glucose drink (7.8 to <11.1 mmo/L)—*IGT*. So, normal glucose tolerance is fasting glucose <6 mmol/L and blood glucose at 120 minute after glucose drink <7.8 mmo/L **(Flowchart 3)**.

Clinical presentation of DM: Spectrum of presentation ranges from asymptomatic, atypical, and typical features.
- Asymptomatic biochemically identified only. A vast majority of asymptomatic DM patients belong T2DM. They remain asymptomatic until blood glucose persistently remains above the renal threshold (approximately 10 mmol/L). So, routine checkup usually picks up this form of diabetes.
- Typical features start with "glycosuria," which means passage of glucose in urine that begins after the blood glucose level has gone above individual's renal threshold for glucose.
  - Typical features (3Ps and 2Ws):
    – Polyurea (increased urination), polydipsia (increased thirst), polyphagia (increased hunger), weight loss, and weakness.
- Atypical manifestations are nonspecific. As a class or type they mostly belong to T2DM, gestational diabetes mellitus (GDM), and other specific type of DM. A short list includes: (1) Nonhealing infection, (2) infertility or repeated pregnancy loss, (3) undue fatigability, (4) pruritus vulvi, etc. **(Flowchart 4)**.

Diagnosis

By documentation of glucose intolerance (raised blood glucose during fasting state or after a glucose challenge)
Diagnostic procedures:
1. *Oral glucose tolerance test (OGTT)*: It can categorize a person into: (i) Normal or (ii) abnormal with subcategory of: (A) Diabetic, (B) IGT, or (C) IFG
2. *Random (unstandardized) blood glucose level*: It is helpful when a person is suspected to be diabetic on clinical feature. Blood sample is preferably avoided within 2 hours of a major meal. It provides information, such as: (i) diabetes is likely if it is >11.1 mmol/L in venous plasma, (ii) diabetes is unlikely if it is <5.5 mmol/L in venous plasma, or (iii) diabetes is uncertain when it is in between the 2.

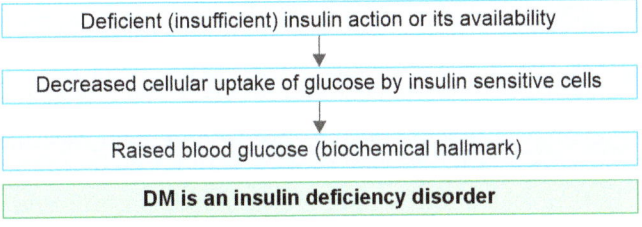

FLOWCHART 3: Diabetes mellitus (DM) occurs due to deficient insulin action or its availability.

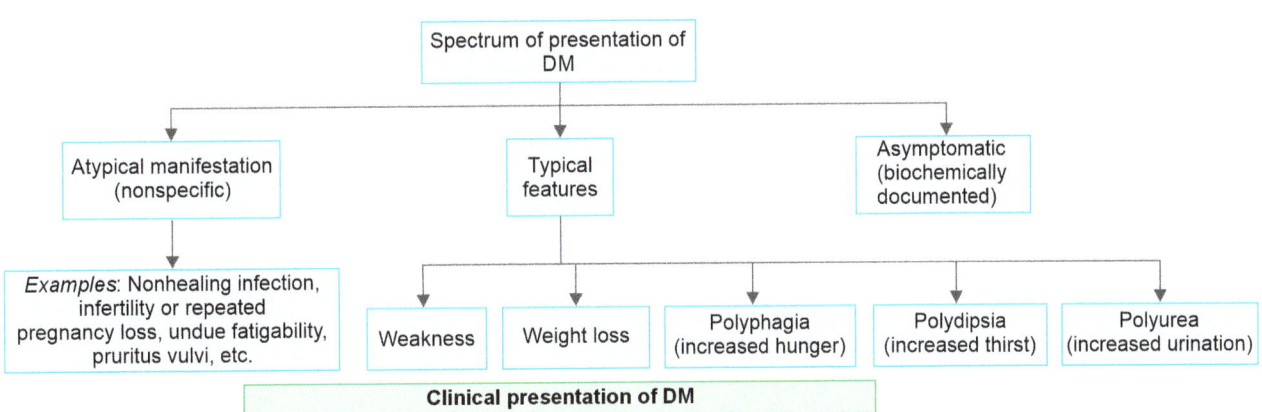

FLOWCHART 4: Spectrum of presentation ranges from asymptomatic, atypical, and typical features.
(DM: diabetes mellitus)

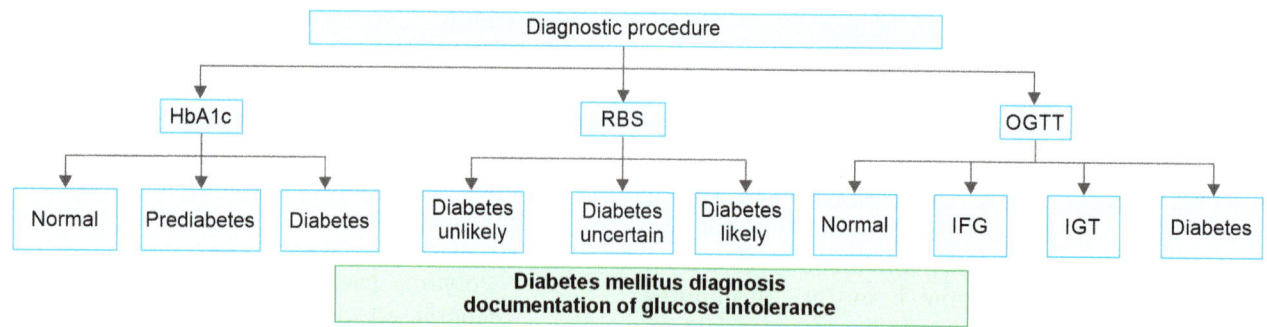

FLOWCHART 5: (1) OGTT, (2) RBS (?), and (3) HbA1c%.
(HbA1c: hemoglobin A1C; IFG: impaired fasting glucose; IGT: impaired glucose tolerance; OGTT: oral glucose tolerance test; RBS: random blood sugar)

TABLE 5: Interpretation of OGTT.

Sample	Whole blood Venous	Whole blood Capillary	Plasma Venous	Plasma Capillary	Result
Fasting or/and	≥7.0	≥7.0	≥7.0	≥7.0	DM
2 hours	>10.0	≥11.1	≥11.1	≥12.2	
Fasting	<6.0	<6.0	<6.0	<6.0	IGT
2 hours	7.8 to <11.1	7.8 to <11.1	7.8 to <11.1	7.8 to <11.1	
Fasting	>6.0–6.9	>6.0–6.9	>6.0–6.9	>6.0–6.9	IFG
2 hours	<7.8	<7.8	<7.8	<7.8	
Fasting	<6.0	<6.0	<6.0	<6.0	Normal
2 hours	<7.8	<7.8	<7.8	<7.8	

(DM: diabetes mellitus; IFG: impaired fasting glucose; IGT: impaired glucose tolerance; OGTT: oral glucose tolerance test)

3. Alternative assay—hemoglobin A1c (HbA1c) level: HbA1c% reflects blood glucose value of preceding 8–10 weeks and is now used an alternative to glucose measurement to determine glucose intolerance/diabetes. A value of HbA1c% 6.5% or more is considered diabetic, <6.0% is normal, and in between is prediabetic (**Flowchart 5**).

Oral Glucose Tolerance Test

Oral glucose tolerance test is considered the diagnostic gold standard for diagnosis of glucose intolerance/DM.

Procedures

- Test is performed in morning after an overnight fasting of 10–14 hours.
- The person is advised to take daily diet containing more than 150 g of carbohydrate for at least previous 3 days. After taking a fasting blood sample a glucose drink is given. Amount of glucose (1) for adult is grams of glucose and (2) for children 1.75 g/kg body weight (maximum 75 g). Dissolve glucose in 250–300 mL of water, and it should be consumed within 5 minutes. The second blood sample is to be collected at 120 minute of the end of glucose drink.
- Glucose levels of the two blood samples are estimated by glucose oxidase method immediately. If preservation is required, it should be preserved with sodium fluoride (6 μg/mL whole blood) and centrifuged, and plasma is frozen until assay. During the test smoking, tea, or stress are not allowed.
- Interpretation of OGTT is given in **Table 5**.

Classification of Diabetes Mellitus

Classification of DM is a remarkably changing subject and currently mostly followed the World Health Organization (WHO) classification of 1990, which is also known as etiology-based classification. Here there are four different classes of DM as follows:
1. T1DM
2. T2DM
3. GDM
4. Secondary DM or other specific type of DM

T1DM: Previously, it was called "insulin-dependent diabetes mellitus (IDDM)/juvenile-onset diabetes." It occurs due to destruction of the insulin-producing beta cells of the islets of Langerhans of pancreas by autoimmune mechanism. From the time of onset of diabetes, there is little or no insulin in the body. Some environmental factors trigger the autoimmune reaction in genetically susceptible individuals.

T2DM: It constitutes major portion of diabetic population. This type of diabetes occurs due to IR and relative insulin deficiency, usually develops with increasing age (previously called IDDM/maturity-onset diabetes). Environmental factors such as obesity and physical inactivity are known strong determinants in genetically susceptible individuals. This type of diabetes usually passes through prediabetic stage (IFG and IGT). At diagnosis a large number of cases of T2DM remain asymptomatic and often present with diabetic specific complications.

GDM: It is glucose intolerance of any degree (IFG, IGT, or DM), which starts or is recognized during pregnancy. Factors include age, obesity, family history of DM, and bad obstetric history. Nowadays universal screening to diagnose GDM cases and very tight glycemic control is advocated to reduce the risk to mother and baby.

Secondary DM or other specific type of DM: Some specific diseases, drugs, or genetic conditions/syndromes are associated with development of chronic hyperglycemia. These forms of diabetes are classified as other specific types of DM. It occurs in persons with known disease, drugs or genetic condition/syndrome associated with secretion and/or action defect of insulin. Examples include:
- Endocrinopathies—Cushing's syndrome, acromegaly, thyrotoxicosis, hyperaldosteronism, and pheochromocytoma
- Drugs—glucocorticoids, adrenocorticotropic hormone (ACTH), diazoxide, diuretics, phenytoin, pentamidine, vaco
- Pancreatic disease—fibrocalculous pancreatic diabetes (FCPD), chronic or recurrent pancreatitis, and hemochromatosis
- Others—genetic defects of the pancreatic beta cells, genetic defects in insulin action, infections, uncommon forms of immune-mediated disease, and other genetic syndrome **(Fig. 16)**.

GENERAL PRINCIPLES IN THE MANAGEMENT OF DIABETES MELLITUS

Management of DM, till date, in general aimed at supporting people to live with minimum or no risk of complication(s).
- This is achievable through some specific goals of blood glucose, blood pressure, lipids, body weight, etc.
- The specific or set goals are termed as targets. "Treat to target" is the principle of management of DM.
- There are algorithms for initiation, maintenance, and switching over to other regimen for Treat to Targets.

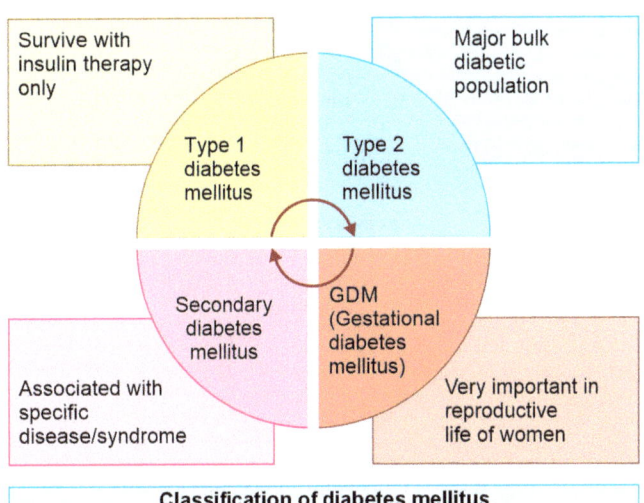

FIG. 16: There are four classes of diabetes mellitus.

Some key points of management of DM are as follows:
- Diabetes mellitus is a life-long disorder. Diabetic education (DE) is an important component to develop knowledge, skill, and attitude of patient and family to take part in the management of DM.
- In T1DM, there is absolute lack of insulin; so, its management is "efficient replacement of the deficiency" and lifestyle is to be synchronized with insulin administration.
- T2DM is a complex disorder. There are factors of glucose intolerance and comorbidities such as hypertension and dyslipidemia. Its treatment consists of glycemic care, modification of modifiable risks, and care of the comorbidities.
- A significant portion of these T2DM patients can achieve and maintain the goals set for management with only lifestyle measures for a reasonable period (if diagnosed early). Drug therapy is added along with the lifestyle changes when the treatment target falls below that is to be achieved. There are a rapidly expanding number of drugs that improve many factors in causation/deterioration of type 2 diabetes—they may be called adjuvants. Principle molecules used for treatment of T2DM are either insulin or insulin secretagogues.
- A prescription for any type 2 diabetic should have adjuvant molecule(s) when there is any definite prospect of risk factor modification.

General Treatment Components of Diabetes Mellitus

Treatment components are: (1) Medical nutrition therapy (MNT), (2) physical exercise, (3) Medication, (4) monitoring of treatment result, and (5) DE of patient and family members **(Fig. 17)**.

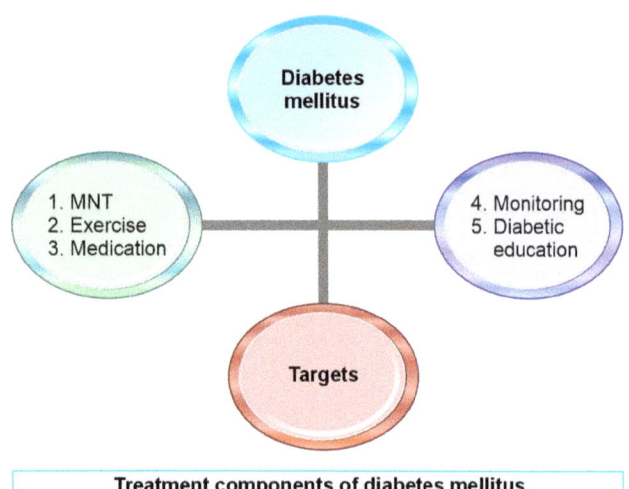

FIG. 17: (1) Medical nutrition therapy (MNT), (2) Exercise, (3) Medication, (4) Monitoring, and (5) Diabetic education.

Aims of Treatment of Diabetes Mellitus

- To relive symptoms of symptomatic patients.
- To maintain glycemic targets round the clock.
- To prevent any acute metabolic derangement, such as hypoglycemia and ketoacidosis.
- To prevent or delay chronic diabetic complications, such as nephropathy and retinopathy.
- To ensure proper growth and development of children with diabetes.
- To maintain women health during pregnancy and lactation.
- To support a productive and socially respectful life for diabetic person.

Steps of Management of Diabetes Mellitus

Step 1—diagnosis: OGTT is the standard test for diagnosis. Other tests: FBG only, HbA1c, and RBS can also be done.

Step 2—factor analysis: Patient factors may influence the choice of initial treatment regimen. They include:
  i. Age and body weight of the person
  ii. Associated medical illness like acute/chronic complications, pregnancy or lactation, major surgery, etc.
  iii. Lifestyle of the person, severity of hyperglycemia, history of previous antidiabetic agents, and socioeconomic condition.

Step 3—informing about treatment targets to patients: Treat to targets is the most important agenda in the management of DM. Treatment targets of DM are glycemic, lipid, and others as follows:
  i. *Targets of blood (plasma) glucose (for adult) are*: (A) Fasting/premeals (6.00 mmol/L), (B) postmeals (2 hours after a main meal <8.00 mmol/L), and (C) HbA1c < 7%

  ii. *Targets of blood lipids are*: (A) Low-density lipoprotein (LDL) cholesterol < 100 mg/dL, (B) HDL cholesterol >40 mg/dL in male) and >50 mg/dL in female), and (C) triglyceride < 150 mg/dL.
  iii. *Blood pressure*: Systolic < 140 mm Hg and diastolic < 80 mm Hg.
  iv. *Body weight*: Body mass index (BMI) < 25 kg/m^2 and WC < 90 cm in male and <80 cm in female.
  v. Diabetic education of patient by teaching, training, and empowerment, so that they can take part in the treatment of DM.

Step 4: Selection and initiation of a treatment regimen: Some key points on selection of regimen of treatment at diagnosis include:
  i. Severity of glucose intolerance (say HbA1c%) is the primary determinant of initial treatment regimen in T2DM.
  ii. Insulin is the single treatment option in in T1DM.
  iii. In GDM if lifestyle fails to achieve the glycemic target, only insulin is added.
  iv. Principles of T2DM are mostly followed in other type of DM.

There are three basic regimens of treatment of DM:
1. *Lifestyle-based treatment regimen* consists of (i) lifestyle (dietary measures and physical activities) and +/–ve adjuvant drugs (excepting insulin and insulin secretagogue).
2. *Secretagogue-based treatment regimen* consists of insulin secretagogue with lifestyle and +/–ve adjuvant drugs but no insulin.
3. *Insulin-based treatment regimen* consists of insulin with lifestyle and +/–ve adjuvant drug(s).

Severity of glucose intolerance in newly detected case of DM is best reflected by HbA1c% and if not available FBG can be used. In T2DM and secondary DM, a case with HbA1c 8-10% (or FBG 11.1-16.7 mmol/L), the initial treatment regimen advocated is the *secretagogue-based one* (provided there is no contraindication). And cases with HbA1c < 8.0% or >10.0%, lifestyle-based and insulin-based treatment are used, respectively. T1DM is always with insulin-based treatment, and GDM is treated by lifestyle, so long blood glucoses are on target and otherwise by insulin-based treatment.

Step 5—monitoring and changing treatment regime: Structured different pre- and postmeal blood glucose testing [self-monitoring of blood glucose (SMBG)] is the principle tool used for adjustment of drug dose and or change in treatment regimen. Other important tools include HbA1c% (if SMBG is not satisfactory) or screening tests for chronic complications of diabetes (retinopathy, nephropathy, and neuropathy).

Lifestyle Modification in Diabetes Mellitus

Lifestyle modification is the important issue of diabetics (also prediabetes). Appropriate lifestyle of diabetics includes their dietary habit, physical activity and exercise, regular monitoring of blood glucose, physical care such as foot and oral care, regular follow-up, etc.

Medical Nutrition Therapy in Diabetes Mellitus

A proper diet is a fundamental element of therapy in all diabetic individuals. An appropriate dietary management is called Medical Nutrition Therapy.

Some important terms relevant to MNT include:
- *Diet*: A proper diet is a fundamental element of therapy is all diabetic individuals. A diet recommended for a diabetic patient is, in fact, a "balanced diet" for anyone.
- *Balanced diet*: A balanced meal is the combination of carbohydrates, fats, proteins, and fibers appropriate for the individual; at the same time, it should provide sufficient vitamins, minerals, and micronutrients.
- *Diet plan*: A diet plan should be individualized according to his/her needs; it must be simple to understand and easy to follow.
- *Dietitian*: All diabetics should be referred to a dietitian for counseling at diagnosis of diabetes and also subsequently if they have problem with their diet adjustment.
- *Special diet*: Special counseling is necessary in children and adolescents, pregnant and lactating women, and other conditions of acute or chronic illnesses where diet is of immense concern.

Goals of MNT in Diabetes
- To have a balanced and regular meal.
- To achieve metabolic goals for blood glucose, lipid, blood pressure, etc.
- To achieve and maintain desirable body weight.
- To ensure adequate nutrition for health and growth for pregnant and lactating mothers, and children.
- To prevent/delay diabetic complications.
- To enjoy the pleasure of eating.

Four Aspects of MNT in Diabetes
- Calorie consumption
- Nutrients in food
- Timing and consistency of meals
- Regular weight management

Calorie requirement of diabetes

The daily calorie requirement is related to existing body weight and activity level but not on diabetic status. Calorie requirement is similar in diabetics and nondiabetics.

Factors determining calorie requirement: The daily calorie requirement is determined primarily by any two factors of the following:
1. Existing body weight
2. Activity level
3. Other factors that influence the caloric requirements are lifestyle, pregnancy, lactation, other illnesses, and age, especially in growing period.

Determination of daily calorie allowance: The following formula is used.

$$\text{Daily calorie allowance (kcal)} = \text{Ideal body weight (IBW)} \times \text{Caloric factor (CF)}$$

Ideal body weight is obtained from standard height–weight charts. It can also roughly be calculated by subtracting 100 from height (in centimeters).

Caloric factor is obtained from a body weight – activity level chart **(Table 6)**.

Components of nutrients

The impact of specific dietary composition on glycemic control and cardiovascular risk remains uncertain in diabetes.

Composition of macronutrient: The optimal macronutrient composition should be individualized depending upon:
- Weight loss goal
- Other metabolic needs (e.g., hypertension, dyslipidemia, nephropathy, etc.) and individual preference **(Table 7)**.

TABLE 6: Caloric factor (CF).			
Body weight	Sedentary	Moderately active	Active
Overweight	20/25	25/30	30/35
Normal weight	30	35	40
Underweight	35	40	45

TABLE 7: Distribution of macronutrient.		
Carbohydrate	Fat	Protein
50–60% of DCI	30% of DCI	10–20% of DCI
Fiber 20–35 g (or 14 g/1,000 kcal)	• Saturated fats < 10% • Trans fats < 1% • Cholesterol < 300 mg	
(DCI: daily calorie intake)		

Carbohydrates, Fat, and Protein

Carbohydrates (Intake of Carbohydrates Those Causes Sudden Rise in Blood Sugar Level should be Limited or Avoided, and Carbohydrates with Lower Glycemic Index and Glycemic Load are to be Selected)

- *Limit or avoid carbohydrates*: Refined or simple carbohydrates, e.g., sugar, glucose, soft drinks, jam, honey, marmalade, sweets, cakes, chocolate, etc., cause sudden rise in blood sugar level. Intake of these should be limited.
- *Select carbohydrates*: Unrefined complex carbohydrates, e.g. bread, cereals, potatoes, rice, etc., are more suitable, as they are digested more slowly in the body and cause less rapid rise in blood sugar levels.

Carbohydrates with lower glycemic index and glycemic load are preferred.

Fats Intake (Fatty Foods have High Calorie, Which Lead to Weight Gain and Increase the Risk of Cardiovascular Disease)

- *Limit or avoid fatty food*: Fats solid at room temperature are high in saturated fat. It is abundantly present in cream, cheese, butter, ghee, animal fat, coconut oil, palm oil, etc.
- Rich sources of trans fat are margarine, French fry, doughnut, pastry, pizza, pie, biscuit/cracker/cookie, etc.
- Dietary cholesterol is high in egg yolk, butter, ghee, etc.

Protein Intake

Protein is essential in meal. A diabetic should receive adequate protein.

Vitamins, Sweeteners, and Alcohol

- *Vitamin and mineral supplements*:
  - There is no sufficient or clear evidence of benefit from vitamin or mineral supplementation in diabetes who do not have underlying deficiencies.
  - Routine supplementation with antioxidants or micronutrients (e.g., chromium, magnesium, and vitamin D) or other herbs/supplements in diabetes is not recommended.
- *Alternative sweeteners*:
  - Sweetening agents, which provide sweetness but little calories, are now approved for use.
  - Non-nutritive sweeteners include aspartame, neotame, saccharin, acesulfame, and sucralose. These are preferred in diabetes. Reduced calorie sweeteners include sorbitol, mannitol, etc. All are safe when consumed within acceptable limit.
- *Alcohol*:
  - Alcohol has various adverse effects in diabetes.
  - Daily intake should be limited to one drink (15 g ethanol) or less in females and two drinks (30 g) or less in males.
  - Alcohol should be avoided in pregnancy, liver disease, pancreatitis, advanced neuropathy, and severe hypertriglyceridemia.
  - Alcohol may cause delayed hypoglycemia, especially in those using hypoglycemic agents.

Weight Management

As most of the people with type 2 diabetes mellitus and prediabetes are overweight or obese, an important aim of MNT in this group is to achieve body weight goals.

This can be achieved by calorie allowance as stated earlier.

Caloric restriction and increase in physical activity are the main strategies of weight losing.

Caloric restriction:
- A moderate caloric restriction (250–500 calories less than average daily intake as calculated from food history) can be done.
- A hypocaloric diet, irrespective of weight loss, is associated with increased sensitivity to insulin and improvement in blood glucose level. Moderate weight loss (5–10%, or 2–8 kg), irrespective of initial weight, an individuals can have a remarkable benefit on blood glucose, dyslipidemia, and hypertension.

Forms of diet have been tried for losing weight:
- Low-fat diet
- Low-carbohydrate diet
- Balanced low-calorie diet
- Mediterranean diet
- Very low-calorie diet

For losing weight calorie restrictions in various forms of diet have been tried. But overwhelming superiority of one over the other has not been proven.

Increase in physical activity: The dietary practice must be supported by an increase in physical activity.

Benefits of weight loss in overweight/obese:
- Decrease in mortality
- Normalization of blood glucose
- Maintenance of blood pressure at normal level
- Improvement in blood lipids (all components)
- Fall in cancer death

Meal timing, composition, and planning: The diet remains a big problem in diabetes care. One of the main reasons for this is lack of nutritional self-management

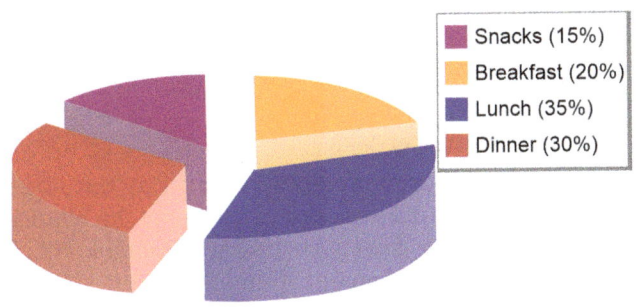

Caloric distribution in meals

FIG. 18: Total daily food intake may be distributed consistently throughout the day as follows: Three main meals—breakfast, lunch, and dinner and 2–3 snacks—mid-morning, afternoon, and bedtime snacks, etc.

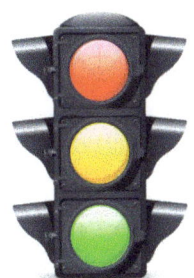

Signal system of food choice

FIG. 19: Signal system classifies foods based on a traffic light system (best suits in buffet party): green—healthy food, yellow—less healthy (try to restrict), and red—least healthy food items (try to avoid).

training. Depending on the individual patient's learning capabilities, clinical needs, level of motivation, and lifestyle, different methods of teaching can be used:
- *Meal timing*: Consistency with meal timing and day-to-day carbohydrate intake is very important, especially in those treated with antidiabetic medications, to avoid erratic blood glucose. Gap between two major meals should not cross 10 hours maximum.
- A meal plan should be based on the individual's usual food intake, integrating with lifestyle pattern, activity level, drugs (if used), and blood glucose results.
- *Meal composition*: Meals, especially carbohydrates, are to be evenly distributed over a day, and should not vary in this regard from day to day. Practicing "carbohydrate counting (carb-counting)" can promote glycemic control by implementing a consistent pattern of carbohydrate consumption in meals and snacks. Total daily food intake may be distributed consistently throughout the day as follows:
  ○ Three main meals such as breakfast, lunch, and dinner and 2–3 snacks such as mid-morning, afternoon, bedtime snacks, etc. **(Fig. 18)**.

Healthy Food Choice Models

Food choice systems are developed to make food selection process more practicable to the lay peoples. Some examples are given here:
- Signal system
- Food pyramid
- Plate model
- Hand Jive method **(Figs. 19 to 22)**

Anthropometric Measurement

Body mass index and WC are two important measurements of overweight and obesity. Overweight and obesity are the risk factors of diabetes and other noncommunicable

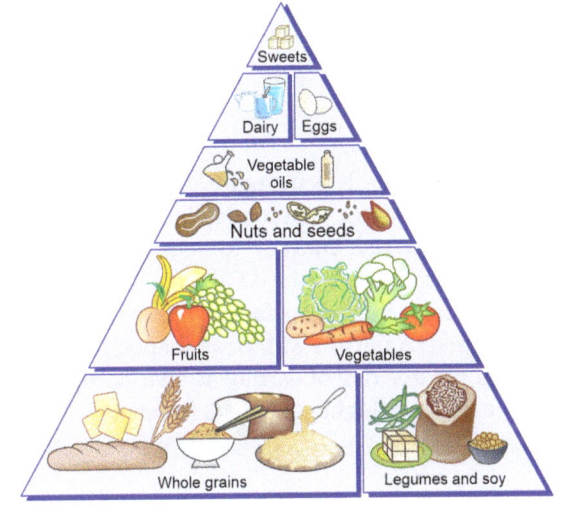

Food pyramid system of food choice

FIG. 20: Potions of a foods (best suits in home settings): Foods with high glycemic index (sweets/fruits)—try to avoid; grains—take less; protein and dairy—moderate; vegetables/fruits (not sweet)—take most.

diseases like hypertension, dyslipidemia, ischemic heart disease, chronic respiratory disease, and certain cancers. Correction of BMI and WC is incorporated as targets of treatment of T2DM.

Body Mass Index

Weight and height measurements are required to determine BMI. The formula for calculation is as follows:

$$BMI = Weight\ in\ kg/(height\ in\ meter)^2$$

According to BMI, one is categorized to underweight, normal, overweight, obese, and morbid obese if BMI < 18.5, 18.5–24.9, 25–29.9, 30–39.9, and >40 kg/m^2, respectively.

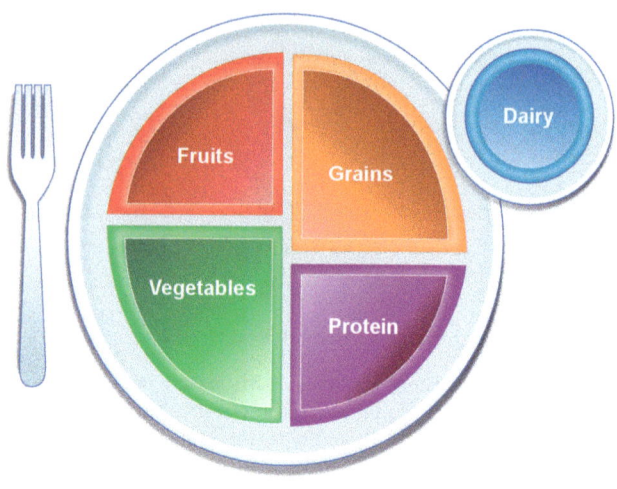

Plate model of food choice

FIG. 21: Potions of a plate (suits in eating anywhere): Grain approximate 25%; protein approximate 25%; and rest with vegetables/fruits (not sweet).

Waist Circumference

Waist circumference is a measure of central adiposity. Central adiposity rather than total adiposity is considered as an important risk marker for cardiovascular and metabolic diseases. Higher the WC greater is the risk. Based on fat distribution the body shape is referred as "pear" or "apple" shaped. A person with pear shaped has a higher WC and so greater risk of cardiovascular complications than apple-shaped (higher gluteal fat) person.

Waist or abdominal circumference is a measure at midway between the costal margin and the iliac crest; it is the smallest circumference at the waist.

Hip Circumference

Hip or gluteal circumference is taken at the largest circumference at the posterior extension of the buttocks, measured over the greater trochanters. Desirable WC: for male <90 cm and for female <80 cm.

Waist–Hip Ratio

Hip circumference (HC) and WC are used to calculate a parameter called Waist–Hip ratio **(WHR)** or abdominal-gluteal ratio. The formula to have WHR is $WHR = WC$ (in cm)$/HC$ (in cm). WHR is considered risky for cardiovascular and metabolic diseases if >0.9 for male and if >0.8 for female **(Figs. 23A to C)**.

Exercise and Diabetes Mellitus

Exercise

Exercise is an important component of treatment of DM. In addition to physical fitness, exercise helps in preventing atherosclerosis and thereby macroangiopathic complications in diabetes. It also improves mental well-being and quality of life.

An exercise plan should be individualized according to his/her physical status, meals, drugs, profession, interest, etc. To start with exercise, one should be gradual in increasing the duration and intensity. For adults over

Handy portion guide

Your hands can be very useful in estimating appropriate portions. When planning a meal, use the following portion sizes as a guide:

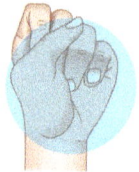

Fruits/grains and starches:
Choose an amount the size of your fist for each of grains and starches, and fruit

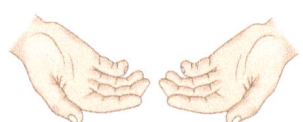

Vegetables:
Choose as much as you can hold in both hands

Meat and alternatives:
Choose an amount up to the size of the palm of your hand and the thickness of your little finger

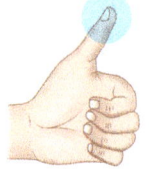

Fats:
Limit fat to an amount the size of the tip of your thumb

Milk and alternatives: Drink up to 250 mL (8 oz) of low-fat milk with a meal

Hand's grip model of food choice

FIG. 22: Hand's grip system (best suits in community education): Vegetable: as much as both hands can hold; meat and alternatives: as size of your hand (thickness your little finger); fruits/grains and starch: amount of your fist. Fats: Limit to the size of your thumb. Milk and alternatives: up to 250 mL.

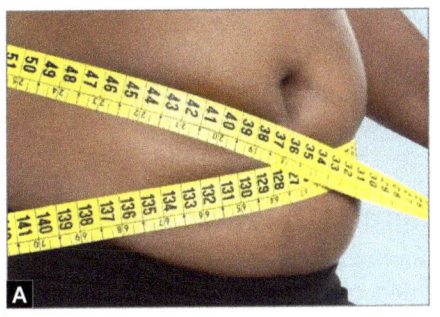
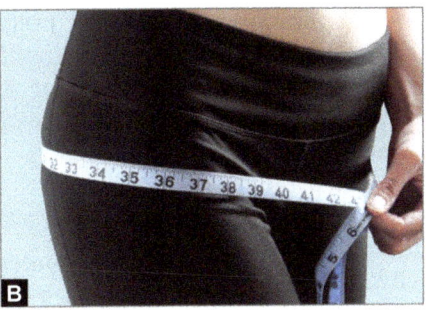

BMI (kg/m^2)	Category
<18.5	Underweight
18.5–24.9	Normal
25–29.9	Overweight
30–39.9	Obese
>40	Morbid obese

A Waist circumference (WC) B Hip circumference (HC) C BMI = Weight in kg/(height in meter)^2

FIGS. 23A TO C: Anthropometry.
(BMI: body mass index)

the age of 18 years, there should be ultimate target of doing aerobic exercise of moderate intensity for at least 150 minutes per week or vigorous intensity for at least 75 minutes per week, or equivalent combination of both types. It can be done in at least 3 days per week, but no more than two consecutive days without exercise. T2DM should perform anaerobic exercise involving all major muscle groups at least 2 days a week.

Intensity of Exercise

Intensity of exercise is assessed by the maximum heart rate (MHR). Formula for MHR is as follows:

$$MHR = 220 - Heart\ rate$$

Intensity of exercise is called: (1) *Vigorous* if heart rate achieved is >70% of MHR; (2) *Moderate* if heart rate achieved is 50–70% of MHR; (3) *Low* if heart rate achieved is <50%.

Prior to recommending any exercise program one should be careful of:
- Coronary heart disease
- Proliferative retinopathy
- Neuropathy and advance renal failure
- Hypoglycemia unawareness, etc.

Exercise: Aerobic and Anaerobic

Aerobic exercise
- Aerobic exercise uses large group of muscles, can be maintained continuously, and is rhythmic in nature.
- This type of exercise overloads the heart and requires oxygen to provide energy.
- Examples include walking, running, stair climbing, swimming, jogging, treadmill, cycling, aerobic dancing, etc.

Benefits of aerobic exercise:
- Maximal oxygen consumption increases.
- Cardiovascular and respiratory function improves.
- Blood supply of muscles and ability to use oxygen increase.
- In people with hypertension lowers resting systolic and diastolic blood pressure.
- Increases HDL cholesterol and reduces LDL cholesterol and triglyceride.
- Reduces body fat and improves weight control.
- Glucose intolerance improves and reduces IR.

Anaerobic exercise
- Anaerobic exercise is a short duration exercise.
- This type of exercise does not require oxygen and can be supported by energy stored in the muscles.
- Examples include weight lifting, sprinting at very fast speed, strength training, etc.

Benefits of anaerobic exercise:
- Muscular strength increases.
- Flexibility of joints improves.
- Body fat improves and lean body mass (muscle mass) reduces.
- Glucose intolerance improves and reduces IR.
- Strength, balance, and functional ability in older adults improve.

Some important points on exercise and DM
- Exercise recommendations for a person with diabetes are same as for a nondiabetic.
- Exercise program includes a proper warm-up and cool-down periods.
  - Warm-up should consist of 5–10 minutes of aerobic activity (e.g., walking) at low intensity level; it prepares heart for exercise.
  - After a short warm-up, muscles should be gently stretched for another 5–10 minutes; it prepares muscles for exercise without injury. This period is called "stretching period."
  - The cool-down period also consists of 5–10 minutes of aerobic activity at low intensity level after main activity session. It gradually brings heart rate down to pre-exercise level.

- Person with T1DM who do not have any complications and blood glucose profile satisfactory can do all levels of exercise, including leisure activities, recreational sports, and competitive professional performances. The emphasis must be given on adjusting therapeutic regimen with level of exercise and diet and avoiding hypoglycemia.
- In children, extra attention needs to be paid to balance glycemic control with activity level and for this the support of parents, teachers, and trainers may be necessary. Their meal and activity in school are impertinent.
- Person with T2DM must view exercise as a vital component for the management. Exercise along with a reduce calorie intake may enhance weight loss. Combination of diet, exercise, and behavioral modifications is the most effective approach to weight control. Normally low to moderate intensity long duration exercise is recommended for weight loss.
- The diabetic patient with peripheral neuropathy and loss of protective sensation should not engage in repetitive weight-bearing exercise, e.g., prolong walking, treadmill, jogging, etc., as these activities may result in blistering, ulceration, and fracture. Non-weight-bearing exercise, e.g., swimming, cycling, rowing, chair exercise, arm exercise, yoga, etc., may be better.
- Person with severe Charcot's joint should avoid weight-bearing exercise, as it can result in multiple fracture and dislocation of ankles and feet even without patient being aware of it.
- In patients who have proliferative and moderate to severe nonproliferative diabetic retinopathy, strenuous activity may precipitate vitreous hemorrhage or fractional retinal detachment. These individuals should avoid anaerobic exercise and physical activities that involves straining, jarring, or Valsalva-like maneuvers, e.g., weight lifting, boxing, heavy competitive sports, etc. In these persons low-impact exercise like swimming (but not diving), walking, or stationary cycling may be recommended.
- Patient with stable coronary heart disease should perform exercise of moderate intensity. Person with uncontrolled hypertension should withhold exercise until control of blood pressure.
- If the person develops symptomatic hypoglycemia or ketosis, exercise should be postponed. If blood glucose is <5.5 mmol/L, the person should take extra 15–30 g of carbohydrate before exercise.
- One should not do exercise during any significant acute illness or uncompensated major chronic illness.
- During pregnancy moderate exercise, e.g., walking at moderate speed for 30 minutes a day at a time or in divided fashion is advised. Vigorous exercise or exercises causing pressure in the abdomen should be avoided.

Drug Treatment of Diabetes Mellitus

Various treatment modes are needed in dealing diabetes, which can be divided into two—nonpharmacological (lifestyle modifications) and pharmacological (oral and injectable agents).

Nonpharmacological approach initially can be sufficient for some cases of T2DM; but all T1DM patients and most of the T2DM require pharmacological agents also.

Drugs used to treat DM are of three categories: (1) Insulin, (2) insulin secretagogue, and (3) adjuvant agents **(Fig. 24)**.

Drugs for Diabetes Mellitus

Drugs for diabetes mellitus are shown in **Flowchart 6**.

Insulin

- After the discovery of insulin in 1921, it has revolutionized the treatment of diabetes. In 1922, the first short of insulin (initially named "isletin", later "insulin") was pushed into human. Commercial production began in 1923. This oldest antidiabetic agent is still the most potent one. With time preparations of insulin and its delivery system are constantly evolving.
- Insulin preparations used for treatment of DM are either human insulin or their analogs. Most of them are designed to adopt blood profile to control blood sugar of diabetic persons.
  ○ Human insulins are grouped into short-, intermediate-, or long-acting one and analog insulins are also grouped into rapid-, long-acting, or

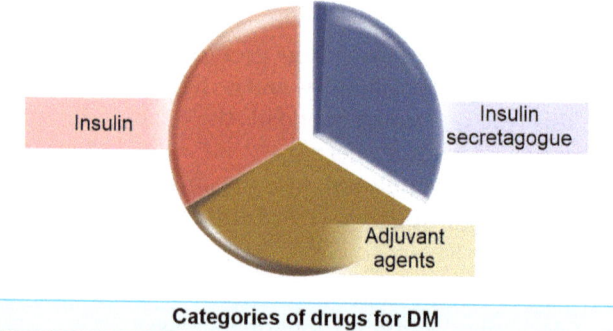

FIG. 24: Three categories of drugs for diabetes mellitus (DM).

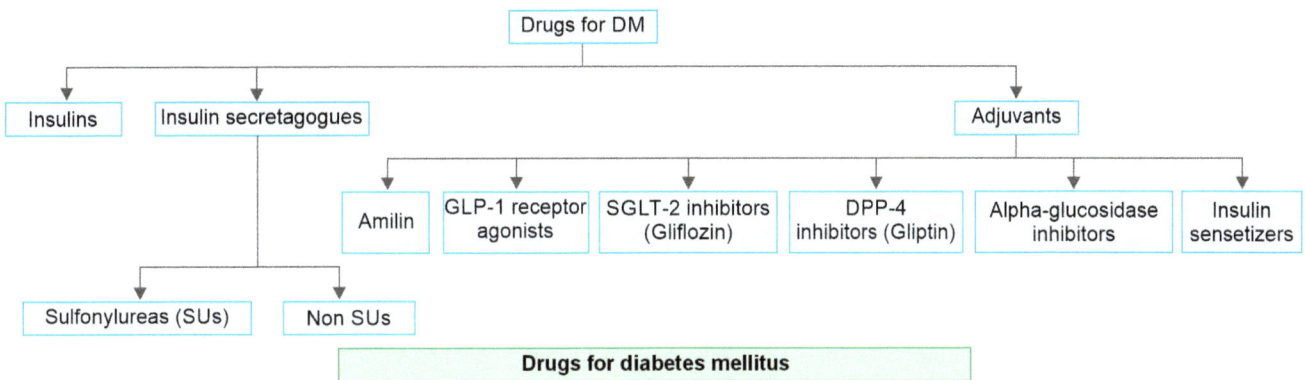

FLOWCHART 6: Three categories of drugs for DM: (1) Insulin, (2) Insulin secretagogue, and (3) Adjuvant agents.
(DM: diabetes mellitus; DPP-4: dipeptidyl peptidase-4; GLP-1: glucagon-like peptide-1; SGLT-2: sodium-glucose cotransporter-2)

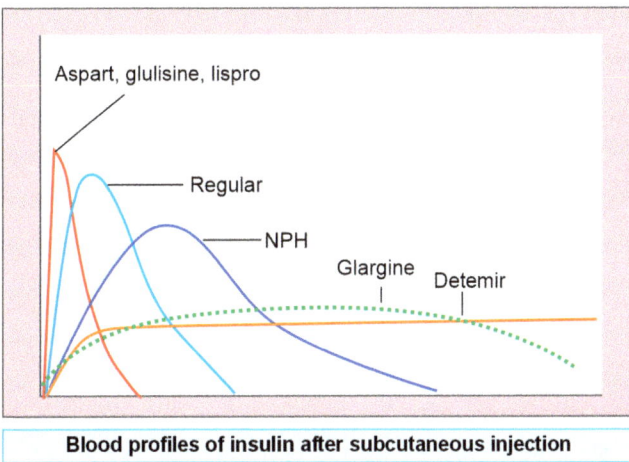

FIG. 25: Three types of insulin: (1) Short acting (regular, aspart, lispro, glulisine, etc.), (2) Basal/long acting (glargine, detemir, etc.), and (3) Intermediate actin [neutral protamine Hagedorn (NPH)].

ultralong-acting one. Premixed precreation of different ratio is also available for both types of insulins **(Fig. 25 and Table 8)**.

Indications of insulin use
- T1DM
- Severe acute complication/illness
- Uncompensated chronic complication/illness
- Pregnancy, lactation, major surgery, and very high blood glucose
- Oral antidiabetic (OAD) or noninsulin agent failure
- Adverse effect with OAD

Insulin regimen
- One injection a day
- Two injections a day
- Multiple injections a day
- Insulin pump

One injection a day regimen:
- One injection of intermediate-/long-acting insulin is given in evening or long-acting insulin analog is given in morning or evening. It serves as basal secretion and ideally its dose is titrated to bring fasting glucose level to the target.
- It is effective only in T2DM as monotherapy or in combination with OADs of adjuvant group **(Fig. 26)**.

Two injections a day regimen:
- Most commonly used regimen.
- Injections are given before breakfast and dinner. Any of the following insulins can be used:
  o Intermediate insulin-only in T2DM
  o Biphasic (premixed) insulin including analog though convenient for patients, sometimes it is difficult to achieve glycemic control with this regimen.
  o Split-mixed (self-mixed) regimen—short-acting insulin or rapid-acting insulin analog is mixed with intermediate-acting insulin in proportions that are adjusted by trial.

When premixed or split-mixed regimen is started twice daily, the total daily dose is divided into morning dose of two-thirds and evening dose of one-third with an aim of providing two-thirds longer acting insulin with one-third shorter acting insulin.

Doses are titrated to bring fasting glucose level by predinner insulin and prelunch glucose level by prebreakfast dose initially and thereafter the postmeal blood glucose. In T2DM combination with adjuvant molecule(s) **(Fig. 27)**.

Multiple injections a day regimen: 3–7 injections per day are used where there is difficulty in achieving optimal control with previous regimens. Intermediate-acting insulin is given at bedtime or long-acting insulin analog

TABLE 8: Action of different type of insulin.

Type	Name			Action onset	Peak action	Duration of action	Time with meal
				Human/conventional insulin			
Short acting	Regular			0.5–1.0 hour	2–4 hours	6–8 hours	0.5–1.0 hour ac (higher BG more interval)
Intermediate acting	NPH	Lente		2–4 hours	6–8 hours	12–18 hours	0.5–1.0 hour ac or bedtime
Long acting	Ultralente			4–6 hours	8–14 hours	24–36 hours	No specific time
				Analog insulin			
Rapid-acting analog	Aspart	Lispro	Glulisine	5–15 minutes	1–1.5 hour	3–4 hours	With meals (within 15 minute ac/pc)
Long-acting analog	Glargine	Detemir		2–4 hours	No peak	24 hours	No specific time
Ultra-long-acting analog	Degludec				No peak	40+ hours (half-life >24 hours)	No specific time
				Premix insulin			
Premix conventional insulin	Short- and intermediate-acting insulin are mixed in different proportions (30/70%; 50/50%; 25/75%)						As indicated for short-acting insulin
Premix analog insulin	Rapid and intermediate acting analogs (protaminated rapid-acting analog) are mixed in different proportions (30/70%; 50/50%; 25/75%, 30/70%; 50/50%; 25/75%)						As indicated for rapid-acting analog

(ac: before meal; pc: after meal)

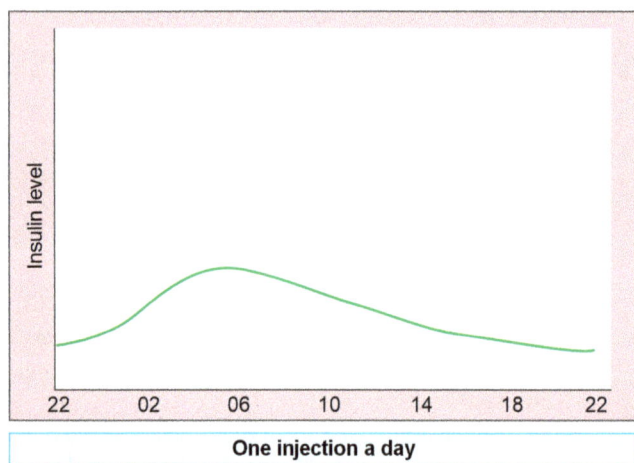

One injection a day

FIG. 26: It serves as basal secretion and ideally its dose is titrated to bring fasting glucose (hepatic glucose output) level to the target. It is effective only in type 2 diabetes mellitus as monotherapy or in combination with adjuvant molecule(s).

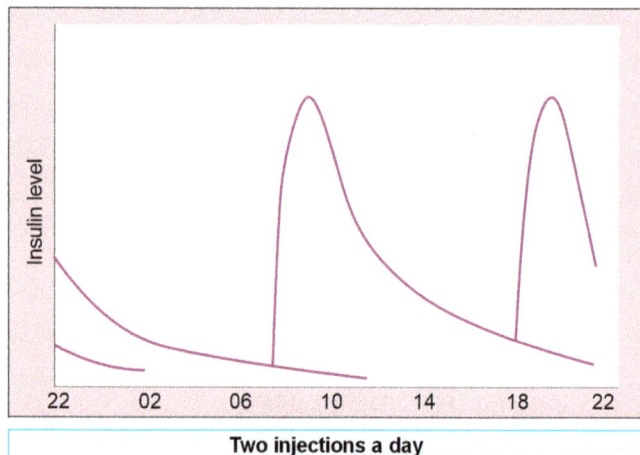

Two injections a day

FIG. 27: Injections are given before breakfast and dinner. Any of the following insulins can be used: Intermediate insulin-only in type 2 diabetes mellitus. Biphasic (premixed) insulin including analog though convenient for patients. Split-mixed (self-mixed) regimen—short- or rapid-acting insulin analog is mixed with intermediate-acting insulin in proportions that are adjusted by trial.

is given at bedtime or morning as basal doses and short-acting insulin or rapid-acting insulin analog is given before each meal as bolus doses (basal-bolus regimen). The total daily dose is divided into 50% longer acting insulin with 50% shorter acting insulin. This is very flexible and ideal for those who are very active and cannot comply with the rigid meal plan or in whom diabetes control is difficult with the above regiments **(Fig. 28)**.

Insulin pump: Continuous subcutaneous insulin infusion (CSII) is delivered through small device delivering insulin at basal rate throughout 24 hours and patient activated boluses during meal times through a subcutaneous cannula. Some of the devices are also equipped with continuous glucose monitoring (CGM) system. Insulin pumps are used only in selected patients **(Fig. 29)**.

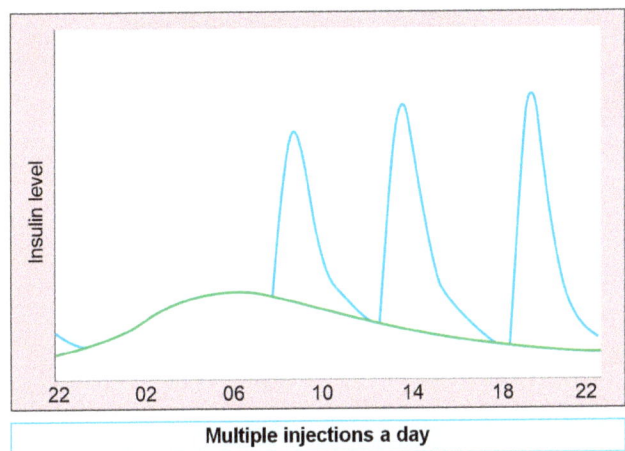

FIG. 28: About 3–7 injections per day are used where there is difficulty in achieving optimal control with other regimens. Intermediate- or long-acting insulin analog is given at bedtime or morning and short-acting insulin is given before each meal as bolus doses (basal-bolus regimen). The total daily dose is divided into 50% longer acting insulin with 50% shorter acting insulin.

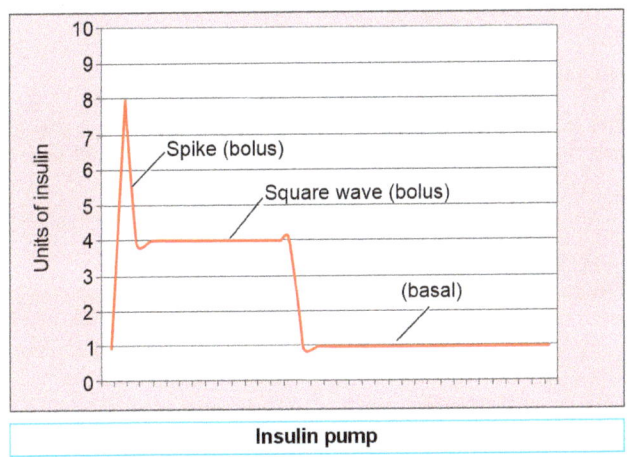

FIG. 29: Device delivers insulin at basal rate throughout 24 hours and patient-activated boluses during meal times through a subcutaneous cannula. Some of the devices are also equipped with continuous glucose monitoring (CGM) system.

Indications of insulin pump use are:
- T1DM
- DKA and hyperglycemic hyperosmolar state (HHS)
- Critical illnesses, e.g., acute myocardial infarction (MI), stroke, etc.
- Prolonged (>12 hours) nothing per oral (NPO) status
- Total parenteral nutrition (TPN)
- Perioperative period
- During delivery
- Uncontrolled hyperglycemia exacerbated by illness or steroid
- Any condition requiring prompt lowering of blood glucose

Insulin Secretagogue

Sulfonylureas (SUs) and glinides are two groups of molecules that are mostly used in the treatment of T2DM. They act by releasing insulin from pancreatic beta cell so named as *insulin secretagogue.*

Sulfonylureas

Sulfonylureas increase the release of insulin from pancreatic beta cells and thus exert a hypoglycemic effect in diabetic as well as nondiabetic persons. First introduced in 1955, these are the oldest oral agents and still in use in large scale in T2DM.

Pancreatic action of SU is initiated by binding to a specific sulfonylurea receptor on the pancreatic beta cells, leading to closure of potassium-dependent ATP (K_{ATP}) channel. With the closure of K_{ATP} channel, there is increase in calcium influx and translocation of secretary granules on the cell surface and extrusion of insulin by exocytosis.

Extra pancreatic effect of SUs: (1) To reduce HGU, (2) to improve insulin-stimulated glucose uptake in muscle, and (3) to stimulate lipogenesis in fatty tissue. But these effects are not significant **(Fig. 30)**.

Metabolism: Sulfonylureas are rapidly absorbed from gut, have extensive plasma protein binding, and almost completely metabolized by liver, excreted in urine and feces.

Sulfonylureas are potent in reducing both pre- and postprandial blood glucose, may cause hypoglycemia and weight gain, and have limitation of use in impaired renal and liver function.

Sulfonylureas are contraindicated in impaired renal and liver function.

Important SUs that are in use for treatment of T2DM include glibenclamide, glipizide, gliclazide, and glimepiride.

Table 9 shows the duration of action, route of elimination, and doses of different SUs in secretagogue-based treatment for T2DM.

Insulin secretagogues:
Nonsulfonylureas/glinides

Mechanism of action of glinides is similar to the SU. But because of their slightly different binding site, pharmacokinetic profile is also different. First introduced in 1983, and is in use in large scale for T2DM. Hypoglycemic action is glucose dependent and hence work better in the presence of hyperglycemia and effect wears off as the plasma glucose concentration returns to the normal range. Therefore, these agents are also called *"prandial glucose regulator."*

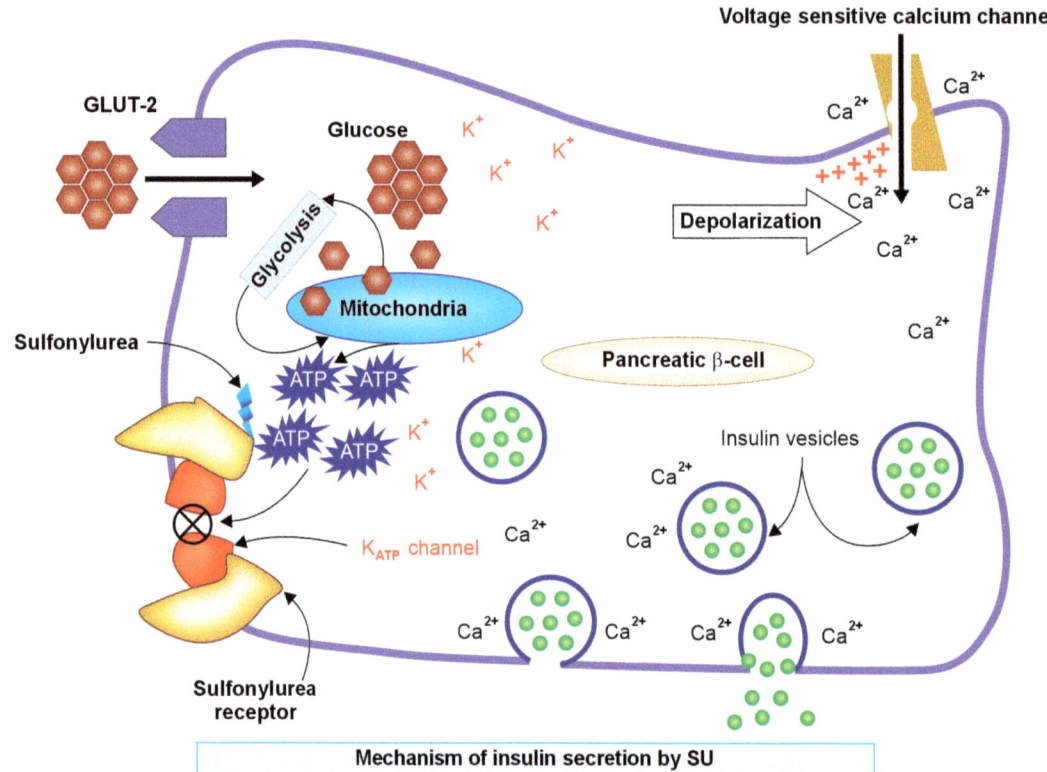

FIG. 30: (1) SU binding to a specific SU receptor on the pancreatic beta cells; (2) Closure of potassium-dependent ATP (K_{ATP}) channel; (3) With the closure of K_{ATP} channel, there is increase in calcium influx and translocation of secretary granules on the cell surface; (4) Extrusion of insulin by exocytosis.
(GLUT-2: glucose transporter 2; SU: sulfonylurea)

SUs	Duration of action	Elimination	Start dose	Maximum dose	Dose adjustment interval
Glibenclamide	24 hours	Bile (>60%) and feces	(1.25–2.5 mg) ×1; 30 minutes ac	20 mg (in 1–2 dose)	Every 2 weeks
Glipizide	4–8 hours	Urine (~70%) and feces	(2.5 mg) ×1; 30 minutes ac	40 mg (in 1–2 dose)	Every 2 weeks
Gliclazide	4–8 hours	Urine (~65%) and feces	(40 mg) ×1; 30 minutes ac	320 mg (in 1–2 dose); MR 120 mg (in one dose)	Every 2 weeks
Glimepiride	24 hours	Urine (~60%) and feces	(1 mg) ×1; 30 minutes ac	8 mg (in one dose)	Every 1–2 weeks

TABLE 9: Duration of action, route of elimination, and doses of different sulfonylureas (SUs) used in treatment for T2DM.

(ac: before meal; MR: modified release preparation; SUs: sulfonylureas; T2DM: type 2 diabetes mellitus)

Metabolism: Glinides are rapidly absorbed from gut, have extensive plasma protein binding, and almost completely metabolized by liver; repaglinide excreted mostly in feces and nateglinide mostly in urine. Glinides are potent in reducing only postprandial blood glucose, do not cause hypoglycemia or weight gain, and can be used in impaired renal and liver function.

Two glinides that are in use for the treatment of T2DM repaglinide and nateglinide are shown in **Table 10**.

Adjuvant Agents in the Treatment of Diabetes Mellitus

In general, they can be added to all types of prescriptions for DM. Choice of particular molecule depends on its mode of action(s) that are beneficial for the individual. Hazards and limits of the molecules are to be considered.

TABLE 10: Duration of action, route of elimination, and doses of glinide in the treatment of type 2 diabetes mellitus (T2DM).

Glinide	Duration of action	Excretion	Start dose	Maximum dose	Dose adjustment interval
Repaglinide	4–5 hours	Mostly in feces (~90%)	(0.5 mg) ×3; 5–10 minutes before meal	12 mg (in three dose)	Every 1–2 weeks
Nateglinide	3–5 hours	Mostly in urine (~80%)	(60 mg) ×3; 5–10 minutes before meal	360 mg (in three dose)	Every 1–2 weeks

TABLE 11: Initiation and dose titration of insulin sensitizers: Metformin in T2DM.

	OAD class: Biguanides		
Name	Starting daily dose	Maximum	Adjustment
Metformin	500 mg ×1 (within meal; buildup the dose weekly)	2,500 mg (in 2–3 doses) ER 2,000 mg (one dose)	Increase (on the buildup) by smallest every 4 weeks

(ER: extended release; OAD: oral antidiabetic; T2DM: type 2 diabetes mellitus)

The molecules are classified on their principle mode of action:
- Insulin sensitizers such as biguanide—metformin and thiazolidinediones (glitazones)—pioglitazone
- Alpha-glucosidase inhibitors such as acarbose
- Dipeptidyl peptidase-4 (DPP-4) inhibitors (gliptin)
- Sodium-glucose cotransporter-2 (SGLT-2) inhibitors (gliflozin)
- GLP-1 receptor agonists—exenatide and liraglutide
- Amilin

Insulin sensitizers
- *Metformin*:
  o Metformin is the only biguanide now in use to treat T2DM and become the first-line treatment option.
  o It has lower risk of hypoglycemia and can be combined with other anti-diabetic drugs including insulin.
  o This does not alter blood glucose levels in nondiabetic persons, but produce an antihyperglycemic effect in persons with diabetes.
  o This is well absorbed on oral administration, not bound to plasma proteins, not metabolized, and is excreted almost unchanged in urine.
  o Precise mechanism of action is not clear, but possibilities include:
    – Inhibition of hepatic neoglucogenesis
    – Increase in insulin sensitivity with peripheral utilization of glucose
    – Delay in absorption of glucose in gut
  o Metformin is started with 500 mg ×1 dose during the largest meal daily and then buildup dose weekly. The maximum dose is 2,500 mg in two to three meals or extended release 2,000 mg in single dose. The dose adjustment should be slow, e.g., monthly.
  o Common side effects of metformin include nausea, vomiting, stomach pain, and diarrhea **(Table 11)**.
- *Thiazolidinediones*:
  o Thiazolidinediones are a class of drugs that improve insulin sensitivity and are useful in T2DM where IR is a major component in the pathogenesis.
  o Mechanism of action of the drugs includes:
    – Reduce HGU
    – Increase peripheral glucose utilization improving insulin sensitivity
  o These have low risk of hypoglycemia.
  o Pioglitazone is started with 15 mg ×1 dose daily and then buildup in every 4-6 weeks. The maximum dose is 45 mg in one dose.
  o Rosiglitazone is started with 4 mg ×1 dose daily or 2 mg ×2 doses daily and then buildup in every 4-6 weeks. The maximum dose is 8 mg in 1-2 doses.
  o Common side effects of pioglitazone and rosiglitazone include weight gain and fluid retention and of rosiglitazone is ischemic heart disease (IHD).

Table 12 shows initiation and dose titration of insulin sensitizers: Thiazolidinediones in T2DM.

Alpha-glucosidase inhibitors
- They competitively block the action of the intestinal enzyme alpha-glucosidase. Normally, intestinal enzyme alpha-glucosidase breaks down oligosaccharides into monosaccharides. Therefore, the inhibitor inhibits the complete digestion of carbohydrate in food.
- They also cause formation of gases due to unabsorbed carbohydrate in the colon.
- Acarbose is poorly absorbed from gut and extensively metabolized in the intestinal wall.
- But miglitol and voglibose are completely absorbed from the gut and excreted unchanged. Three drugs of

TABLE 12: Oral antidiabetic (OAD) class: Thiazolidinediones.

OAD	Starting daily dose	Maximum	Adjustment
Pioglitazone	15 mg (in one dose)	45 mg (in one dose)	Increase by smallest every 4–6 weeks
Rosiglitazone	4 mg/2 mg (in 1–2 doses)	8 mg (in 1–2 doses)	

TABLE 13: Alpha-glucosidase inhibitors.

OAD	Elimination	Starting daily dose	Maximum	Adjustment
Acarbose	• Feces (~98%) • Urine (~2%)	25–50 mg × (one to three doses within meal)	300 mg × (three doses)	Increase by smallest dose every 6 weeks
Miglitol	Urine (~100%)	25–50 mg × (one to three doses within meal)	300 mg × (three doses)	Increase by smallest dose every 6 weeks
Voglibose	Urine (~100%)	2 mg × (one dose with meal)	2–3 mg × three times	Increase by smallest dose every 6 weeks

(OAD: oral antidiabetic)

TABLE 14: OAD class: DPP-4 inhibitor (gliptin).

OAD	Elimination	Starting daily dose	Maximum	Adjustment
Sitagliptin	Urine (~80%)	100 mg (one dose)	100 mg (one dose)	• 50 mg if CCr < 50 mL/min • 25 mg if CCr < 30 mL/min
Vildagliptin	Urine (~80%)	50 mg (one to two doses)	100 mg (two doses)	50 mg if CCr < 50 mL/min
Linagliptin	Bile (~80%)	5 mg (one dose)	5 mg (one dose)	Full dose in renal failure
Saxagliptin	Urine (~60%)	2.5 mg (one dose)	5 mg (one dose)	2.5 mg if CCr < 50 mL/min
Alogliptin	Urine (>70%)	25 mg (one dose)	25 mg (one dose)	

(CCr: creatinine clearance; DPP-4: dipeptidyl peptidase-4; OAD: oral antidiabetic drug)

this class are currently available: Acarbose, miglitol, and voglibose.

Table 13 shows initiation and dose titration of alpha-glucosidase inhibitors for T2DM.

DPP-4 inhibitors (Gliptin)
- DPP-4 inhibitors are incretin mimetics.
- *Mechanism of action*:
  o DPP-4 inhibitors inhibit action of the DPP-4 enzyme.
  o So, there is delayed clearance of gut hormone incretins.
  o Incretin level remains higher for longer time.
  o Incretins lower blood glucose by reduce hepatic glucose production (HGP).
- *Common side effects of DPP-4 inhibitors include*:
  o Gastrointestinal problems—including nausea, diarrhea, and stomach pain
  o Flu-like symptoms—headache, runny nose, and sore throat
  o Skin reactions—painful skin followed by a red or purple rash
  o Pancreatitis

Currently available classes are: Sitagliptin, vildagliptin, linagliptin, and saxagliptin.

Table 14 shows initiation and dose titration of DPP-4 inhibitors for T2DM.

SGLT-2 inhibitors (Gliflozin)
- SGLT-2 reabsorbs the filtered glucose in renal tubules. Gliflozin inhibits SGLT-2 in the proximal tubules. So, the reduced reabsorption of filtered glucose from the tubular lumen and lower the renal threshold for glucose.
- The reduction of filtered glucose reabsorption and lowering of renal threshold. Therefore, there occurs increased urinary excretion of glucose and ultimately reduction of plasma glucose concentration.

Currently available classes are: Dapagliflozin, canagliflozin, and empagliflozin **(Table 15)**.

Glucagon-like peptide-1 receptor agonists
- GLP-1 receptor agonists affect glucose control through several mechanisms, including:
  o Enhancement of glucose-dependent insulin secretion
  o Slowed gastric emptying

TABLE 15: OAD class: SGLT-2 inhibitors.

OAD	Elimination	Starting daily dose	Maximum	Adjustment
Dapagliflozin	Urine (~10%)	5 mg × one dose	10 mg × one dose	Increase by every 4 weeks
Canagliflozin	Urine (~100%)	100 mg × one dose	300 mg × one dose	Increase by every 4 weeks
Empagliflozin	Urine (~100%)	10 mg × one dose	25 mg × one dose	Increase by every 4 weeks

(OAD: oral antidiabetic drug; SGLT-2: sodium-glucose cotransporter-2)

- o Reduction of postprandial glucagon
- o Reduce food intake
- These agents do not usually cause hypoglycemia.
- Side effects include GI upset and pancreatitis

Exenatide and liraglutide are two injectable GLP-1 receptor agonists currently in use for T2DM treatment.

- Starting dose of exenatide is 10 μg in two doses with meals [within 15 minute before meal/after meal (ac/pc)]
- Increment of dose: After 4 weeks
- Maximum dose: 20 μg/day
- Once-weekly exenatide (2 mg) is now available.
- Start dose of liraglutide is 0.6 units daily (no specific time)
- Increment of dose: After 1 week
- Maximum dose: 1.8 units/day

Amilin analogs

- Amilin analogs control glucose through several mechanisms, including:
  - o Slowed gastric emptying
  - o Reduction of postprandial glucagon
- Amilin analogs may cause hypoglycemia.
- Side effects include GI upset and upper respiratory tract infection.
- Pramlintide is the only amilin analog currently in use for T1DM and T2DM treatment.

For T1DM: Starting dose of pramlintide is 15 μg in three doses with meals; increment of dose: after 1 week and maximum dose: 60 μg/day.

For T2DM: Starting dose of pramlintide is 60 μg in three doses with meals; increment of dose: after 1 week and maximum dose: 60 μg/day.

Pancreas Transplantation for Diabetes Management

- Pancreas transplantation may be an option in the management of diabetes only in patients with serious progressive complications, e.g., end-stage renal disease, having or planning for kidney transplantation.
- It may also be done if there is history of frequent, acute, and severe metabolic complications (hypoglycemia, marked hyperglycemia, and ketoacidosis), incapacitating clinical and emotional problems with exogenous insulin therapy, and consistent failure of insulin-based management to prevent acute complications.

Procedures are of three different types:
1. Islet transplantation
2. Pancreas transplantation
3. Pancreas plus kidney transplantation

Islet transplantation is an evolving technology; it can be performed only in research settings.

Pancreas transplantation has a higher rate of insulin independence and morbidity than islet transplantation **(Flowchart 7)**.

Prescription for Diabetes Mellitus
Role of Three in Diabetology

1. Diabetic patients are of three types—(i) DM without any complication of DM; (ii) DM with complication of DM, and (iii) DM without any complication of DM but other comorbidity(s).
2. Diabetic prescription recipients are of three types—(i) require first time prescription; (ii) require follow-up prescription for dose adjustment, and (iii) require new regimen.
3. Diabetic prescription drug regimens are of three types—(i) insulin; (ii) insulin secretagogue, and (iii) adjuvant drugs **(Flowchart 8)**.

Prescription for DM is influenced by many factors and one of them is type/class of diabetes. We shall discuss it on the class basis—for T1DM, T2DM, GDM, and Secondary DM.

Prescription for T1DM

It is done by insulin synchronizing with his/her lifestyle. Structured SMBG plays a key role in successful treatment of T1DM. Multiple insulin injection regimen and use of insulin pump have brighten the treatment aspect of challenge of T1DM treatment.

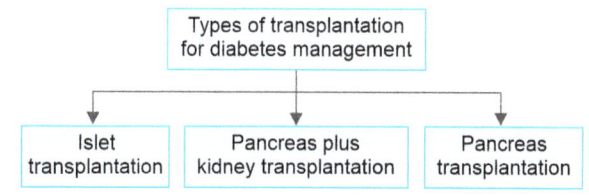

FLOWCHART 7: Transplantation for diabetes management.

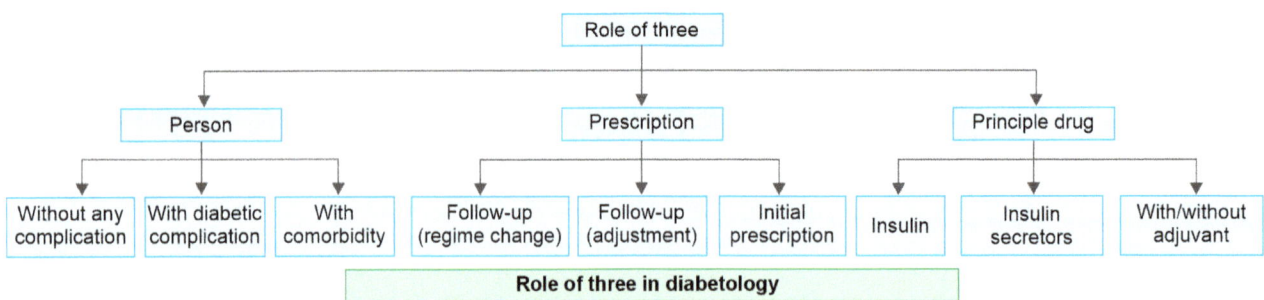

FLOWCHART 8: Three types of persons, prescription, and drug regimens.

Prescription for T2DM

Initial prescription for T2DM:
- Initial prescription for a person without any diabetic complication and mild hyperglycemia (FBG < 11.1 mmol/dL or HbA1c <8%) should be on lifestyle only but specific adjuvant molecule(s) for obvious risk factor(s) may be added, e.g, metformin for obesity.
- Initial prescription for a person without any diabetic complication and moderate hyperglycemia (FBG > 11.1–16.7 mmol/dL or HbA1c < 8–10%) should be on low dose of long-acting SU (e.g., glimepiride/modified release gliclazide) with lifestyle so that raised hepatic glucose output, i.e., FBG is effectively controlled. Specific adjuvant molecule(s) can either be initiated from beginning or can be started after the FBG is controlled.
- Initial prescription for a person without any diabetic complication and severe hyperglycemia (FBG > 16.7 mmol/dL or HbA1c > 10%) should be on low dose of long-acting/basal insulin with lifestyle so that raised hepatic glucose output, i.e., FBG is effectively controlled. Specific adjuvant molecule(s) and/or short-acting insulin for postmeal surges may be started after the FBG is controlled.
- Initial prescription for a person with specific diabetic complication(s) and mild hyperglycemia should be on lifestyle only. And regarding specific adjuvant molecule(s) for obvious risk factor(s) may added provided are not contraindicated for the complication(s).
- Initial prescription for a person with any diabetic complication and moderate/severe hyperglycemia should be on intermediate/long acting insulin with lifestyle so that raised hepatic glucose output, i.e., FBG is effectively controlled. Specific adjuvant molecule(s) and or short acting insulin for postmeal surges may be started after the FBG is controlled.
- Initial prescription for a person with comorbidity(s) needs to follow the same principle of treatment based on severity of hyperglycemia with/without diabetic complication(s) enshrining management of the comorbidity.

Follow-up prescription for T2DM:
A follow-up prescription primarily depends on the achievement by the current prescription.
- If the current prescription achieved targets effectively (pre- and postmeal blood glucose on target), follow-up prescription should be as it was.
- If the current prescription achieved targets partly (fasting/premeal blood glucose on target but postmeal high and HbA1c% on target), follow-up prescription should be adjusted for postmeal surge by: Addition/ increasing of short-acting insulin of an insulin-based prescription.
  - Addition of an appropriate adjuvant molecule with the meal(s) of an insulin secretor/lifestyle-based prescription.
  - The current prescription failed to achieve targets (fasting/premeal blood glucose, postmeal high and HbA1c high), follow-up prescription should be done by:
- Increasing dose of basal/long-acting insulin of an insulin-based prescription to control fasting blood sugar first than if require adjust postmeal surge (called dose adjustment)
  - Increasing dose of long-acting sulfonylurea of a secretagogue-based prescription to control fasting blood sugar first than if require adjust postmeal surge (called dose adjustment).
  - If present dose of sulfonylurea is maximum in a case of OAD failure, change with insulin regime prescription (called regimen shift)
  - If present prescription is on lifestyle with adjuvant molecule(s), change with a prescription of secretagogue regimen (called regimen shift).

Prescription for GDM

Initial prescription for GDM:
- Initial prescription for a lady with minimum hyperglycemia (FBG normal and postmeals normal or <8.0 mmol/L) should be on lifestyle only.
- Initial prescription for a lady with mild hyperglycemia (FBG normal and postmeal(s) >8.0 mmol/L) should

be on lifestyle plus short-acting insulin(s) for specific meal(s).
- Initial prescription for a lady with moderate/severe hyperglycemia [FBG and post meal(s) raised] should be on low dose of long-acting/basal insulin with lifestyle so that raised hepatic glucose output, i.e., FBG is effectively controlled and on follow-up add short-acting insulin for postmeal surges if they persist.

Follow-up prescription for GDM:
- If the current prescription achieved targets (fasting/premeal and postmeal blood glucose on target), follow-up prescription should remain unchanged.
- If the current prescription achieved targets partially (fasting/premeal blood glucose on target but postmeal high), follow-up prescription should be adjusted for postmeal surge by addition/increasing of short acting insulin for the meal(s).
- If the current prescription failed to achieve targets (fasting/premeal blood glucose, postmeal high), follow-up prescription should be done by adding/increasing dose of basal/long-acting insulin to control fasting blood sugar first than if require adjust postmeal surge by adding/increasing dose of short action insulin for the meal(s).

Prescription for secondary DM

Prescription for secondary DM will be on similar to that T2DM along with the treatment of primary cause (when available).

Acute Metabolic Complications of Diabetes Mellitus

The complications of DM may be acute or chronic. The acute complications are related to immediate and rapid changes in metabolism that arise within a short time (hours to weeks). These are: (1) DKA, (2) hyperosmolar non-ketotic Coma (HONK), (3) lactic acidosis, and (4) hypoglycemia **(Flowchart 9)**.

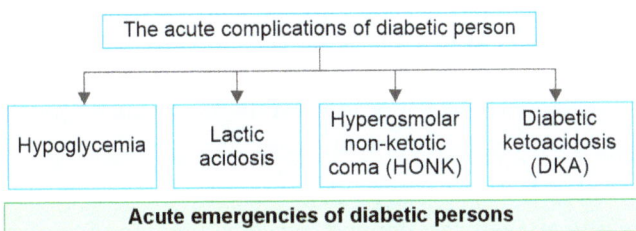

FLOWCHART 9: Four types of acute complications seen in diabetic person.

Diabetic Ketoacidosis

Diabetic ketoacidosis is a medical emergency in diabetic patients. It is commonly found in T1DM. But it also occurs in other types of diabetes during stressful situations. It results from lack of insulin and rise in counter-regulatory hormones that lead to hyperglycemia and subsequent lipolysis.

Causes of DKA
- Undiagnosed diabetes omission of insulin dose
- Injudicious reduction of insulin dose, illness, especially acute infection
- Trauma, pregnancy, etc.

Clinical features of DKA
- DKA develops rapidly (hours to days)
- Symptoms of uncontrolled diabetes precede
- Weakness, vomiting, impairment of level of consciousness, and acute abdomen
- Dehydration is the most obvious clinical feature with dry skin and tongue, low BP, and rapid weak pulse
- Acidotic breathing is characteristic; there may be acetone smell in breath.

Diagnosis of DKA by biochemical features
- Blood glucose—usually >15 mmol/L
- Acidosis—arterial pH < 7.3; plasma bicarbonate <15 mEq/L
- Ketone bodies in blood and urine are greatly increased.
- Serum osmolality is variable.

Principle of DKA management
- Hospitalization
- Clinical assessment
- Determination of blood glucose, electrolytes, arterial blood gas with pH, osmolality, complete blood picture, urea, etc. Blood or urine test for ketone body.

Treatment institution is to be done immediately without waiting for laboratory reports.
- Fluid replacement should be initiated promptly. Normal saline is a choice and rate should be high but should not be overloaded for cardiac status.
- Insulin pump or by microinfusion set should start at rate of 3–6 units of regular insulin per hour and adjustment is made so that fall of blood glucose is in between 3 and 4 mmol/h. Shift to subcutaneous insulin if blood glucose comes to 14 mmol/L.
- Potassium replacement is not started so long serum K^+ is >5.5 mmol/L; 20 mmol K^+ infusion is given to each liter of fluid if serum K^+ is 5.5–3.3 mmol/L and 40 mmol K^+ infusion is given to each liter of fluid if serum K^+ is <3.3 mmol/L.

- Bicarbonate is used very slowly and cautiously in severe acidotic (pH < 7.0) cases only.
- Monitoring—clinically, biochemically, and treatment of identified precipitating causes.
- Proper nursing care

Complications of DKA
- Cerebral edema
- Circulatory failure
- Thromboembolism
- DIC
  Overall mortality from DKA is 2% or less.

Hyperosmolar Non-ketotic Coma (HONK) (Another Name—Hyperglycemic Hyperosmolar State)

HONK is a combination of severe degree of hyperglycemia, dehydration, and hyperosmolality, without significant ketonuria; usually seen as complication of elderly T2DM patients. Here residual insulin reserve prevents ketosis.

Causes of HONK
- Lack of proper treatment of diabetes
- Any acute stress, e.g., infection, stroke, MI, and trauma
- Compromised fluid intake drugs, e.g., glucocorticoids, diuretics, etc.

Clinical features of HONK
- HONK develops slowly (days to weeks).
- Symptoms of uncontrolled diabetes precede.
- Dehydration is profound; impairment of consciousness is common.

Diagnosis of HONK by biochemical features
- Blood glucose—usually >30 mmol/L
- Hyperosmolality—effective serum osmolality >320 mOsm/kg
- Arterial pH > 7.3; plasma bicarbonate < 15 mEq/L (no acidosis)
- Absence of significant ketonemia or ketonuria

Principe of HONK management
- Hospitalization
- Clinical assessment
- Determination of blood glucose, osmolality, electrolytes, arterial blood gas with pH, and complete blood picture
  Treatment is to be started immediately without waiting for laboratory reports.
  Treatment and monitoring protocols are similar to that of DKA in some issues as follows:
- Rapid change in plasma osmolality should be carefully checked and avoided.
- Insulin requirement is less in HONK than in DKA.
- Bicarbonate use is not required here.
- Proper nursing care is very important as the patients are usually older with more comorbidities.

Complications of HONK are similar to that of DKA:
- Cerebral edema
- Circulatory failure
- Thromboembolism disseminated intravascular coagulation (DIC), etc.
  Overall mortality is higher for HONK and is 10-20%.

Lactic Acidosis

Impaired tissue oxygenation, leading to increased anaerobic metabolism, is usually responsible for lactic acidosis.

In DM, lactic acidosis can be precipitated by:
- Biguanide therapy, although the risk is very low, or
- Sometimes in DKA, probably due to hypervolemia
- It can also be precipitated by alcoholism, severe infection, hepatic failure, and malignancy.

Features of lactic acidosis
- The onset may be rapid (minutes to hours) or progressive (several days).
- Patients present with severe dehydration, marked acidosis, mild (or no) ketonuria, etc.
- Diagnostic feature: Plasma lactate concentration exceeds 4 mEq/L.

Treatment of lactic acidosis
- Fluid replacement
- Acidosis correction
- Improvement of tissue perfusion
- Blood sugar control, correction of precipitating factors
- Supportive measures
  Mortality is very high, may be up to 75% in severe cases.

Hypoglycemia

Hypoglycemia is defined with blood glucose level below 70 mg/dL (4.0 mmol/L) with clinical features of neuroglycopenia and autonomic over activity.

Some diabetics, especially those with high blood glucose, may develop clinical features (particularly autonomic) of hypoglycemia at a higher blood glucose level due to relative hypoglycemia.

Hypoglycemia is a very common phenomenon in diabetes. It occurs much in T1DM than T2DM.

Clinical features of hypoglycemia

Clinical features depend on hormonal and neural response to hypoglycemia and called autonomic features and neuroglycopenic features, respectively.

TABLE 16: Clinical features of hypoglycemia.

Autonomic features "warning symptoms"	Neuroglycopenic features
• Sweating • Palpitation • Tremor • Irritability • Hunger	• Headache • Confusion • Visual disturbances • Behavioral abnormality • Drowsiness • Convulsion • Coma

TABLE 17: Severity of hypoglycemia.

Severity	Mild-to-moderate hypoglycemia	Severe hypoglycemia
Autonomic features	• Sweating • Palpitation • Tremor • Irritability • Hunger	Absent
Neuroglycopenic features	• Headache • Visual disturbances	• Confusion • Drowsiness • Abnormal behavior • Convulsion • Coma

Autonomic features (also called "warning symptoms"). They are due to response of adrenal glands and sympathetic nervous system to the low blood glucose. Symptoms include sweating, palpitation, tremor, irritability, and hunger.

Neuroglycopenic features: These are due to disturbance of central nervous system form low glucose availability. Symptoms include headache, confusion, difficulty of visual, abnormal behavior, drowsiness, convulsion and coma **(Table 16)**.

Table 17 describes severity of hypoglycemia (based on clinical features).

Hypoglycemia may vary from mild to severe. In severe hypoglycemia, the affected individual requires assistance of another person and cannot be treated with oral carbohydrate due to confusion or impaired consciousness.

Unaware hypoglycemia: Hypoglycemic attacks without any warning sign are seen in individuals with long-standing type 1 diabetes, autonomic neuropathy, medication (like nonselective beta-blockers), or very strict glycemic control.

Nocturnal hypoglycemia:
- Features of nocturnal hypoglycemia:
  o Hypoglycemia at night, usually occurring between 2 and 4 AM
  o Patients or their relatives may be awakened due to trembling or sweating.
  o Sometimes the patient may have morning headache, dizziness, forgetfulness, and confusion.
  o Confirmation of the suspected condition is made by blood test at appropriate time.

Causes of hypoglycemia in a diabetics
- Administration of too much insulin
- Excess intake of insulin secretagogues
- Delay or omission of a meal
- Doing more exercise than usual
- Overindulgence in alcohol
- Severe impairment of renal or hepatic function

Treatment of hypoglycemia
Treatment of hypoglycemia is according to its severity and type.

Treatment of mild-to-moderate hypoglycemia:
- Most cases are treated by the patient him/herself or by a family member.
- Symptoms subside by 15 g glucose or equivalent food, e.g., a glass of soft drink or fruit juice or snacks or meal (if it is due to missed meal). These measures are usually adequate to raise blood glucose and remain above the safe limit (5.5 mmol/L). If not, food/drink is repeated every 15 minutes until the patient is stable.
- If recurrent hypoglycemia follows, hospitalization is to be considered as in a case of severe hypoglycemia. Treatment modification may be required.

Treatment of severe hypoglycemia:
- Diagnosis is made with a finger prick. Injection glucagon 1 mg intramuscularly or subcutaneously may be given. 50–100 mL of 25% dextrose is given intravenously, for which hospitalization may be required.
- If hypoglycemia is due to longer acting antidiabetic medications, then 10% dextrose infusion should be started to prevent recurrent hypoglycemia. Ongoing activity of the antidiabetic medication may lead to recurrence of hypoglycemia; so food ingestion is to be ensured after initial recovery.
- If recovery does not occur, search for additional causes and modification in the treatment should be done.

Treatment of nocturnal hypoglycemia:
- Reduction of evening dose of insulin
- Changing the time of evening insulin dose with dinner time
- Bedtime snacks may help.
- The adjustments are made according to the blood glucose monitoring chart.

Treatment of unaware hypoglycemia:
- Frequent blood glucose monitoring is mandatory for the severe hypoglycemia.
- Patient and family education is required to prevent and manage future episodes.

Consequences of hypoglycemia
- Recurrent hypoglycemia may cause behavioral change and cognitive impairment.
- In T2DM—increased incidence of life-threatening cardiovascular events and mortality (cardiovascular and all cause).
- In T1DM—increased mortality (4–10% of deaths)

Chronic Complications of Diabetes Mellitus

Diabetes mellitus is a chronic disease. It has wide range of debilitating chronic complications.

Chronic complications produce changes in small or large vessels of the body. Accordingly, these complications are grouped into two types:
1. If smaller vessels, e.g., capillaries, are affected: Microvascular complications or microangiopathy and
2. If large vessels are affected: Macrovascular complications or macroangiopathy

Hyperglycemia is the principle risk factor to develop micro- and macroangiopathies in a diabetic individual. Both the lesions result in *organ dysfunctions*. Early detection of these angiopathies and proper glycemic management can prevent or halt these processes. It is considered as a major challenge in diabetic care.

Magnitude and pattern of complications are changing with time. During preinsulin era, life expectancy was very short for such acute metabolic complications, like ketoacidosis or HONKs. With the discovery of insulin and other drugs, lives of diabetic patients have been prolonged, and chronic complications are rising, some of which lead to premature death or considerable morbidity.

Complications may even present at detection of diabetes. Routine/annual health checkup programs pick up significant diabetic subjects with chronic complications. Many studies have shown that the morbidity as

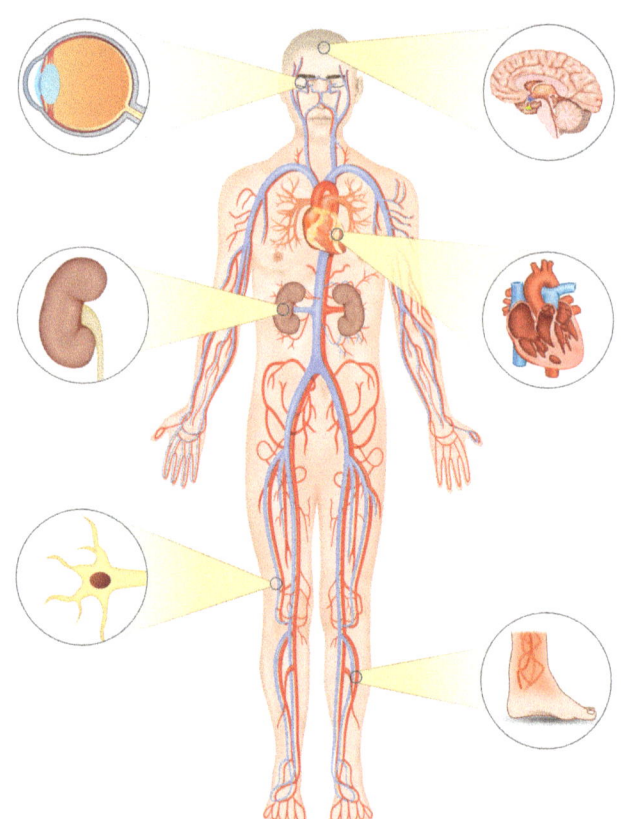

Risk of developing chronic complications in diabetes mellitus

FIG. 31: Organs affected by microangiopathy: Kidney—nephropathy five times than nondiabetics. Eye—retinopathy—blindness 25 times than nondiabetics. Peripheral nerves—neuropathy in >50% cases. Organs affected by macroangiopathy: Heart leads to coronary artery disease (CAD) two to three times than nondiabetics. Brain leads to cerebrovascular disease (CVD) six times than nondiabetics. Lower limbs amputation—20 times than nondiabetics.

well as mortality risks associated with diabetes can be reduced by treating to its targets **(Fig. 31)**.

Organ affected by microangiopathy:
- Kidneys lead to nephropathy.
- Eyes lead to retinopathy.
- Peripheral nerves lead to neuropathy.

Organ affected by macroangiopathy:
- Heart leads to coronary artery disease (CAD).
- Brain leads to cerebrovascular disease (CVD).
- Lower limbs lead to peripheral vascular disease (PVD).

Screening for Chronic Complications in Diabetic

Flowchart 10 shows the screening for chronic complications in diabetic.

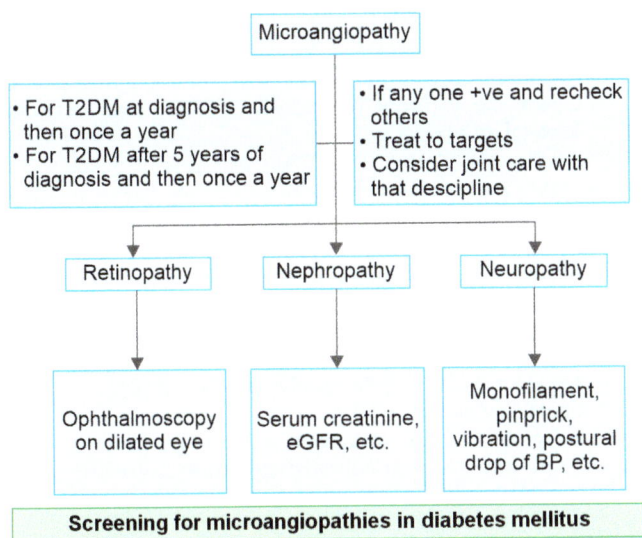

Screening for microangiopathies in diabetes mellitus

FLOWCHART 10: Type 2 diabetes mellitus: At diagnosis and then yearly. Type 1 diabetes mellitus: 5 years after diagnosis and then yearly. (1) Ophthalmoscopy; (2) Albuminuria and estimated glomerular filtration (eGFR) calculation; (3) Touch, pain, and vibration senses.

INSULINOMA

Patients with insulinoma present with symptoms of hypoglycemia that include diplopia, blurred vision, palpitations, or weakness. Other symptoms include confusion, abnormal behavior, unconsciousness, or amnesia. The classical presentation of pancreatic insulinoma is described by Whipple triad which consists of: (1) Fasting hypoglycemia (<50 mg/dL), (2) symptoms of hypoglycemia, and (3) immediate relief of symptoms after the administration of IV glucose **(Fig. 32)**.

The biochemical diagnosis is established in 95% of patients during prolonged fasting when the following parameters are found: (1) Serum insulin levels >10 μU/mL (normal <6 μU/mL), (2) glucose levels of <40 mg/dL, and (3) C-peptide levels >2.5 ng/mL (normal <2 ng/mL).

Apart from insulinoma, patient reporting with spontaneous hypoglycemia may be due to (1) reactive hypoglycemia, (2) hormone deficiency states like adrenal insufficiency, hypopituitarism of hypothalamic disease, (3) non-beta-cell tumors, or (4) critically ill patient.

Imaging studies for localization of insulinoma include: (1) Computed tomography (CT) scan, (2) magnetic resonance imaging (MRI), (3) endoscopic ultrasonography (EUS), and (4) arterial calcium stimulation with hepatic venous sampling (ASVS).

- *CT of insulinoma of pancreas*: Typically, insulinomas are hypervascular and show a greater degree of enhancement than pancreatic parenchyma during arterial and capillary phases of contrast bolus.

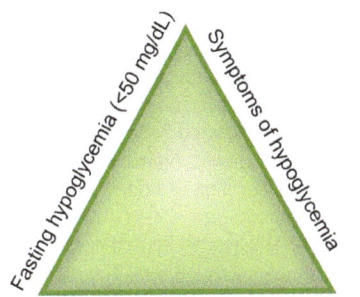

FIG. 32: Whipple triad of insulinoma.
(IV: intravenous)

- MRI of insulinoma of the pancreas: Insulinoma demonstrates low signal intensity on T1-weigted images and high signal intensity on T2-weigted images.
- EUS is highly accurate in the preoperative localization of insulinomas. The appearance of insulinomas is quite characteristic, with most tumors homogeneously hypoechoic, rounded in shape, and with distinct margins.
- ASVS: It is most sensitive technique for the precise localization of insulinomas. For atypical insulinomas, preoperative localization of insulinomas by ASVS is particularly important. Insulinomas are seen as well-defined, round, or oval vascular blushes that are of increased vascularity compared with the surrounding normal pancreatic parenchyma.

Treatment modalities for pancreatic insulinomas are either surgical or medical.

Most patients with benign insulinomas can be cured with surgery. Although other techniques for the management of insulinomas include: (1) Injection of octreotide, (2) EUS-guided alcohol ablation, (3) radiofrequency ablation (RFA), or (4) embolization of an insulinoma of the pancreas.

After identification of an insulinoma, surgery is indicated for all localized tumors.

The choice of procedure will depend on the features of the tumor mass, such as type, size, and localization.

- Typically, surgical resection, including (1) enucleation, (2) partial pancreatectomy, or (3) middle pancreatectomy.
- Laparoscopic resection has often been performed for insulinomas that are benign, small, and/or located in the body or tail of the pancreas.
- Radical resection should be considered for patients in whom the lesion is not single, not well-capsulated, >4 cm in diameter, and involves or is near the main pancreatic duct.
- Nonresectable malignant insulinomas are tried with other techniques, such as (1) injection of octreotide, (ii) EUS-guided alcohol ablation, (3) RFA, or (4) embolization of an insulinoma of the pancreas.

FURTHER READINGS

1. Anatomy and Physiology by ©2017 Rice University. Textbook content produced by OpenStax. [online] Available from https://openstax.org/ [Last accessed September, 2023].
2. Standring S (Ed). Gray's Anatomy: The Anatomical Basis of Clinical Practice, 41st edition. [online] Available from https://www.amazon.com/Garys-Anatomy-Henry-Gray/dp/B00DXO9JRA) [Last accessed September, 2023].
3. Barrett K, Barman S, Yuan J, Brooks H (Eds). Ganong's Review of Medical Physiology, 26th edition. [online] Available from https://www.amazon.com/Ganongs-Review-Medical-Physiology-Twenty/dp/1260122409 [Last accessed September, 2023].
4. Melmed S, Koenig R, Rosen C, Auchus R, Goldfine A. Williams Textbook of Endocrinology, 14th edition. [online] Available from (https://www.elsevier.com/books/williams-textbook-of-endocrinology/bresnahan/978-0-323-55596-8 [Last accessed September, 2023].
5. Gardner D, Shoback D (Eds). Greenspan's Basic and Clinical Endocrinology, 10th edition. McGraw Hill; 2017. [online] Available from https://www.amazon.com/Greenspans-Basic-Clinical-Endocrinology-Tenth/dp/1259589285 [Last accessed September, 2023].
6. Coleman W, Tsongalis G (Eds). Molecular Pathology: The Molecular Basis of Human Disease, 2nd edition. [online] Available from https://www.elsevier.com/books/molecular-pathology/coleman/978-0-12-802761-5 [Last accessed September, 2023].
7. DeFronzo RA, Ferrannini E, Zimmet P (Ed). International Textbook of Diabetes Mellitus, 2 Volume Set, 4th edition. Wiley-Blackwell; 2015. [online] Available from (https://www.wiley.com/en-us/International+Textbook+of+Diabetes+Mellitus%2C+2+Volume+Set%2C+4th+Edition-p-9780470658611) [Last accessed September, 2023].
8. Ashraf Ali Z. (2022). Insulinoma Guidelines. [online] Available from https://emedicine.medscape.com/article/283039-guidelines [Last accessed September, 2023].

CHAPTER 7

Disorders of Growth and Development

- Introduction to growth and development (anatomy and applied embryology; physiology)
  - Disorders of growth and development
- Short stature
  - Causes of short stature
- Tall stature
  - Pituitary gigantism
  - Nonendocrine causes of tall stature
- Obesity
  - Prader–Willi–Lambert (PWL) syndrome
  - Laurence–Moon–Biedl syndrome
  - Alström–Hallgren syndrome
  - Froehlich's syndrome (other name adiposogenital dystrophy)
  - Hyperostosis frontalis interna
  - Multiple lipomatosis
- Pubertal development and disorders
  - Pubertal growth spurt
  - Precocious puberty
  - Turner's syndrome (other names: Ullrich–Turner's syndrome, Bonnevie–Ullrich–Turner's syndrome)
  - Klinefelter's syndrome
  - Testicular feminization syndrome
  - Reifenstein syndrome (other name: Lub syndrome, Gilbert–Dreyfus syndrome, or Rosewater syndrome)

The chapter is about Growth and Development, which begins with an introduction to normal growth and development. It covers short stature, tall stature, pubertal disorders, and obesity. It also covers disorders, such as Turner's syndrome, Klinefelter's syndrome, and Testosterone resistance syndrome. This chapter consists of 37 Figures, 7 Tables, and 7 Flowcharts to illustrate its text.

INTRODUCTION TO GROWTH AND DEVELOPMENT (ANATOMY AND APPLIED EMBRYOLOGY; PHYSIOLOGY)

Growth and development means process of attaining an adult individually from his/her conception, i.e., unicellular stage of life.

Growth can be defined as a phenomenon of persistent increase in the size of an organ or of a cell. It is a basic characteristic of all living bodies. It occurs with energy expenditure by various metabolic processes. Growth means the increase in mass and size of a body. Development means the process where a particular organism acquires mental and physiological growth in addition to the physically growth.

For human it is an enormous phenomenon where in intrauterine phase there is approximately 44×10^7 times increase in mass and 3,850 times increase in length. And in postnatal phase, there is 20 times increase in mass and 3–4 times increase in length.

Determinants of height/length of an individual are genetic and environmental. Factors in intrauterine phase include endocrine, maternal, uterine, and chromosomal. And factors in postnatal life include endocrine (growth

Factors/hormones	Time (years)																		
	0 (before birth)	1	2	3	4	5	6	7	8	9	10	11	12	13	14	15	16	17	18+
Maternal, uterine, and chromosomal																			
Thyroid hormone																			
Growth hormone																			
Sex hormones																			
Growth velocity in (cm/year)	25		12.5	8	6		Growth spurt early in girls. A boy gain 30–31 cm and a girl gain 27.5–29 cm during puberty which is approximately 17% of their final height												

FIG. 1: Relative importance of different hormones during normal growth.

hormone, thyroid, and pubertal hormones mostly), genetic, racial and hereditary factors, nutritional status, and psychological factors.

The relative importance of different hormones during normal growth is shown diagrammatically in **Figure 1**.

▪ Disorders of Growth and Development

Most of the disorders of growth and developments are either related to height (short or tall stature) and puberty (delayed or precocious puberty). Disorders of height may either due to endocrine or nonendocrine causes but pubertal disorders are due to endocrine cause **(Flowchart 1)**.

To study the growth and development, physician has to be accounted with the use of growth charts. They are for linear growth/height and weight gain from birth to completion of growth (18 or 20 years). These are nomograms and are influence race/genetic of the population. Therefore, ideally every population should have their own but for practical limitation we have mentioned charts of Centers for Disease Control and Prevention (CDC) **(Figs. 2 and 3)**.

SHORT STATURE

Definition: An individual is of short stature when (1) abnormally low height/length (<3 standard deviation (SD) below for age); (2) abnormally low growth velocity (<2.5 SD below for age during 2–9 years); or (3)

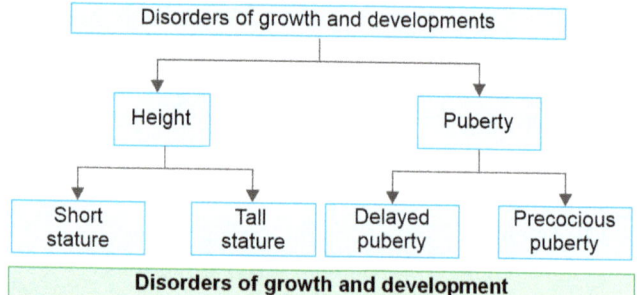

FLOWCHART 1: Disorders of height may either due to endocrine or nonendocrine causes but pubertal disorders are due to endocrine cause.

abnormally low height corrected for midparental height (<2.5 SD below).

▪ Causes of Short Stature

Short statue can be caused by endocrine and nonendocrine disorders. Endocrine disorders causing short stature may be either due to growth hormone deficiency or other hormonal diseases. Among the nonendocrine cases, it may have related to skeletal development defect, part of syndrome, or due to other effects. **Table 1** summarized the causes of short stature.

Endocrine Causes of Short Stature
- Growth hormone deficiency disorders
- Congenital growth hormone deficiency may be isolated deficiency or as a part of panhypopituitarism **(Fig. 4)**.

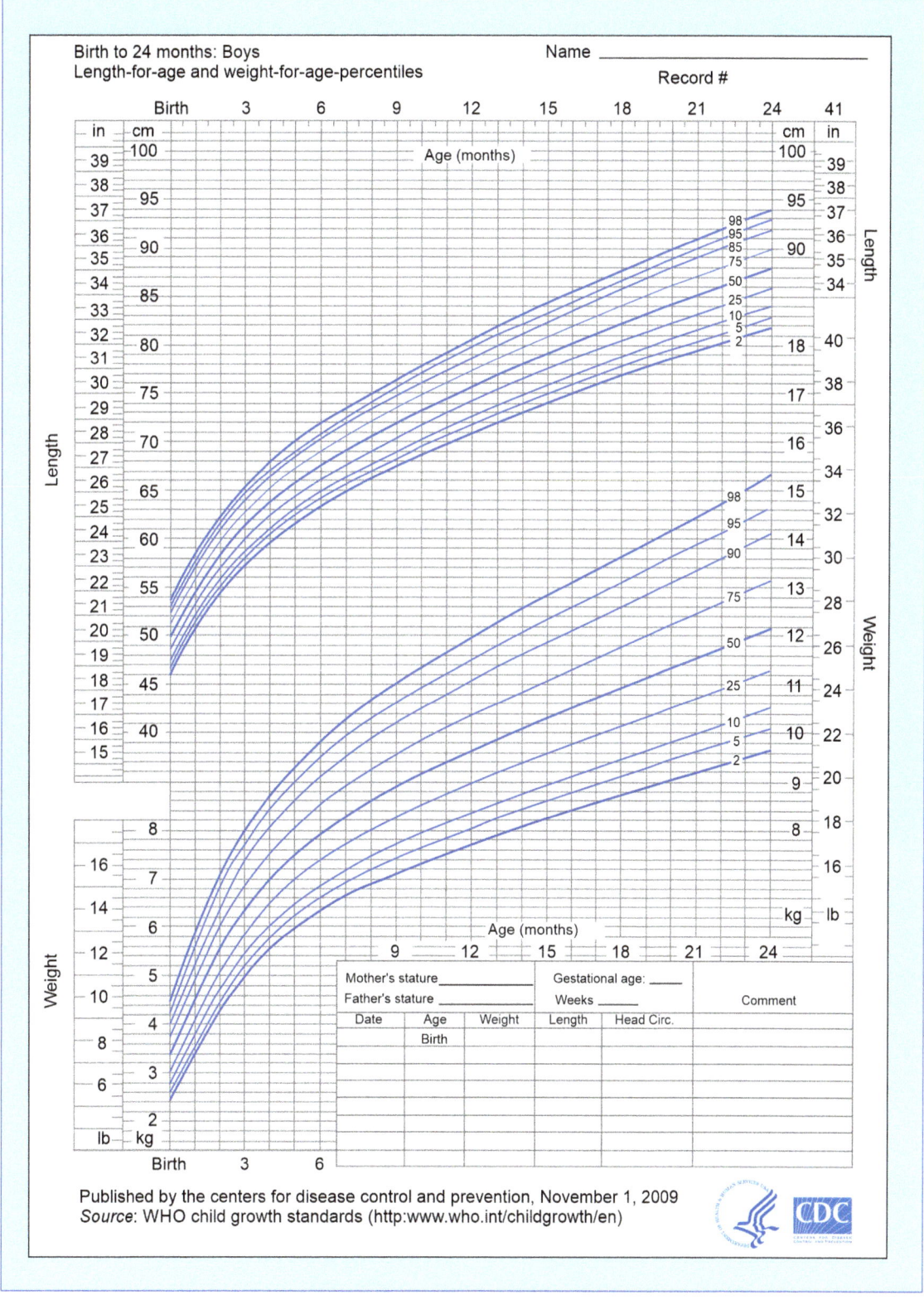

A

Growth chart of boys in first 2 years of life (approximately 12.5 cm length is gained)

FIGS. 2A TO D: *Continued*

128 CHAPTER 7: Disorders of Growth and Development

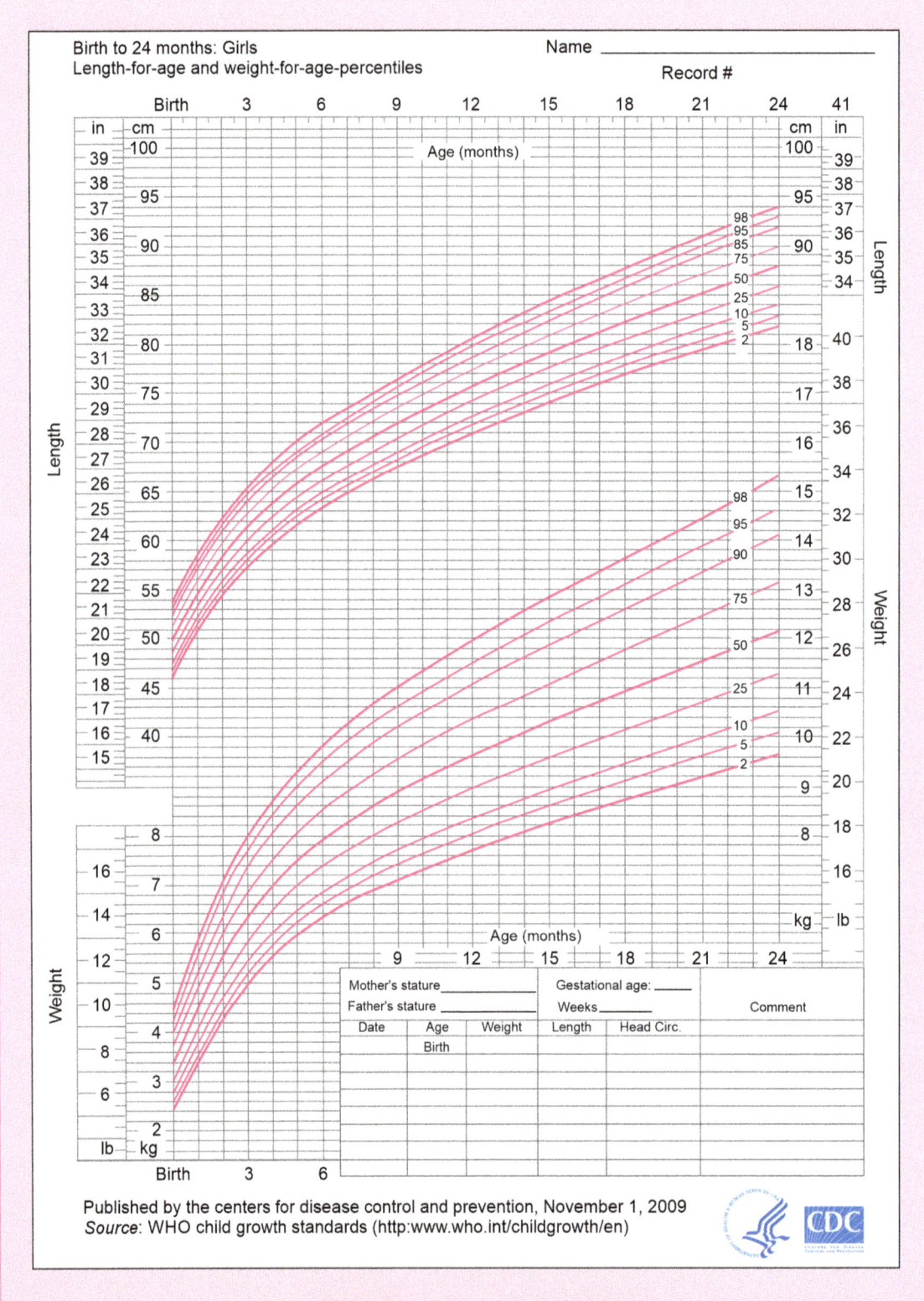

Growth chart of girls in first 2 years of life (approximately 12.5 cm length is gained)

B

FIGS. 2A TO D: *Continued*

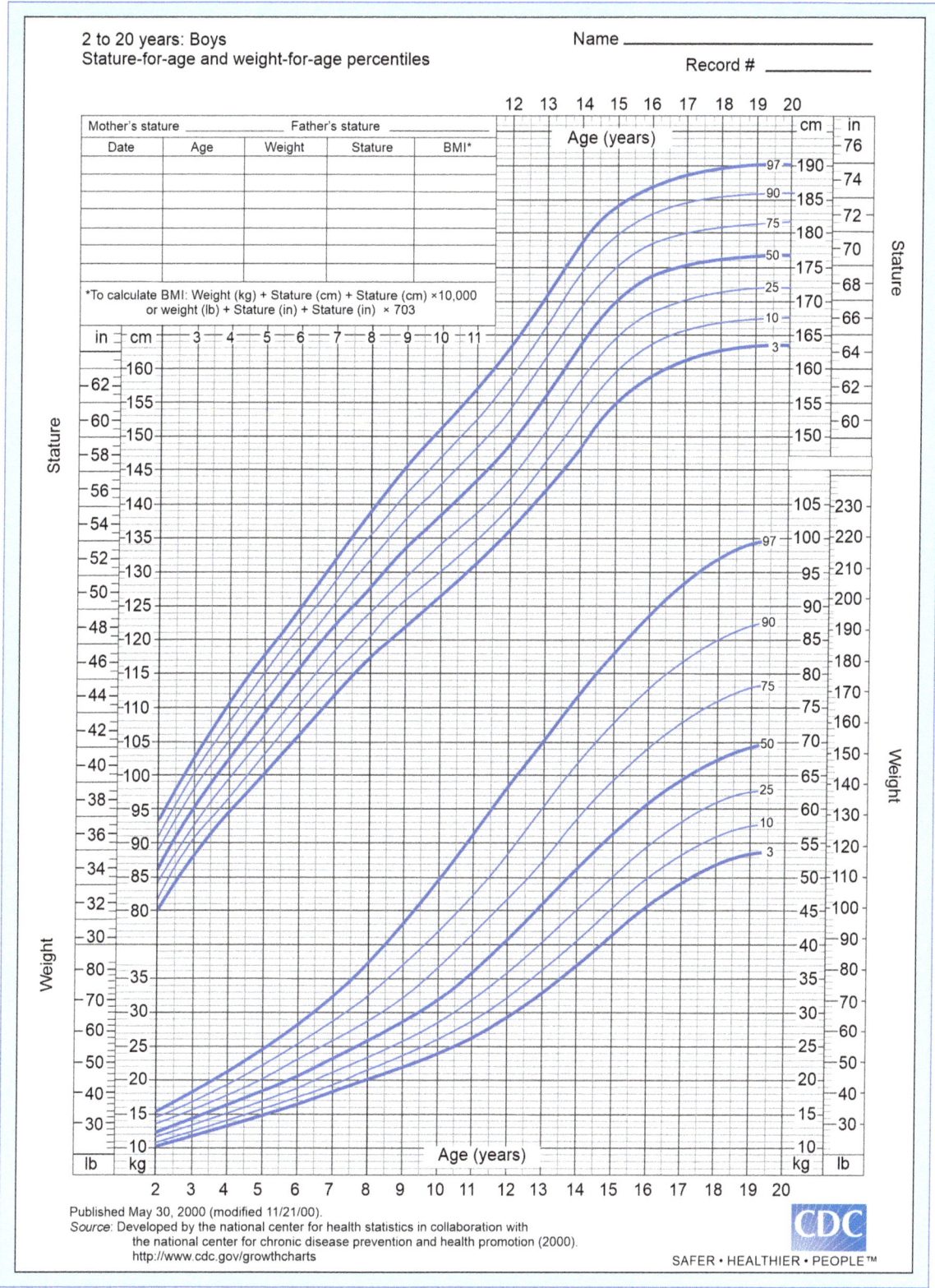

Growth chart of boys in first 2–20 years of life (approximately >100 cm length is gained)

FIGS. 2A TO D: Continued

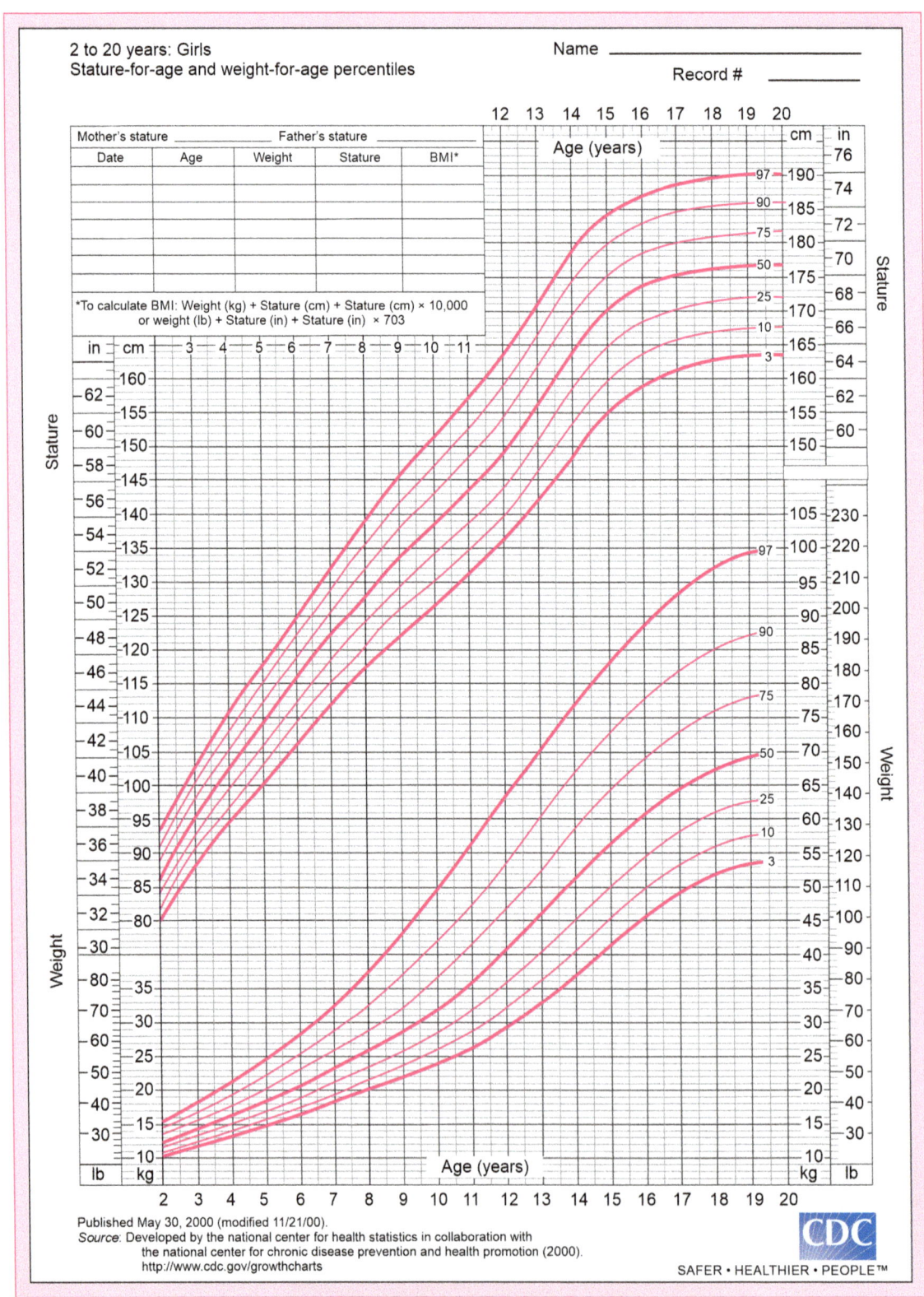

Growth chart of girls in first 2–20 years of life (approximately > 100 cm length is gained)

D

FIGS. 2A TO D: Nomograms used for study growths in children.

CHAPTER 7: Disorders of Growth and Development **131**

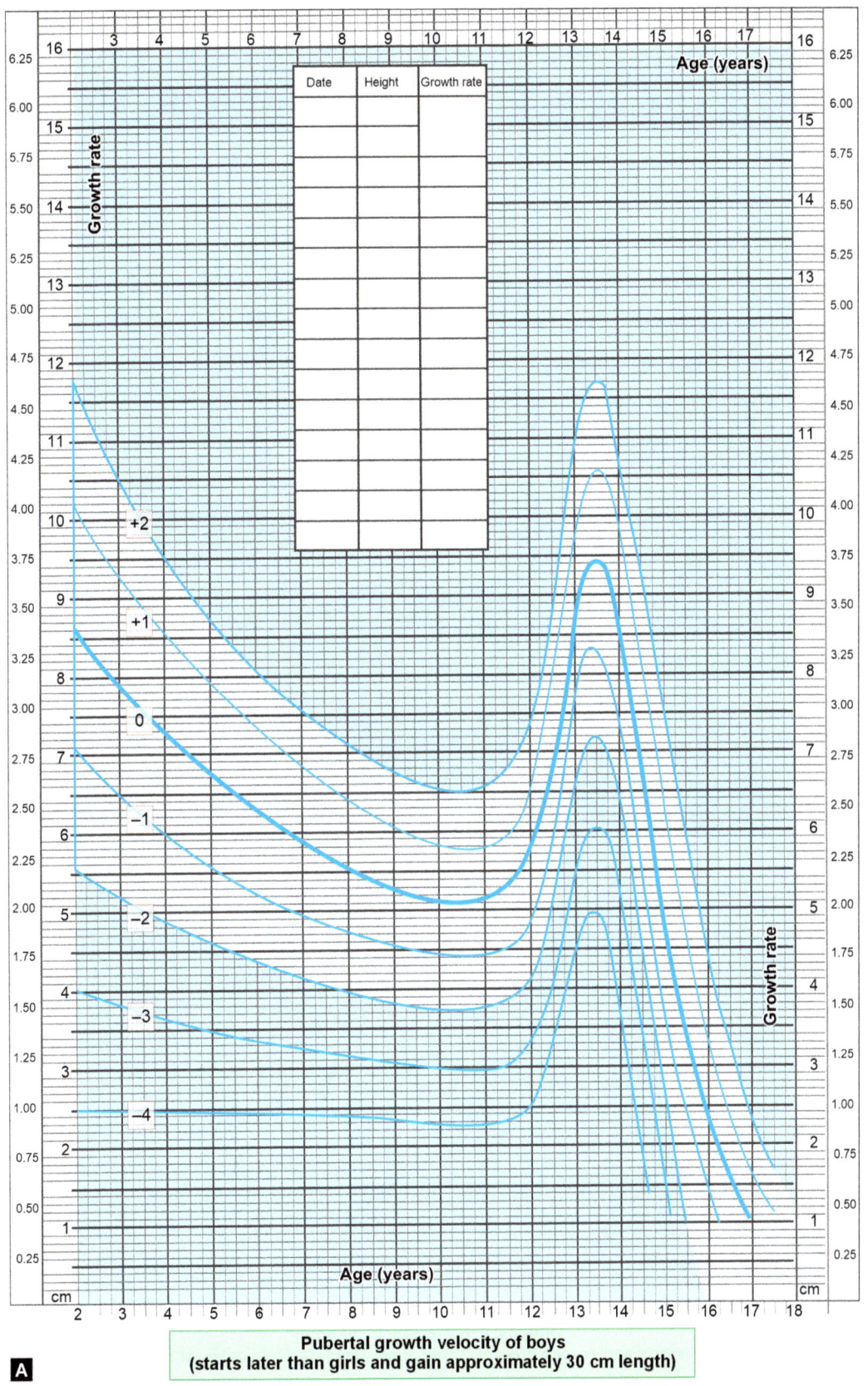

A

Pubertal growth velocity of boys
(starts later than girls and gain approximately 30 cm length)

FIGS. 3A TO C: *Continued*

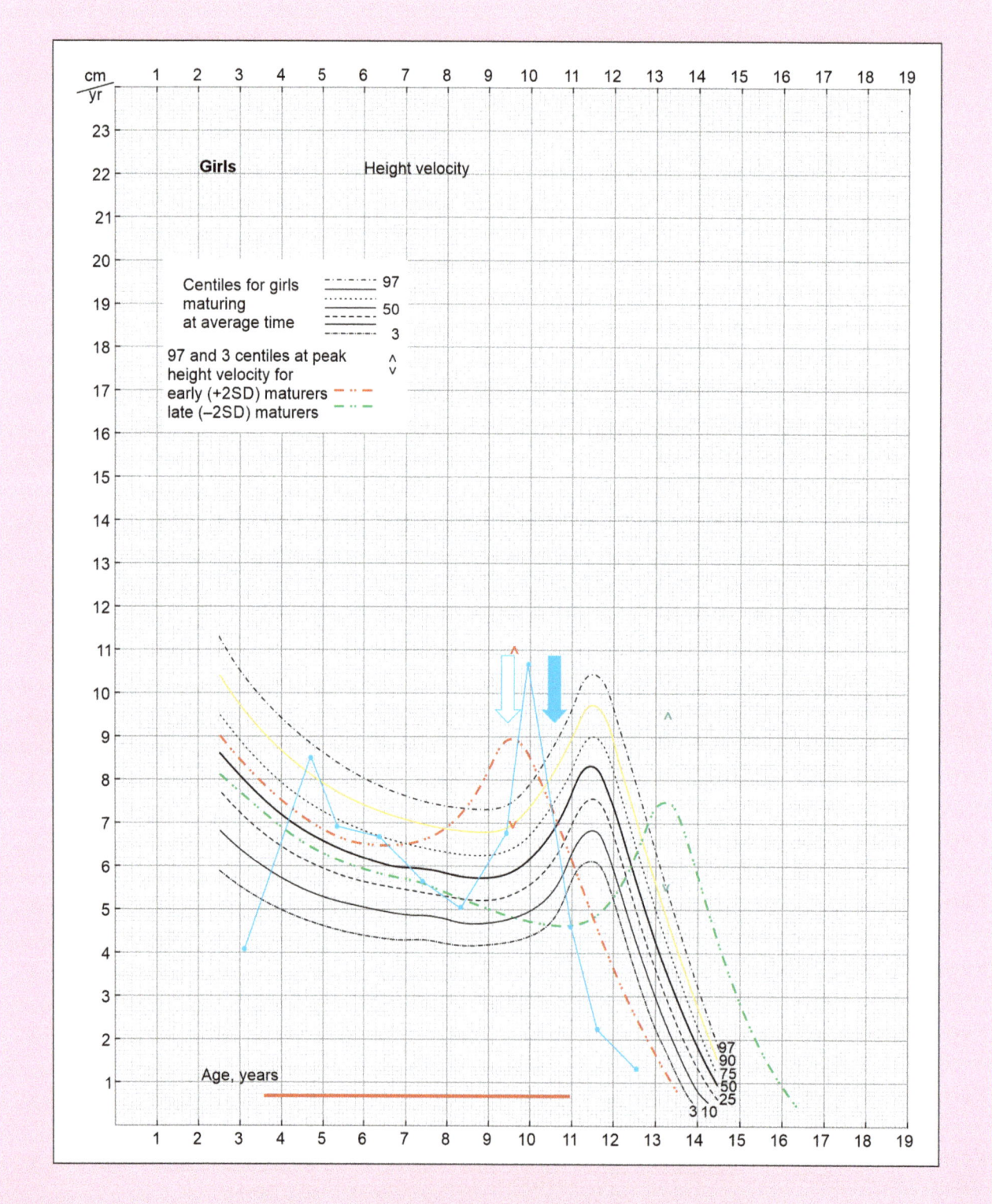

FIGS. 3A TO C: *Continued*

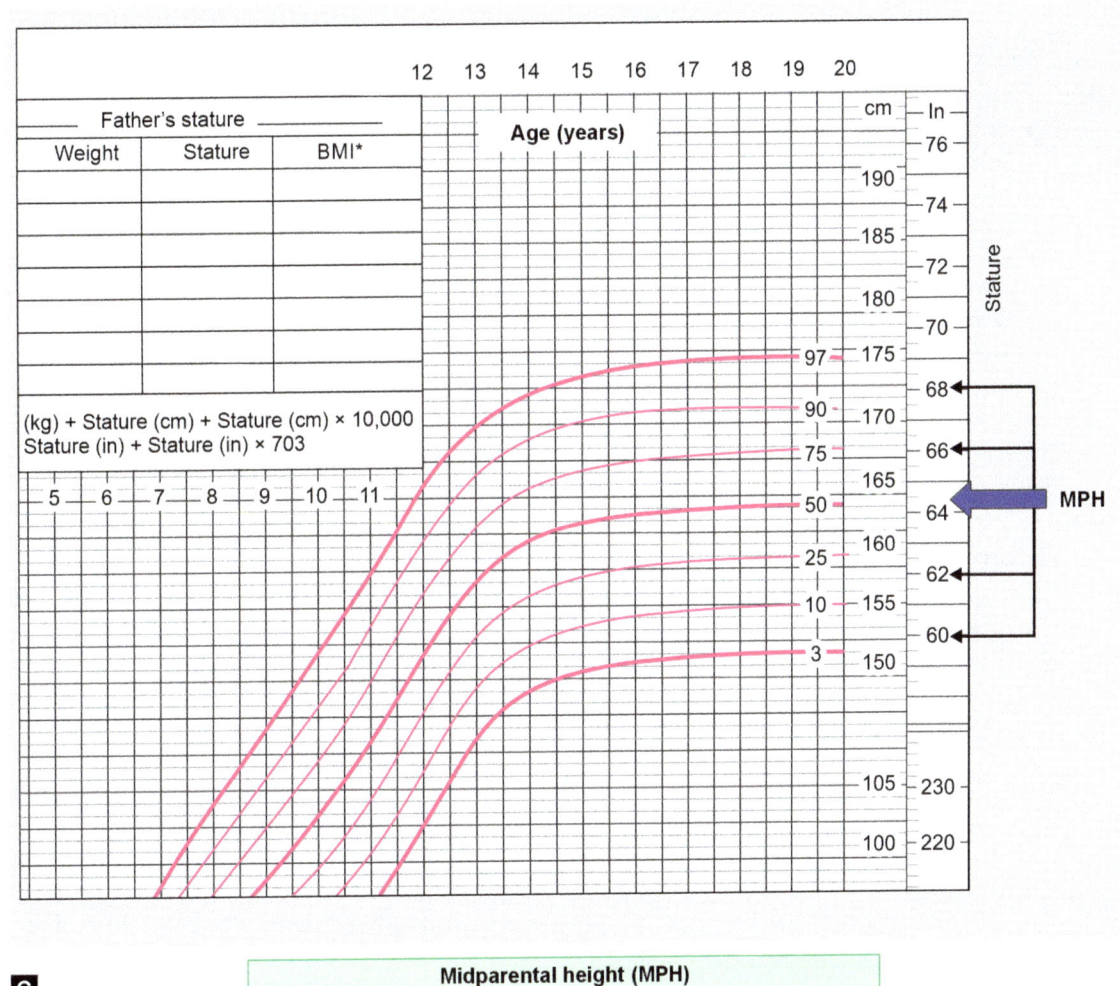

FIGS. 3A TO C: The midparental percentile calculates the expected height of an individual given their parents' heights. (1) The first stage is to take a mean of the parental heights. (2) The midparental height is calculated in males, by adding 7 cm to the mean of parental heights; in females by subtracting 7 cm. This gives the height expected at 18 years for the child. This measurement aids distinction between genetic and constitutional growth disturbances.

TABLE 1: Cause list of short stature.		
Group	**Causes/Diseases**	
Endocrine causes	Growth hormone (GH) deficiency	• Congenital growth hormone deficiency. *Example*: Isolated GH deficiency • Acquired growth hormone deficiency. *Example*: Craniopharyngioma, histiocytosis, cranial irradiation, and brain surgery • Variants of growth hormone deficiency. *Example*: Laron syndrome, Pygmy people, growth hormone insensitivity syndrome (GHIS)
	Other hormone defects	• Hypothyroidism • Cushing's syndrome • Diabetes mellitus • Diabetes insipidus • Panhypopituitarism

Continued

Continued

Group	Causes/Diseases
Nonendocrine causes	• Constitutional short stature (CSS) • Genetic short stature (GSS) • Intrauterine growth retardation (IUGR) • Genetic syndrome with short stature. *Example*: Turner's syndrome, pseudo-Turner's syndrome, Prader–Willi–Lambert (PWL) syndrome, Laurence–Moon–Biedl (LMB) syndrome, and pseudohypoparathyroidism • Chronic diseases. *Example*: Congenital heart disease, chronic renal failure, thalassemia, sickle cell disease, liver disease, celiac disease, Crohn's disease, and chronic diarrhea • Psychological short stature • Skeletal disorders. *Example*: Achondroplasia, hypochondroplasia, epiphyseal dysplasia, and rickets

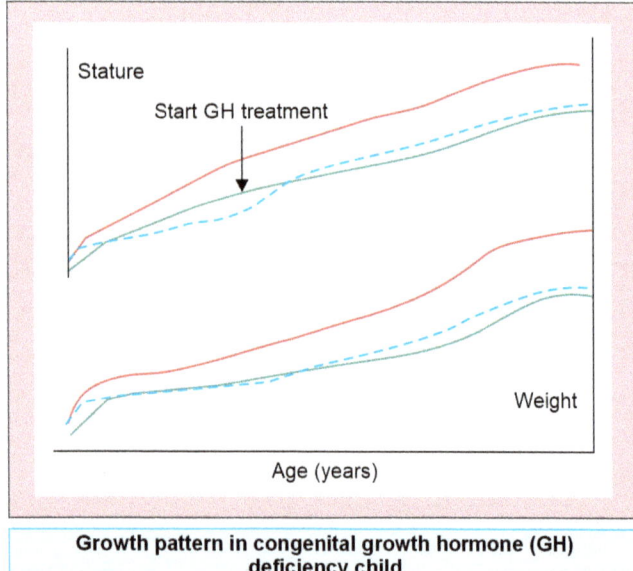

Growth pattern in congenital growth hormone (GH) deficiency child

FIG. 4: Growth curves start going down between 1 and 3 years. Start of replacement therapy returns to normal but in lower centiles.

The common clinical features are:
○ Normal birth weight
○ May have breach presentation at delivery
○ Neonatal hypoglycemia (including seizer)
○ Decreased growth rate soon after birth, obvious in 1-2 years of age
○ Child is short, obese with immature facial appearance.
○ Bone maturity (bone age) is delayed.
○ Microphallus is seen often in boys.
○ Midline anatomical defects such as cleft palate may be seen.
• Acquired growth hormone deficiency in early life (childhood) due to craniopharyngioma, histiocytosis, cranial irradiation, brain surgery, etc. may result in short stature.

• *Variants of growth hormone deficiency*:
  ○ Biologically inactive growth hormone
  ○ Laron short stature
  ○ Pygmy:
    – Biologically inactive growth hormone features are:
      ▪ Serum growth hormone levels normal but somatomedin/insulin-like growth factor (IGF) level low
      ▪ They response with growth hormone treatment—somatomedin/IGF level and growth velocity improves
    – Laron short stature is the predominant feature. Laron syndrome (LS) is an autosomal recessive (AR) disorder. It is due to either growth hormone insensitivity or growth hormone receptor deficiency (GHRD). They can produce insulin-like growth factor 1 (IGF-1; somatomedin) in after growth hormone [GH; human growth hormone (hGH); somatotropin] injection. Classically, the Laron are severe short stature, obesity, craniofacial abnormalities, micropenis, and hypoglycemia. Some of them have low serum IGF-1 despite elevated basal serum growth hormone. Growth hormone receptor gene mutations by molecular genetic testing can confirms the diagnosis. The genetic origins of these individuals seen in Mediterranean, South Asian, and Semitic ancestors **(Fig. 5)**.
    – Pygmy features are:
      ▪ Mostly they are seen in some specific populations of Africa, Oceania, and Myanmar.
      ▪ Pubertal growth spurt (PGS) is absent.
      ▪ Serum growth hormone is higher than normal but somatomedin/IGF level is low.
      ▪ They do not response with growth hormone treatment.
      ▪ Adult males are <150 cm.

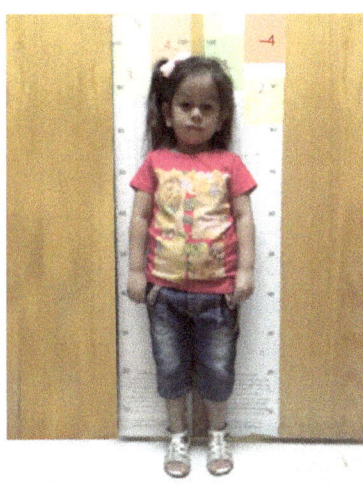

Laron syndrome
(growth hormone insensitivity/
growth hormone receptor deficiency)

FIG. 5: Laron short stature features are: (1) Autosomal recessive disorder; (2) Birth length is less; (3) Birth weight is normal; (4) Serum growth hormone is higher than normal but somatomedin/insulin-like growth factor (IGF) level is low. They do not response with growth hormone treatment—somatomedin/IGF level and growth velocity do not improves.

- Other endocrine disorders responsible for short stature include childhood and congenital hypothyroidism, Cushing's syndrome, diabetes mellitus, diabetes Insipidus, etc.
  - Hypothyroidism of children due congenital or acquired hypothyroid, constitute a significant bulk of short stature. Common features include decreased growth rate may have idiotic facial appearance with low IQ. Their bone maturity (bone age) is delayed. Timed detection and treatment provides best result (see also Chapter 3).
  - Cushing's syndrome (excess glucocorticoid) in children often decrease growth rate prior to expression of other signs symptoms. It occurs both in endogenous (spontaneous) and exogenous (steroid therapy) and is because steroid prevents somatomedin effects on growing cartilage (see also Chapter 5).
  - Diabetes mellitus or diabetes insipidus in child affects growth mostly by severity of disorder and good control improves the final height.

Nonendocrine Causes of Short Stature

- Constitutional short stature (CSS)
- Genetic short stature (GSS)
- Intrauterine growth retardation (IUGR)

- Genetic syndrome with short stature
- Chronic diseases lead to short stature
- Psychological short stature
- Skeletal disorders with short stature

Constitutional short stature characteristic features are **(Fig. 6)**:
- Family incidence common
- Body built thin
- Birth weight and length normal
- Gradual decrease in height gain from second to fourth year of life
- Bone age is returned but proportionate for height
- Delay in onset of puberty
- Final height normal/lower normal

Genetic short stature characteristic features are **(Fig. 7)**:
- Family history positive
- Bone age is normal
- Onset of puberty is normal
- Low genetic height potential
- Corrected height for midparental height is normal.

Intrauterine growth retardation:
- During pregnancy, IUGR is defined by ultrasonographic examination. The most common definition used is fetal weight below the 10th percentile for gestational age according to (national) fetal growth graph. Postnatal characteristic features include (1) Small for gestational age (SGA) infant (exclude prematurity); (2) Body built

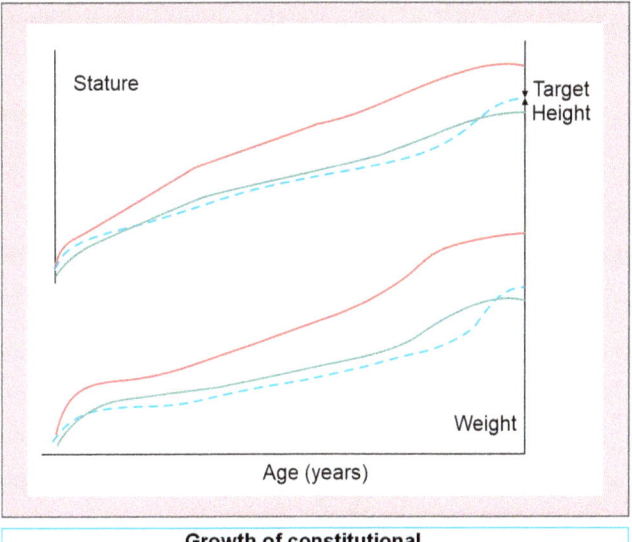

Growth of constitutional
short stature (CSS) children

FIG. 6: Characteristic features constitutional short stature (CSS) are: (1) Family incidence common; (2) Body built thin; (3) Birth weight and length normal; (4) Gradual decrease in height gain from second to fourth year of life; (5) Bone age is returned but proportionate for height; (6) Delay in onset of puberty; (7) Final height normal/lower normal.

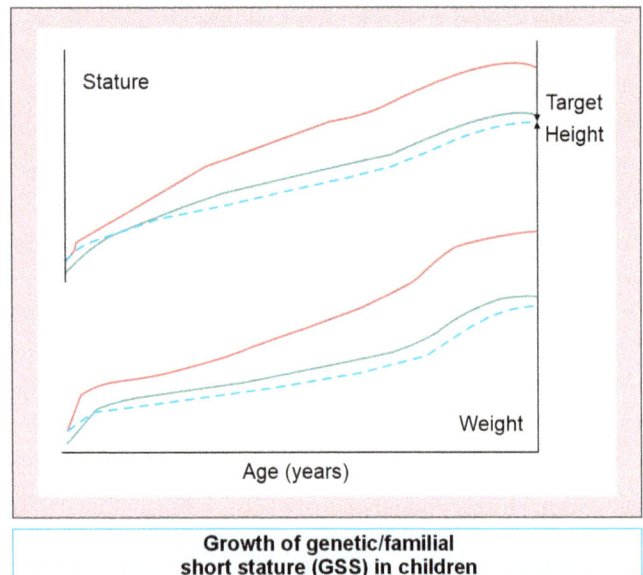

Growth of genetic/familial short stature (GSS) in children

FIG. 7: Characteristic features of GSS are: (1) Family history positive; (2) Bone age is normal; (3) Onset of puberty is normal; (4) Low genetic height potential; (5) Corrected height for mid-parental height is normal.

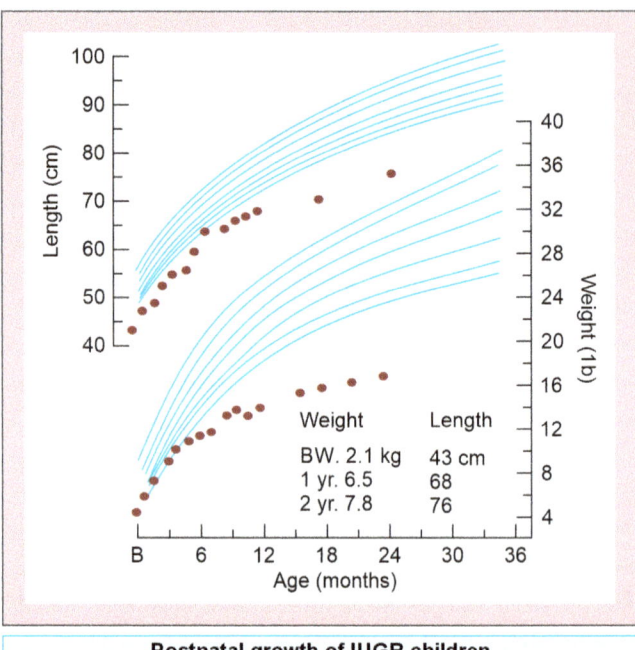

Postnatal growth of IUGR children

FIG. 8: Intrauterine growth retardation (IUGR) postnatal features are: (1) Family history of short stature is negative; (2) Small for gestational age (SGA) infant; (3) Body built thin; (4) Bone age is normal; (5) Onset of puberty is normal.

thin; (3) Bone age is normal; (4) Onset of puberty is normal; (5) No catchup growth so final height is low; (6) Normal growth hormone level, and (7) Family history of short stature is negative.
- There are several maternal factors that can be responsible for IURG. Factors include (1) general factors, such as age, weight, uncontrolled hypertension, glucose intolerance, race of mother; (2) socioeconomic factors, such as mother's nutrition status, tobacco (active and passive), alcohol, drugs, and coffee consumption. Therefore, there is scope of primary prevention of IURG by preconception planned pregnancy practice **(Fig. 8)**.

Genetic syndrome with short stature: Characteristic features are stigmata of the syndrome and short stature (see later part of this chapter):
- Turner's syndrome
- Pseudo-Turner's syndrome
- Prader-Willi-Lambert syndrome
- Laurence-Moon-Biedl syndrome (LMB)
- Pseudohypoparathyroidism and pseudopseudo-hypoparathyroidism (see Chapter 4).

Chronic diseases lead to short stature: Congenital heart disease, chronic renal failure, thalassemia, sickle cell disease, liver disease, celiac disease, Crohn's disease, chronic diarrhea, etc. in childhood may decrease growth velocity and lead to short stature.

Psychological short stature (PSS): It is a disorder of short stature or growth failure and/or delayed puberty. It occurs due to emotional deprivation, a pathologic psychosocial environment, or both.

The victims show following features:
- They are from families where they were ignored or severely disciplined
- History of caloric deprivation or physical battering may be present
- They develop buzzer eating and drinking habits
- Children may have functional hypopituitarism
- Diagnosis depends on improved behavior or catch-up growth in hospital or in a foster home **(Fig. 9)**.

Skeletal disorders such as skeletal dysplasia and rickets produce short stature:
- Achondroplasias
- Hypochondroplasia
- Epiphyseal dysplasia
- Rickets (see Chapter 4)

Investigations for a child with short stature are grouped into three categories (1) Observation of growth velocity, (2) Screening studies, and (3) Full investigation. Selection of investigation category depends on his/her attained height and growth velocity. **Table 2** summarized the investigation categories to evaluate a short stature.

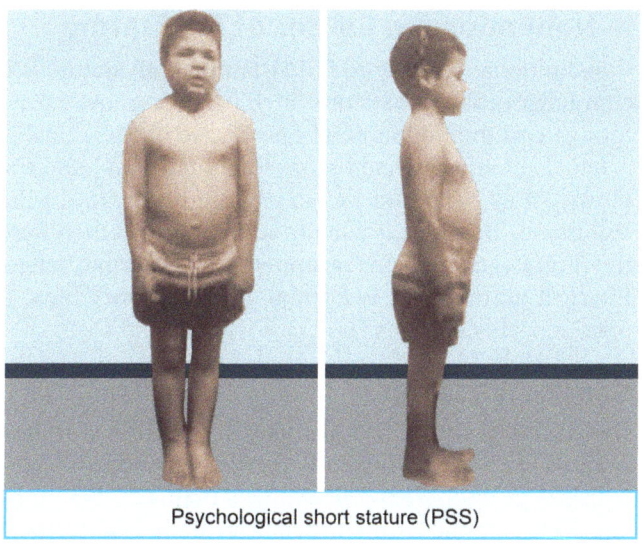

FIG. 9: Diagnosis depends on improved behavior or catch-up growth in hospital or in a foster home.

TABLE 3: Causes of tall stature.	
Group	Disease
Endocrine causes	• Pituitary gigantism (growth hormone excess before epiphyseal closure) • Thyrotoxicosis (thyroid hormone excess before epiphyseal closure) • Sexual precocity (temporary due to premature exposure to sex hormone) • Hypogonadism (eunuch due to delay of epiphyseal closure due to lack of sex hormone)
Nonendocrine causes	• Constitutional tall stature (CTS) • Genetic tall stature (GTS) • Cerebral gigantism • Marfan's syndrome • Beckwith–Wiedemann syndrome • Homocystinuria • Extra-Y syndrome

TABLE 2: When to initiate investigation of a short child?	
Findings	Actions
Height between mean and 2 standard deviation (SD) below the mean for age	Observe growth velocity
Height between mean and 2 SD below the mean for age and Growth velocity less than 3rd percentile for age	Screening studies
Height below 2 SD the mean for age or Growth velocity less than 3rd percentile for age	Full investigation

Screening studies for short child are:
- Detailed history and physical examination
- Evaluation of available developmental data
- Renal function ability to acidify and to concentrate urine
- *Biochemical test*: Creatinine, electrolytes, calcium, phosphorus, alkaline phosphatase, thyroid function status, and IGF-1
- X-ray for bone age and Sella
- Karyotype for girls

TALL STATURE

An individual is of tall stature when (1) abnormally tall height/length (>2.5 SD above for age); (2) abnormally high growth velocity (>2.5 SD above for age during 2–9 years), or (3) abnormally high height corrected for midparental height (>2.5 SD above).

Causes of tall stature: **Table 3** summarized the causes of tall stature.

Pituitary Gigantism

Pituitary gigantism is due to growth hormone excess if it occurs prior to fusion of the epiphyseal growth plates. Therefore, it starts in growing children. Serum growth hormone and IGF-1 are raised and results in rapid and excessive linear growth and so becomes very tall in adult. It is a rare disorder. Pituitary gigantism typically is a sporadic and isolated condition. Sometime, it may be a component of some familial syndrome, for example:
- McCune–Albright syndrome (MAS)
- Multiple endocrine neoplasia type 1 (MEN1)
- Multiple endocrine neoplasia type 4 (MEN4), etc.

Nearly half of patients with pituitary gigantism have a known underlying genetic cause; therefore, these patients should be considered for genetic counseling and screening.

Once growth hormone hypersecretion has been established, prompt initiation of treatment should start to control levels of growth hormone and IGF-1.

Somatotropinomas in pituitary gigantism are usually large. Surgery or medical therapy alone might be difficult to cure; therefore, multimodal approaches are common in pituitary gigantism. Multiple surgeries and radiotherapy in patients with pituitary gigantism often lead to hypopituitarism. Long-term follow-up is required **(Fig. 10)**.

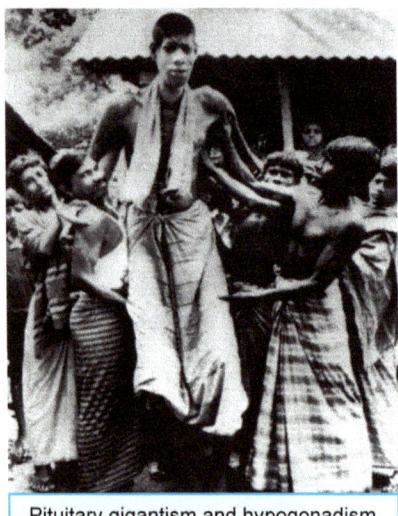

FIG. 10: *Parimal Chandra* Barman born in 1962 in Bangladesh was considered the tallest person in the world in 1991 at 2.51 m (8 ft 3 inch). Parimal had a growth hormone (GH)-secreting pituitary tumor causing his incredible growth spurt. He had hypogonadism due to mass effect of the tumor resulting in eunuchoid body proportions.

Nonendocrine Causes of Tall Stature

Constitutional tall stature (CTS)/familial tall stature is a common cause of tall stature. Their height is above 2.5 SD for age and the midparental height also above +2.5 SD. A female child is affected more than male child and the mother may have had her unusual tall stature during childhood. The bone is usually advanced; and therefore, the final height remains at upper side of normal range. Physical examination is normal and laboratory tests, if obtained, are negative **(Fig. 11)**.

Genetic Tall Stature

Genetic tall stature (GTS) characteristic features are: Their parents are tall. The height is consistently above 2.5 SD for age but midparental height less than +2.5 SD. Bone age is close to the chronological age. There is absence of signs relating to other causes of tall stature. Final height is tall. Final height can be reduced by promoting early epiphyseal closure with estrogen (girls) and testosterone (boys) **(Fig. 12)**.

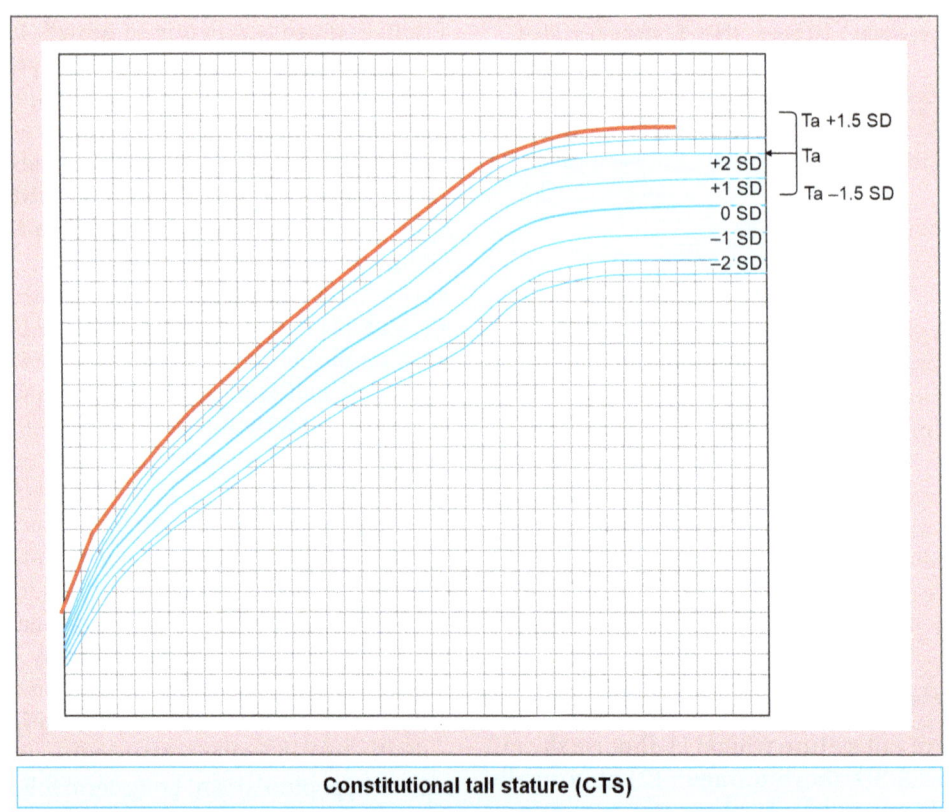

FIG. 11: Constitutional tall stature (CTS) characteristic features are: (1) Taller than peers; (2) Growth velocity within normal range for bone age; (3) Bone age is usually more than the chronological age; (4) Final height usually within normal adult range.

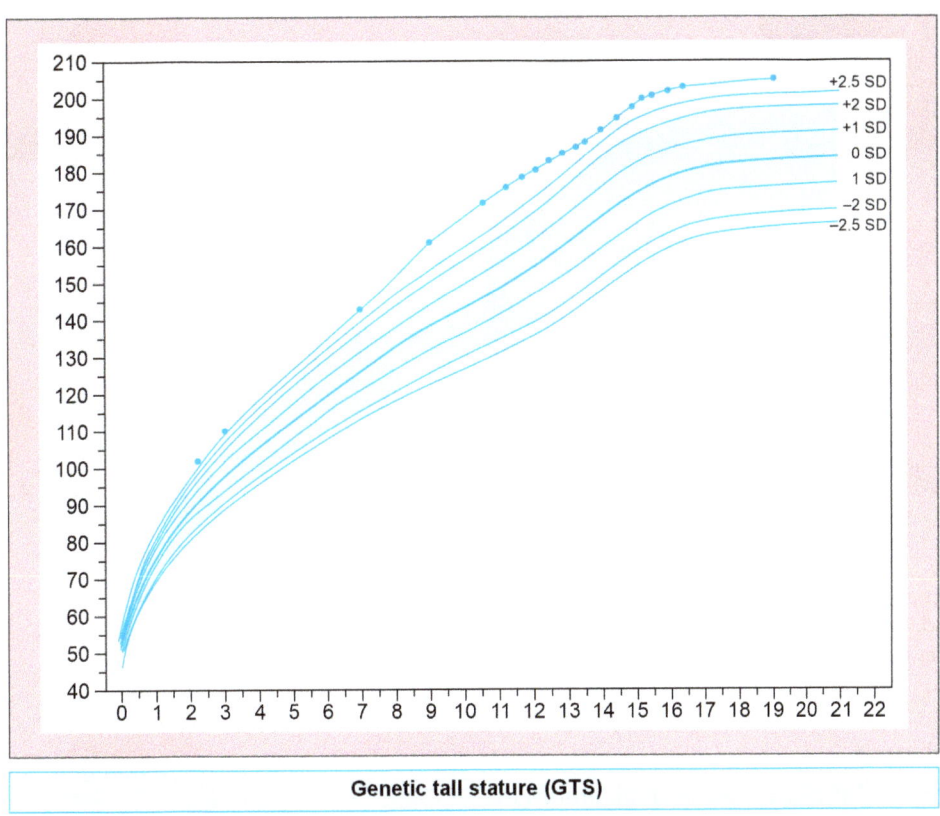

FIG. 12: Genetic tall stature (GTS) characteristic features are: (1) Genetic height potential is high (parents are tall); (2) Growth/height is more than +2.5 SD; (3) Bone age is close to the chronological age; (4) Absence of signs relating to other causes of tall stature; (5) Final height is more than +2.5 SD which can be reduced by estrogen (girls) or testosterone (boys).

Cerebral Gigantism

Cerebral gigantism or Sotos syndrome is a rare genetic disorder caused by mutation in the *NSD1* gene on chromosome 5. It is characterized by birth with macrosomia (weight >4 kg) with length and weight >97th percentile. The overgrowth usually continues till 4–5 years of age; thereafter, it becomes normal. The bone is advanced; so, the final adult height is in the upper normal range. Other features include prominent forehead, high-arched palate, hypertelorism, mental instability, etc. There is no laboratory or radiological feature of cerebral gigantism **(Figs. 13A and B)**.

Beckwith–Wiedemann Syndrome (BWS)

Its other name is fetal overgrowth syndrome. Its feature includes macrocephaly, macroglossia, omphalocele, hepatosplenomegaly, and hypoglycemia due to pancreatic B-cell hyperplasia. Bone age is advance and adult height is usually within normal range. In some cases of Beckwith–Wiedemann syndrome (BWS), genetic study documented duplication of paternal *IGF-2* gene which may be linked with overexpression of IGF-2 in BWS **(Fig. 14)**.

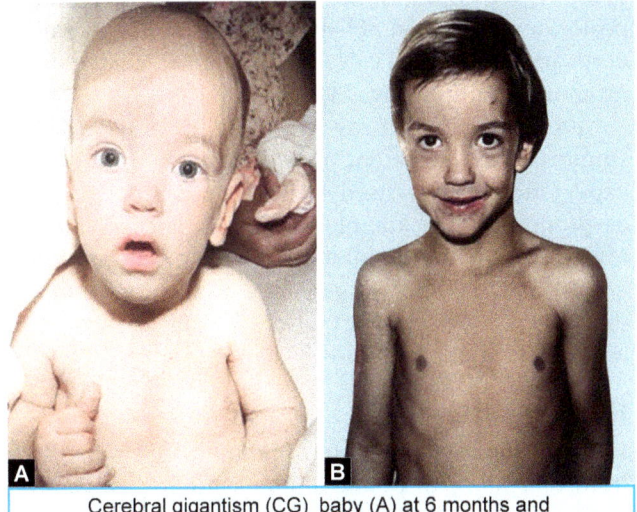

Cerebral gigantism (CG) baby (A) at 6 months and (B) 4 years 6 months

FIGS. 13A AND B: Cerebral gigantism (CG) Characteristic features are: (1) macrosomia (birth weight >4 kg) with length and weight >97th percentile; (2) The growth velocity high till 4–5 years of age and then returns to the normal rate; (3) The bone is advanced so the final adult height is in the upper normal range; (4) Other features include prominent forehead, high-arched palate, hypertelorism, mental instability, etc.

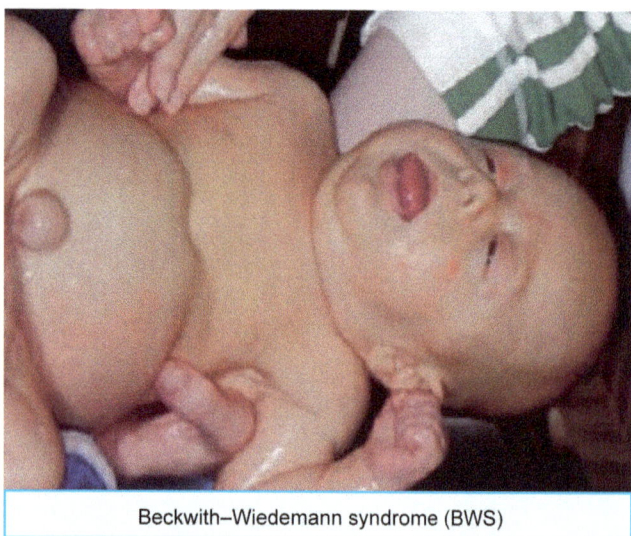

Beckwith–Wiedemann syndrome (BWS)

FIG. 14: Beckwith–Wiedemann syndrome (BWS) is characterized by macrocephaly, macroglossia, omphalocele, hepatosplenomegaly, and hypoglycemia due to pancreatic B-cell hyperplasia; Bone age is advance; Adult height is usually within normal range.

Marfan's Syndrome

Marfan's syndrome (MS) is an autosomal dominant disorder due to defective fibrillin gene on chromosome 15. In MS, there is defect in synthesis of fibrillin. MS is characterized by tall and thin built, eunuchoid body proportions, long thin spider like figure (arachnodactyly), pectus excavatum, joint laxity, high-arched palate, posterior subluxation of lens, aneurism of the ascending aorta, prolapse mitral valve, etc. Diagnosis is often based on clinical features **(Fig. 15)**.

There is no known cure for MS till date. With proper supportive management, they may have a normal life expectancy. Drugs used in MS are β-blockers such as propranolol or atenolol. And if β-blockers are not tolerated, calcium channel blockers or ACE inhibitors are used. Sometimes surgery may be required to repair the aorta or replace a heart valve. They are also advised to avoiding strenuous exercise.

Homocystinuria

Homocystinuria is an amino acid metabolism resulting from deficiency of cystathionine synthase. It is an AR disorder. Its gene is located on chromosome 21. Its characteristic features are tall body, eunuchoid body proportions, mental retardation, arachnodactyly, inferior subluxation of lens, etc. Mark tendency of arterial thrombosis resulting in myocardial infarction.

Laboratory findings includes (1) urine cyanide nitroprusside test positive and (2) in urine homocysteine present. Megaloblastic anemia is supportive finding. Methylenetetrahydrofolate reductase (MTHFR) enzyme

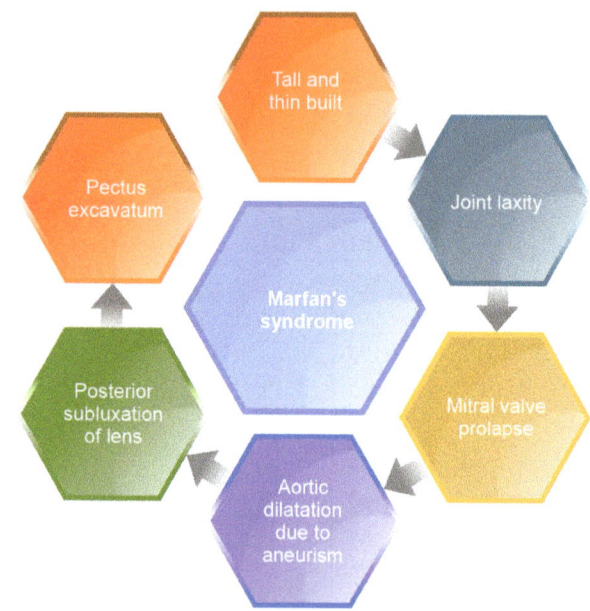

FIG. 15: Features of Marfan's syndrome.

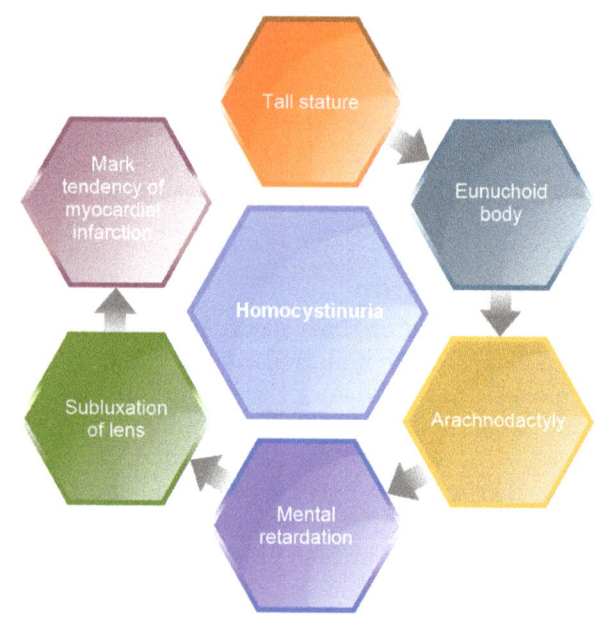

FIG. 16: Features of homocystinuria.

activity of cultured fibroblast or leukocytes is to confirm diagnosis. MTHFR activity of chorionic villus culture or amniocyte culture is used for prenatal diagnosis. Deoxyribonucleic acid (DNA) analysis is used for family screening.

Treatment of homocystinuria is supplementation of folic acid, vitamin B6, and vitamin B12, methionine in addition to put them on a special protein-restricted diet to reduce the blood levels of homocysteine and methionine. Early initiation of betaine (trimethylglycine) treatment is also showing effective **(Fig. 16)**.

Extra-Y Syndrome OR 47,XYY Syndrome

It is characterized by taller stature. Most individuals have normal male feature due to normal testosterone levels and normal male sexual development. They are able to be father. Children can have delayed development of motor skills such as sitting and walking. Their muscle tone is weak (hypotonia). Other signs and symptoms include attention-deficit or hyperactivity disorder, depression, anxiety, autism, etc. Physical features may include fatty belly, macrocephaly, macrodontia, pes planus, fifth fingers that curve inward (clinodactyly), widely spaced eyes (ocular hypertelorism), and scoliosis **(Fig. 17)**.

OBESITY

Obesity is a complex disease involving an excessive amount of body fat. Clinical measurement of adipose mass is difficult; therefore, some indices on weight and height relations are used for this purpose.

For growing children, height age is determined by putting his/her height at 50th percentile of age-height chart and then looking the weight at age-weight chart. Weight above 2.5 SD is leveled as obese **(Fig. 18)**.

For adult most popularly body mass index (BMI) is used.

It is defined by formula BMI = (Weight in kg)/(Height in meter)^2

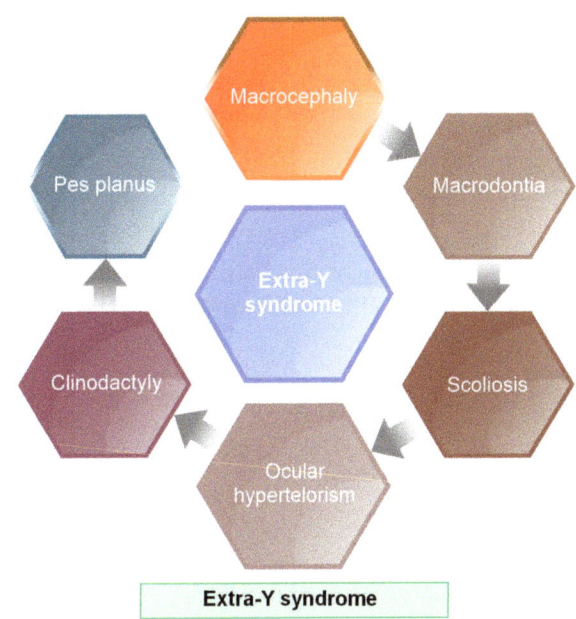

FIG. 17: Extra-Y syndrome or 47,XYY syndrome characterized by several features. They include increased belly fat, macrocephaly, macrodontia, pes planus, fifth fingers that curve inward (clinodactyly), widely spaced eyes (ocular hypertelorism), and scoliosis.

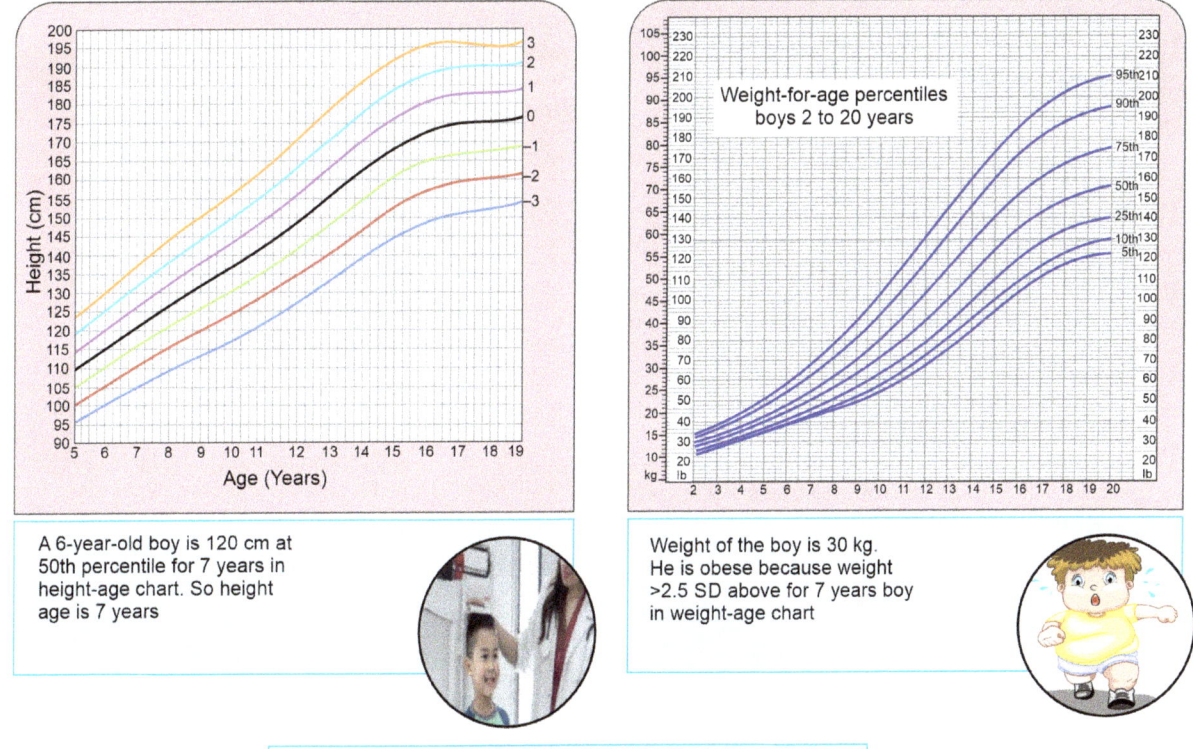

A 6-year-old boy is 120 cm at 50th percentile for 7 years in height-age chart. So height age is 7 years

Weight of the boy is 30 kg. He is obese because weight >2.5 SD above for 7 years boy in weight-age chart

Obesity in children

FIG. 18: Obesity = weight >2.5 standard deviation (SD) for height age.

Normal range of BMI for adult male and female are 20–25 and 19–24, respectively.

There is a percent BMI system where 22.1 and 20.6 is taken as 100% for male and female respectively and obesity is graded as shown in **Table 4**.

Other methods of body fat measurements include (1) under water body weight and (2) skinfold thickness measurement by constant tension skin calipers, bioelectrical impedance analysis, etc.

Types of obesity:
- Based on pattern of fat distribution (1) Gynecoid (around hip) or (2) Android (around waist) **(Fig. 19)**
- Based on time of onset (1) neonatal, (2) childhood, (3) peripubertal, or (4) adult **(Fig. 20)**
- Based on pattern of adipose mass (1) hypertrophic-hyperplastic adipose cell number and size increases as in peripubertal onset obesity or (2) Hyperplastic type—adipose cell size increases as in adult onset obesity **(Fig. 21)**.

Causes of obesity are described in **Table 5**.

TABLE 4: Percent body mass index (BMI) system.	
% BMI	Grade (interpretation)
>140	Morbid obese
130–139	Very obese
120–120	Obese
80–119	Normal
<80	Lean

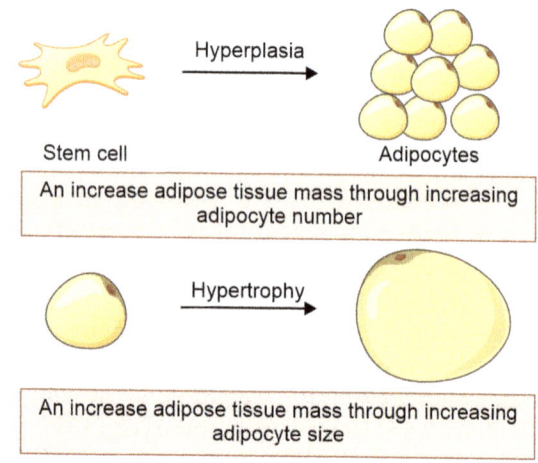

FIG. 21: Two types of obesity based on adipose mass: (1) Hypertrophic-hyperplastic and (2) Hyperplastic type.

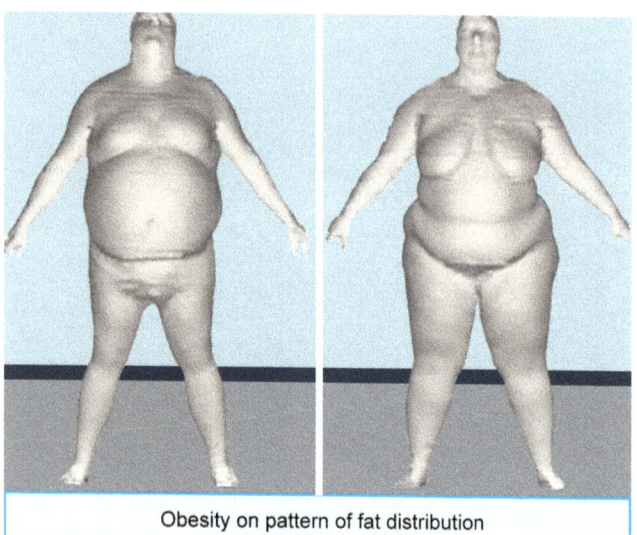

FIG. 19: Two types: (1) Android (around waist/pear shape) or (2) Gynecoid (around hip/apple shape).

TABLE 5: Cause/diseases for obesity.	
Group	Cause/diseases for obesity
Endocrine	• Cushing's syndrome • Hypothyroidism • Hyperinsulinemia (insulinoma) • Hypogonadism associated obesity as in Turner's syndrome, Klinefelter's syndrome, etc.
Nonendocrine	• Exogenous obesity • Syndrome associated obesity as in syndrome X, Prader–Willi–Lambert syndrome, Laurence–Moon–Biedl syndrome, Alström–Hallgren syndrome, Froehlich's syndrome, hyperostosis frontalis interna, and multiple lipomatosis

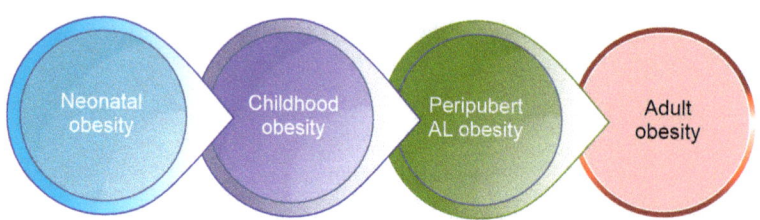

FIG. 20: Type of obesity based on time of onset.

For the endocrine disorders associated with obesity, diagnostic workup and management are given in respective chapters of disorder.

Exogenous obesity is caused by consuming more food than the person's activity level warrants, leading to increased fat storage. They are neither associated with endocrine disorders nor with specific genetic syndrome. The factors influencing obesity are genetic trend of obesity and socioeconomic affluence of consuming high caloric and fatty diet.

Metabolic syndrome (other name syndrome X, insulin resistance syndrome, and dysmetabolic syndrome): It is a collection of risk factors for developing heart disease, stroke, and diabetes, etc. It is characterized by (1) android obesity, (2) hypertension, (3) type 2 diabetes mellitus or impaired glucose tolerance (IGT), (4) dyslipidemia [very low-density lipoprotein (VLDL) and triglyceride (TG) high and low high-density lipoprotein (HDL)], and (5) hyperinsulinemia **(Fig. 22)**.

■ Prader–Willi–Lambert (PWL) Syndrome

It is a genetic disorder caused by a loss of function of specific genes on chromosome 15. It is characterized by (1) obesity, (2) hypotonia, (3) small hands and feet (acromicria), (4) almond-shaped eyes, (5) short stature, (6) mental retardation, (7) delayed puberty, (8) diabetes mellitus, and (9) deletion or translocation of chromosome 15 **(Fig. 23)**.

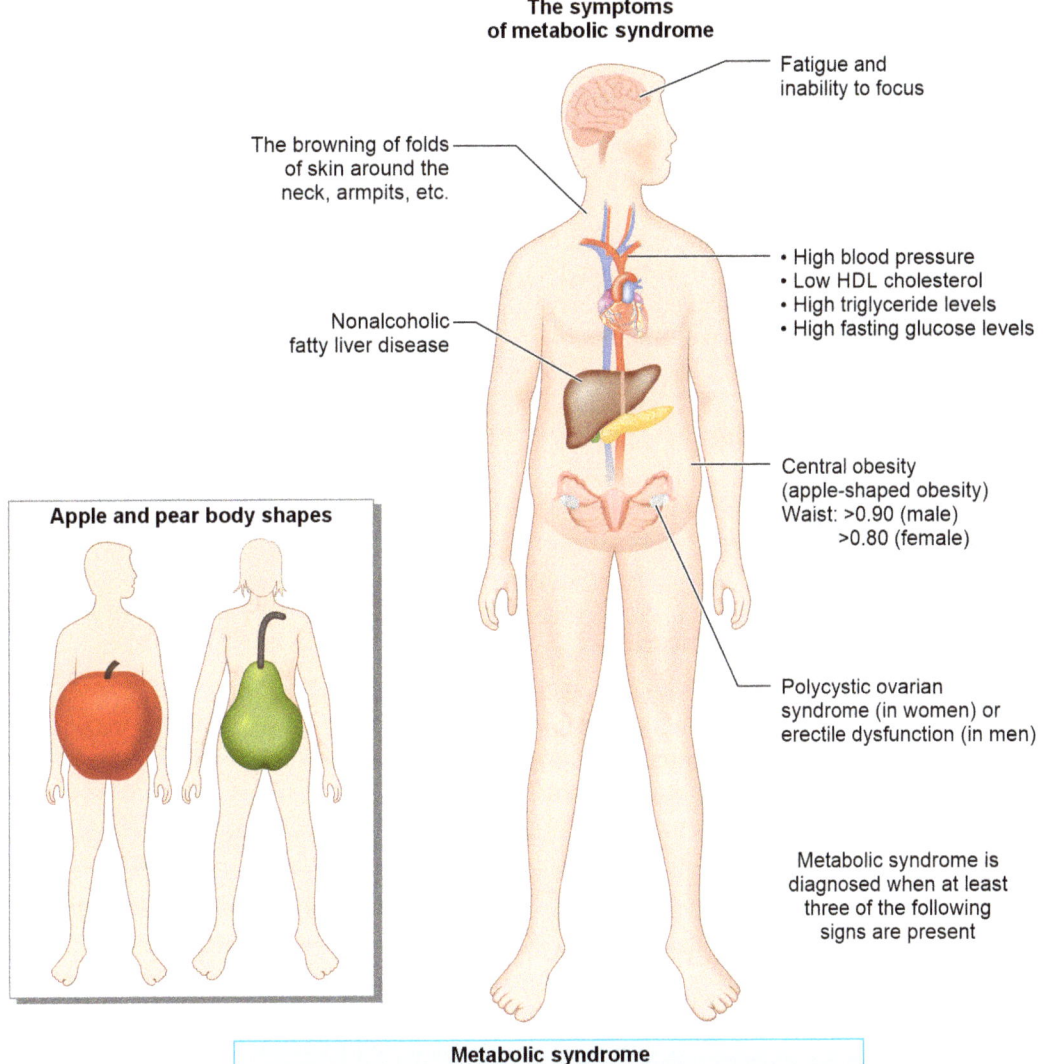

FIG. 22: Characterized by (1) Android obesity; (2) Hypertension; (3) Type 2 diabetes mellitus or impaired glucose tolerance (IGT); (4) Dyslipidemia [very low-density lipoprotein (VLDL) and triglyceride (TG) high and low high-density lipoprotein (HDL)].

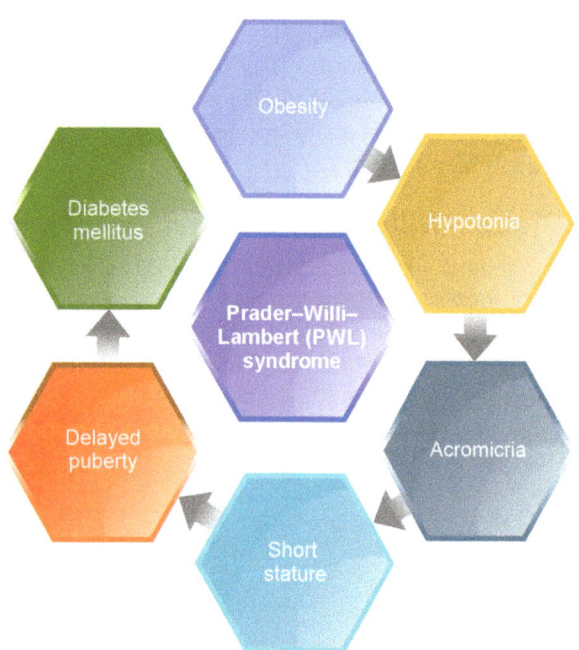

FIG. 23: Features of Prader–Willi–Lambert (PWL) syndrome.

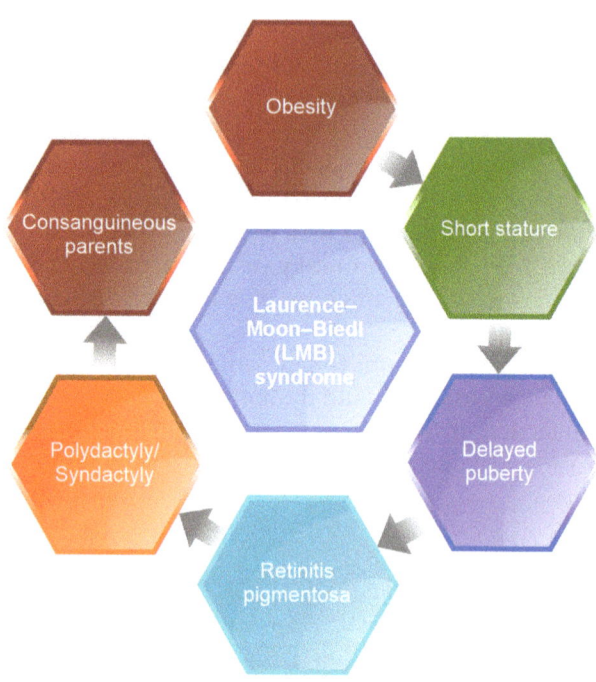

FIG. 24: Features of Laurence–Moon–Biedl (LMB) syndrome.

Laurence–Moon–Biedl Syndrome

It is a rare AR disorder associated. It is characterized by (1) obesity, (2) retinitis pigmentosa, (3) polydactyly/syndactyly, (4) short stature, (5) delayed puberty/hypogonadism, and (6) usually issue of a consanguineous couple **(Fig. 24)**.

Alström–Hallgren Syndrome

Features of Alström syndrome include (1) progressive loss of vision and hearing, (2) dilated cardiomyopathy, (3) childhood obesity, (4) type 2 diabetes, and (5) short stature **(Fig. 25)**.

Froehlich's Syndrome (Other Name Adiposogenital Dystrophy)

It is due to endocrine abnormalities developed from damage to the hypothalamus. It is characterized by (1) android obesity, (2) short stature, (3) microphallus and hypogonadism, (4) adiposogenital dystrophy, (5) decreased visual acuity, (6) diabetes insipidus, and (7) mental retardation **(Fig. 26)**.

Hyperostosis Frontalis Interna

It is characterized by (1) obesity, (2) females are affected more with hirsutism, (3) variety of neuropsychiatric complaints with (4) small rounded exostosis arising from the inner table of frontal bone.

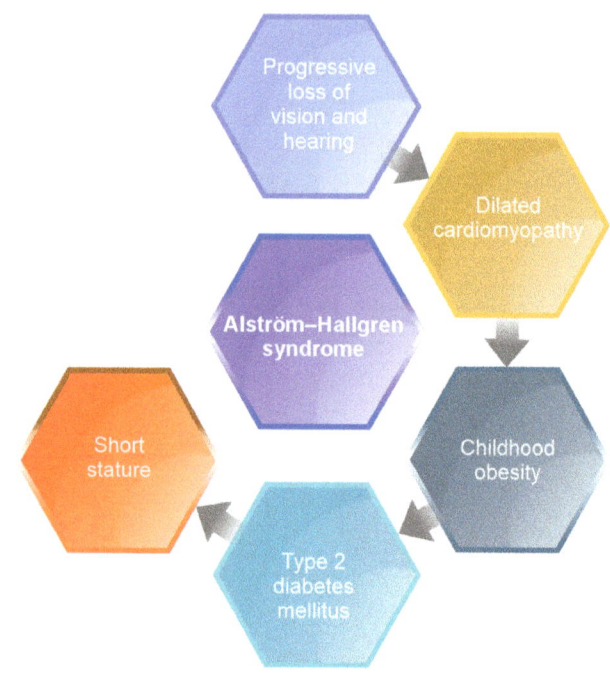

FIG. 25: Features of Alström–Hallgren syndrome.

Multiple Lipomatosis

It is characterized by (1) obesity; (2) noncapsulated lipomas in the nape of neck, supraclavicular or deltoid region (bull neck appearance); (3) lipomas anywhere

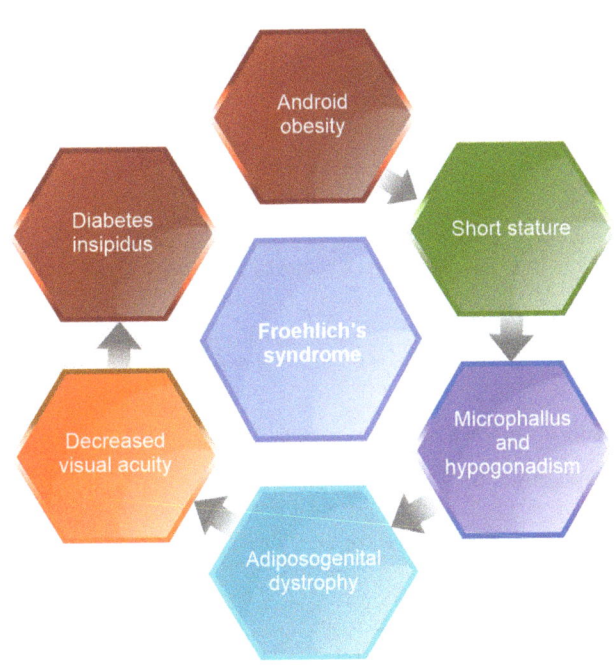

FIG. 26: Features of Froehlich's syndrome.

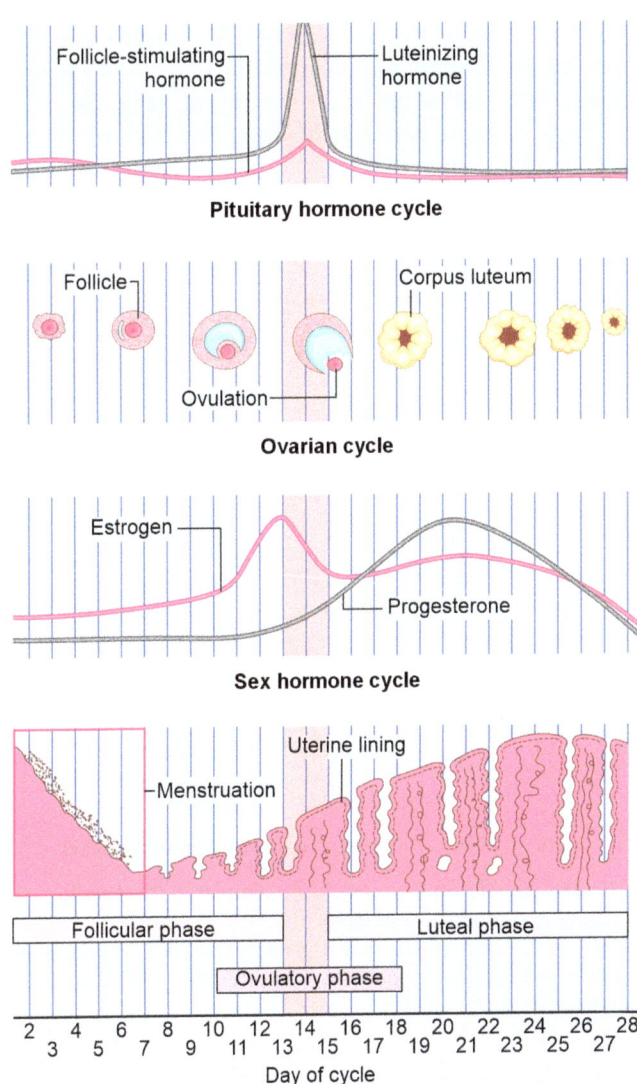

Female secondary sex characters and menstrual cycle

FIG. 27: Estrogens from ovarian follicles provide a positive-feedback on hypothalamus or pituitary gland. Pituitary provides midcycle LH surge. This surge induces ovulation from one of the most matured follicle and converts that follicle into a corpus luteum (CL). CL provides progesterone in the circulation for approximately 14 days.

in the body; and (4) may be associated with (i) hypertriglyceridemia, (ii) hyperuricemia, (iii) hyperinsulinemia, and (iv) renal tubular acidosis.

PUBERTAL DEVELOPMENT AND DISORDERS

Puberty is the growth and developmental state where an individual gets maturity of reproductive capacity. The physical as well as metal changes during puberty are due to sex steroids/hormones that start secreting from testes or ovaries. These secretions are controlled by pituitary and hypothalamic hormones. Approximately 95% of the physical changes of puberty start in boys between 9 and 14 years and in girls between 8 and 13 years. First sign in boys is enlargement of testes [testicular volume (TV) >3 mL] and that in girls is breast development (breast stage >2). Hormonal changes start ahead of physical changes. Activation of the gonadotropin-releasing hormone (GnRH) pulse from hypothalamus is the initial biochemical marker of onset of puberty. Soon concentration of luteinizing hormone (LH) and follicle-stimulating hormone (FSH) from pituitary rises in blood.

In girls, estrogens from ovarian follicles (OF) of ovaries provide a positive-feedback on hypothalamus or pituitary gland to provide LH surge (called midcycle LH surge). This surge induces ovulation from one of the most matured follicle and converts that follicle into a corpus luteum (CL) that start providing progesterone in the circulation for approximately 14 days after which it loses its capacity.

Cyclical exposure to estrogens and progesterone responsible to induce and maintain menstrual cycle and other secondary sex characters. The first menstrual bleeding called *menarche*; it occurs at about 13 years of age. It generally takes 2–3 years from the breast stage 2 **(Fig. 27)**.

In boys, LH stimulates the Leydig cells to grow and produce testosterone. FSH and testosterone causes the growth of the seminiferous tubules and spermatogenesis. Testosterone maintains male secondary sex characters. The first appearance of sperm in urine is called *spermarche*;

it occurs at about 13.5 years of age. Male voice starts by appearance of Adam's apple at about 13 years of age and gets mature to adult quality by next 2 years **(Fig. 28)**.

Physical changes are body hairs, breast development of girls, and genitalia of boys during puberty. There are scoring systems which are of great clinical importance.

The Tanner's method of scoring grades each of the three components into five grades/stages is shown in **Flowcharts 2 to 4 and Figures 29 to 31**.

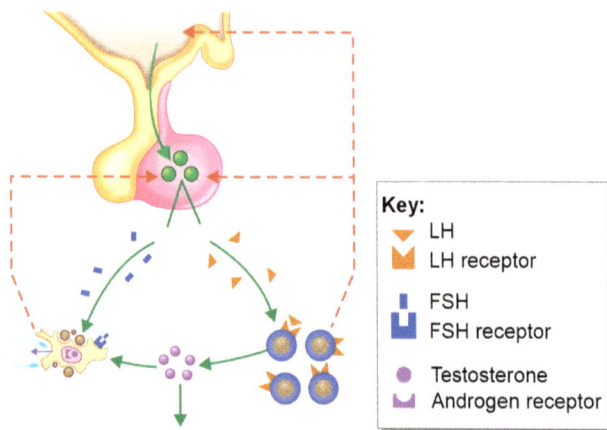

FIG. 28: Luteinizing hormone (LH) stimulates the Leydig cells to grow and produce testosterone. Follicle-stimulating hormone (FSH) and testosterone cause the growth of the seminiferous tubules and spermatogenesis. Testosterone maintains male secondary sex characters.

Stage 1: Vellus hairs on pubis similar to those of abdomen, till onset of puberty

Stage 2: Sparse growth of long, slightly pigmented downy hairs, slightly curled, at the base of penis/along labia between 10.4 to 12.2 years of age

Stage 3: Darker, coarser, and more curled. Spread sparsely over junction of pubis between 12.2 to 13.5 years of age

Stage 4: Adult type hairs, small area covered. No spread to the medial aspect of thigh between 13.0 to 14.2 years of age

Stage 5: Adult in quantity and type with horizontal upper border 14.0 to 14.9 years of age

FLOWCHART 2: The Tanner's grades of pubic hair development.

Note: Pubic hair development in girls is influenced by both adrenal and ovarian androgens. Appearance of facial hairs in boys and axillary hairs in boys and girls coincide pubic hair stage 3.

Stage 1: Testes, scrotum, and penis of about same size and proportion as in childhood, till onset of puberty

Stage 2: Enlargement of scrotum and testes. Scrotum skin reddens and change in texture by 11.2 years of age

Stage 3: Enlargement of penis, at first mainly in length. Further growth of testes and scrotum by 12.9 years of age

Stage 4: Increase in penile with growth in breadth and development of glans, testes, scrotum and scrotum darker by 13.8 years of age

Stage 5: Ganitalia adult and shape by 14.7 years of age

FLOWCHART 3: The Tanner's grades of genitalia development in boys.

Note: To proceed from genital stage 2–5, it requires about 3.5 years.

Stage 1: Papilla is elevated only

Stage 2: Breast budding—breast and papilla elevated as a small mount. Enlarge areola diameter

Stage 3: Further enlargement and elevation of breast and areola, with no separation of their contours

Stage 4: Secondary mount over the breast by areola plus papillary projection. Menarche is preceded by this stage

Stage 5: Mature stage projection of papilla due to regression of areola to the general contour of the breast

FLOWCHART 4: The Tanner's grades of breast development in girls.

Note: In boys, breast development (up to stage 2) occurs in normal adolescent (around genitalia stage 4) and majority regresses by next 2 years.

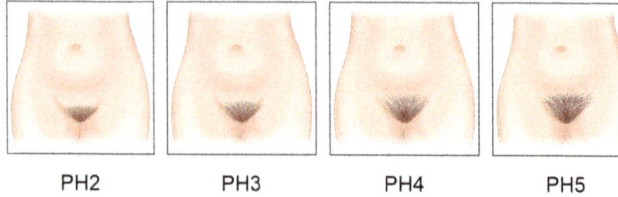

PH2   PH3   PH4   PH5

FIG. 29: The Tanner's grades of pubic hair development.

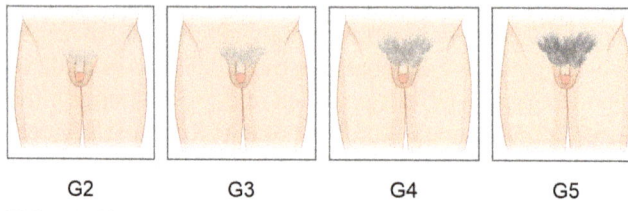

G2   G3   G4   G5

FIG. 30: The Tanner's grades of genitalia development in boys.

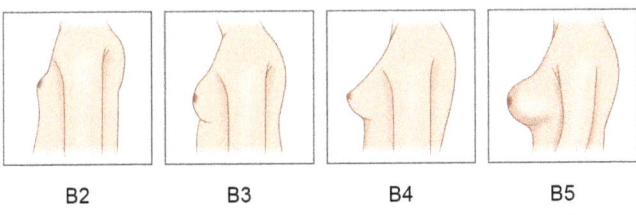

FIG. 31: The Tanner's grades of breast development in girls.

Pubertal Growth Spurt

The overall height gain during puberty is about 28 cm in boys and 25 cm in girls. An accelerated growth velocity called growth spurt is attained during puberty due to combined effects of gonadal steroids and raised growth hormone secretion. The rise of growth hormone secretion in girls occurs in earlier in puberty than in boys. Girls show growth spurt at start of puberty and complete major part of their growth prior to menarche. Peak growth velocity is about 1.3 years prior to menarche. Boys shows growth spurt at genital stage 3. Peak growth velocity is between genital stage 4 and 5 **(Fig. 32)**.

Precocious Puberty

Premature or early puberty is called precocious puberty. It is defined by appearance of pubertal milestones abnormally earlier (>3.5 SD before the mean age).

In boy, milestones are (1) testicular volume >4 mL before 8.5 years; (2) pubic hairs stage 2 before 9 years, or (3) pubic hairs stage 3 before 10 years.

In girl, milestones are (1) breast stage 2 before 8 years; (2) pubic hairs stage 3 before 8.5 years, or (3) menarche before 9.5 years.

There are two types of precocious puberty:
1. Complete/central/true precocious puberty due to premature activation of hypothalamo-pituitary axis, so it is gonadotropin dependent.
2. Incomplete precocious puberty due to premature sexual maturity without hypothalamo-pituitary participation, so it is gonadotropin independent. Incomplete precocious puberty can either (1) Isosexual means change of same sex [congenital adrenal hyperplasia (CAH) or virilizing tumors in boys/large follicular cyst/granulosa cell tumor/use of estrogen pill or cream in girls] or (2) heterosexual means changes of opposite sex (CAH or virilizing tumors in girls).

Table 6 summarizes the causes of precocious puberty.

Complete/Central/True Precocious Puberty (Gonadotropin Dependent)

Children with CPP can be classified into four different groups:
1. Idiopathic precocious puberty (IPP) group constitute the major portion. They are characterized by (1) always

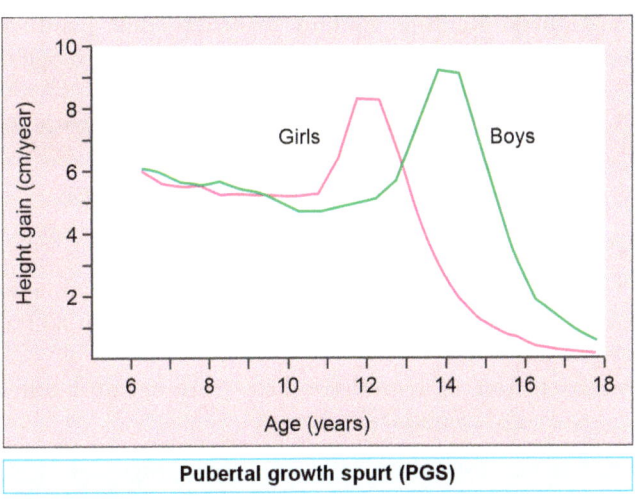

Pubertal growth spurt (PGS)

FIG. 32: In girls, growth spurt at start of puberty and complete major part of their growth prior to menarche. Peak growth velocity is about 1.3 years prior to menarche. In boys, growth spurt at genital stage 3. Peak growth velocity is between genital stage 4 and 5.

TABLE 6: Causes of precocious puberty.

Complete/central/ true precocious puberty (gonadotropin dependent) Endocrine	• Idiopathic precocious puberty (IPP) • Constitutional completes precocious puberty (CCPP) • *Central nervous system disorders*: Example—craniopharyngioma, Astrocytoma, Pineal tumors, encephalitis, miliary tuberculosis, McCune–Albright syndrome, tuberous sclerosis, Sturge–Weber syndrome, prosencephaly, craniostenosis, microcephaly, hydrocephalus, Tay–Sachs disease, etc. • *Severe hypothyroidism*: Van Wyk–Grumbach syndrome
Incomplete precocious puberty (gonadotropin independent)	• *Tumor-secreting gonadotropins*: Example—hepatoma/hepatoblastoma, germinoma of nervous system, teratoma/chorioblastoma of gonads, pineal gland, or mediastinum • *Autonomous androgen secretion*: Example—virilizing adrenal carcinoma, interstitial cell tumors of testes, and Leydig cell hyperplasia • Congenital adrenal hyperplasia (CAH) • Use of exogenous gonadal hormones

isosexual progression, (2) family history is usually absent, (3) girls are affected more than boys, and (4) no definite pathology can be identified.
2. Constitutional precocious puberty (CPP) groups are relatively rare. They are characterized by (1) family history of early puberty is common, (2) rarely due to AR trait, (3) vary rarely due to autosomal dominant trait (in boys only).

3. Central nervous system disorders that produce precocious puberty show features of the neurological lesion.
4. Van Wyk-Grumbach syndrome has clinical features of severe hypothyroidism.

Diagnosis criteria of CPP include documentation of:
- Bone age more than the height age
- Height is more than the chronological age
- Serum gonadotropins (LH and FSH) and gonadal hormone (estrogen/testosterone) are within pubertal range.
- Exclusion of hypothyroidism, tumors, and other causes of incomplete precocity

Treatment of precocious puberty: Aim of treatment is to inhibit puberty and to treat the underlying cause(s).

Puberty inhibition is done by GnRH analog therapy. Prolonged activation of GnRH receptors by GnRH leads to desensitization and consequently to suppressed gonadotropin secretion. Commercially available formulations for treatment of CPP are leuprolide, goserelin, histrelin, triptorelin, etc. Leuprorelin (leuprolide acetate) and goserelin formulations are available for once in every 4 weeks and every 12 weeks for treatment. Triptorelin formulation is used as an injection once in every 6 months. A subcutaneous implant of histrelin is given once in every 12 months.

Delayed Puberty

Delayed puberty is absence of pubertal milestones within the time range. It is defined by absence of any sign of puberty in boy of 14 years and in girls of 13 years. The initial sign of puberty in boy is enlargement of testes (TV >3 mL) and in girls is breast enlargement (breast stage 2).

Depending on etiopathology, there are three types of delayed puberty:
1. Constitutional delayed puberty (CDP) due to nonactivation of gonadotropins (FSH and LH) for no obvious cause. They are short but height is appropriate for bone age.
2. Hypogonadotropic hypogonadism due to midline developmental defects such as Kallmann syndrome. Height is normal if there is no growth hormone deficiency is their but become eunuchoid if not treated in time.
3. Hypergonadotropic hypogonadism due to non-functioning gonads such as Turner's syndrome. Height is usually short with stigmata of disorder.

Table 7 summarizes the causes of delayed puberty.

Management of delayed puberty: General principle of management of delayed puberty is establish the cause(s) and to treat accordingly. For CDP, induction of puberty is done sex hormone—for boys injectable testosterone and for girls initially with oral estrogens for 3-4 months and then cyclical estrogen and progesterone.

Turner's Syndrome (Other Names: Ullrich–Turner's Syndrome, Bonnevie–Ullrich–Turner's Syndrome)

- It is the most common form of hypogonadism named after Henry Turner, who first described its physical features in 1938. Chromosome study subsequently established that it results from missing of one sex

TABLE 7: Causes of delayed puberty.	
Hypogonadotropic hypogonadism	• *Hypopituitarism*: Isolated gonadotropin deficiency, growth hormone deficiency, multiple pituitary hormone deficiency, etc. • *Tumors*: Craniopharyngioma and chromophobe adenoma • *Central nervous system disorders*: Example—histiocytosis X, tuberculosis, sarcoidosis, postradiation, etc. • *Developmental defects*: Stepto-optic dysplasia, cleft lip/palate, and Kallmann syndrome • *Chronic illness*: Chronic renal failure, chronic diarrhea, congenital heart disease, and thalassemia/sickle cell anemia • *Others*: Anorexia nervosa, strenuous exercise, hypothyroidism, Prader–Willi syndrome, and Laurence–Biedl–Moon syndrome
Hypergonadotropic hypogonadism	• *Syndrome of gonadal dysgenesis*: Turner's syndrome and its variants, 46,XX gonadal dysgenesis, Klinefelter's syndrome and its variants • Androgen insensitivity syndrome either complete form—testicular feminization syndrome or incomplete form—Reifenstein syndrome • Bilateral gonadal failure due to radiation, chemotherapy, or infections like mumps, chickenpox, etc. • *Primary testicular defects*: Biosynthetic defects of testosterone, gonadotropin resistance, anorchia/vanishing testes, and cryptorchidism • *Others*: Noonan's syndrome, Sertoli cell-only syndrome, myotonia dystrophica, ataxia telangiectasia, Bloom's syndrome, etc.

chromosome (45,XO) or of a variant of it such as 45,XO/46, XX mosaic; 46,XXq-; 46,XXp; 46,XXqi; 46,Xpi, and 46,XXr.

NB: (-) = deletion, (i) = isochromosome, and (r) = ring chromosome.
- Gonadal dysgenesis and skeletal developmental defects are two components seen along with varieties of somatic abnormalities are seen in this syndrome.
- Gonadal dysgenesis results in female phenotype and primary pubertal failure
- Skeletal developmental defects account for short stature with other deformities **(Flowcharts 5 to 7)**

Short stature is due to:
- Impaired growth of long bones leading to short height
- Hypoplasia of vertebrae leading to short neck
- Deformed vertebrae leading to scoliosis
- Compromised longitudinal axis leading square appearance of chest
- Usually they attain a mean height of 142 cm with a range of 133–153 cm **(Flowchart 5)**

Other bone deformities include:
In upper extremities:
- Increased depth of inner lip of trochlea resulting in increased carrying angle called cubitus valgus
  - Short fourth metatarsal bone leading to a depressed knuckle called knuckle sign
  - Lateral and dorsal bowing of the radius coupled with carpal crowding and distal dislocation of the ulna resulting in Madelung or Bayonet deformity of wrist **(Flowchart 6)**
- *In lower extremities*: Knocked knee
- *In the face*:
  - *Small lower jaw*: Micrognathia
  - Abnormal palatal arch
  - Low set ears
  - Immature facial skeleton **(Flowchart 7)**

Organ abnormalities in:
- *Cardiovascular abnormalities*:
  - Coarctation of the aorta
  - Bicuspid aortic valve
  - Aortic dissection
  - Hypertension
- *Renovascular abnormalities*:
  - Horseshoe kidney
  - Double collecting system (double ureter)
  - Ectopic kidney
  - Aberrant vascular supply to kidneys
- *Gastrointestinal abnormalities*:
  - Intestinal telangiectasia
  - Hemangiomatosis
  - Phlebectasia
  - Dilated veins or venules
  - Inflammatory bowel disease
- *Endocrine and metabolic abnormalities*:
  - Autoimmune thyroid disorders
  - Polyglandular autoimmunity
  - Type 2 diabetes mellitus

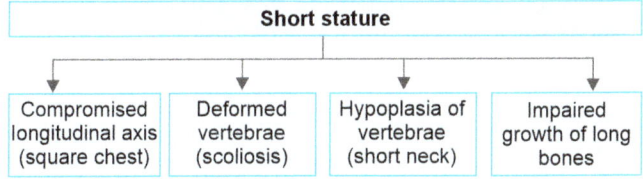

FLOWCHART 5: Features of Turner's syndrome (skeletal).

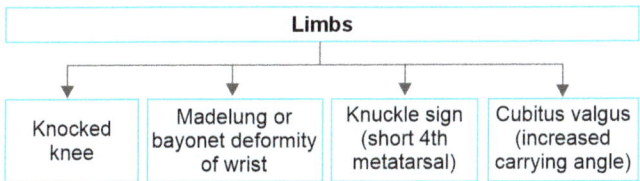

FLOWCHART 6: Features of Turner's syndrome (limbs).

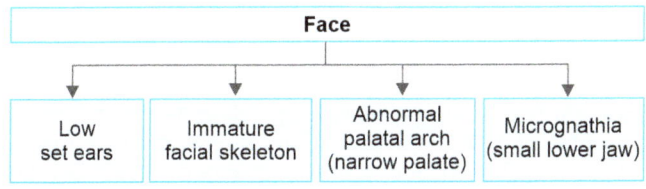

FLOWCHART 7: Features of Turner's syndrome (facial).

Presentation during fetal life: Fetal lymphedema is the hall mark of Turner's syndrome. In severe cases—spontaneous abortion; however, in mild cases baby remains viable and born with deformities such as:
- Webbed neck (pterygium colli)
- Low posterior hairline
- Rotation and malformed ears
- Swelling of hands and feet at birth which usually resolves in the first year of life
- Nail dysplastic or absent
- Hypoplasia of nipple or breast **(Fig. 33)**

Growth pattern of Turner's syndrome is shown in **Figure 34**.

Treatment

The key issues of management of a Turner's syndrome baby are (1) growth promotion, (2) feminization, and (3) long-term medical management.

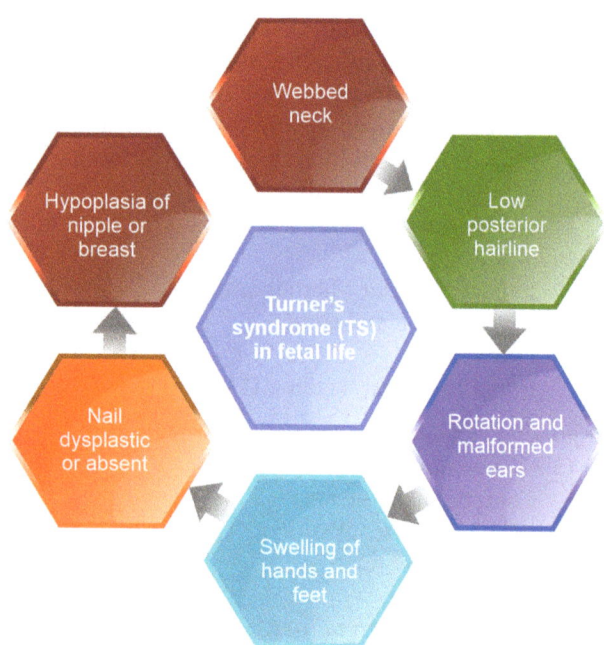

FIG. 33: Presentation of Turner's syndrome during fetal life.

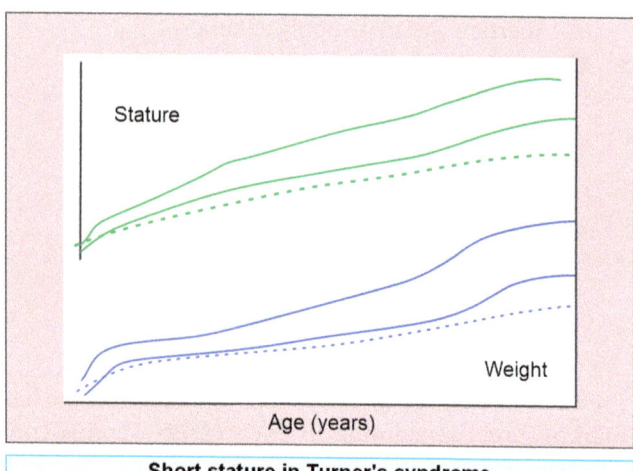

Short stature in Turner's syndrome

FIG. 34: Growth in Tuner's syndrome: (1) Mildly retarded in intrauterine life [length at birth ~ −1 standard deviation (SD)]; (2) Normal growth pattern during first 2 and 3 years; (3) Marked low growth velocity during 3–13 years; (4) No growth spurt there after (mean adult height 142 cm).

Growth promotion: Significant improvement in final height (usually 12-15 cm of growth) may be made by use of growth hormone or oxandrolone or in combination of both. Earlier the initiation of the therapy better is the outcome. Usual dose of growth hormone of 0.3 mg/kg/week administered as daily subcutaneous injections and that of oxandrolone 0.05 mg/kg/day. Combination therapy should be considered for cases reporting late childhood.

Feminization therapy: This should be initiated after initiating growth promotion therapy and after the chronological age appropriate for puberty induction. Estrogen therapy should be the initial continuous therapy for 3–6 months with conjugate estrogen 0.3 mg/day orally followed by cyclical estrogen and progesterone therapy. Conjugate estrogen 0.625 mg/day orally for 21 days than 7 days' gap for each 28 days cycle. Progesterone—medroxyprogesterone (5 mg/day) orally from 12th or 15th day to 21st day of each cycle.

Klinefelter's Syndrome

Definition: It is the most common form of primary hypogonadism in male named after Klinefelter, who first described its physical features in 1942. Chromosome study subsequently established that it results from chromosomal disorder of 47,XXY or of a variant of it such as 46/47,XXY mosaic; 48,XXXY; 49,XXXXY, or 49,XXYY.

Dysgenesis of seminiferous tubules is the principle abnormality of Klinefelter's syndrome. During puberty at adolescent, they show following features:
- Poor to normal virilization with gynecomastia (breast Tanner's stage >2)
- Small and hard testicle (TV <6 mL)
- Azoospermia is almost universal.
- *Tall stature*: Upper segment < lower segment but arm span is not increased (modified eunuchoid)

Postpubertal testosterone and FSH and LH levels vary. Usually testosterone is low and FSH and LH are high **(Fig. 35)**.

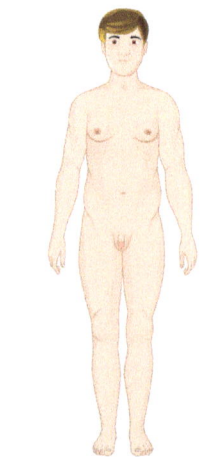

Klinefelter's syndrome

FIG. 35: Poor to normal virilization with gynecomastia (breast Tanner's stage >2). (1) Small and hard testicle (testicular volume <6 mL); (2) Azoospermia is almost universal; (3) Tall stature—upper segment < lower segment but arm span is not increased (modified eunuchoid).

Diagnosis: Karyotype finding is the confirmatory of test of Klinefelter's syndrome. It is usually preceded by physical stigma those appear at adolescence. It can be done in early childhood with long legs, abnormal small testis, and/or children with difficulties with hearing, speech, or language. Early detection and treatment can prevent features SUCH AS gynecomastia and eunuchoidism.

Treatment
- Androgen replacement therapy in deficient cases to completes incomplete puberty and maintains therapy with injectable testosterone
- Mammoplasty for large or psychologically disturbing gynecomastia

Testicular Feminization Syndrome

Testicular feminization syndrome (TFS) is an X-linked recessive form of pseudohermaphroditism. Its other name is complete androgen insensitivity syndrome. Karyotype is 46,XY with mutation in X chromosome in band Xq11-q12 that codes for the androgen receptor.

During puberty at adolescent they show following features:
- Female with poor development of labia
- Blind-ending vagina
- Fully developed breast
- Paucity of body hairs
- Primary amenorrhea
- Gonads (testis) may be intra-abdominal, inguinal, or palpable in labia
- There is absent of mullerian depravities (uterus and fallopian tubes) **(Fig. 36)**.

Pathology: Resistance to all actions of testosterone and dihydrotestosterone.

Postpubertal testosterone and FSH and LH levels vary. Usually testosterone is normal or high for adult male and estrogen high for adult male.

Karyotype: Normal male (46,XY)

Treatment: To assign as a female
- Removal of the gonads
- Construction of vaginal and cyclical estrogen and progesterone therapy
- Androgen supplement (to prevent osteoporosis and anemia)

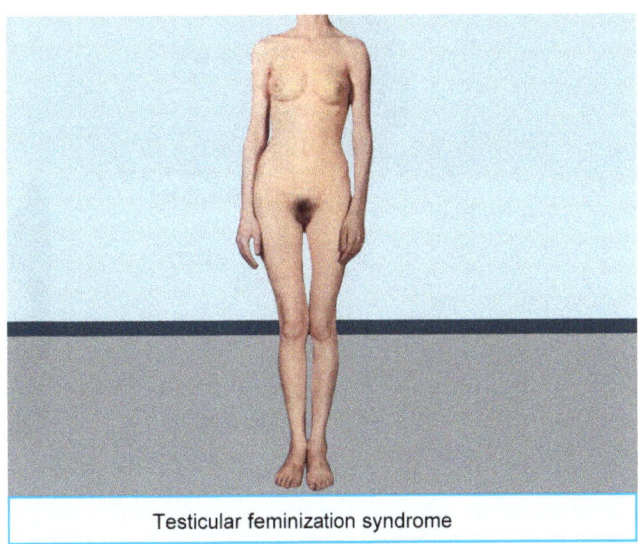

Testicular feminization syndrome

FIG. 36: (1) Female with poor development of labia; (2) Blind-ending vagina; (3) Fully developed breast; (4) Paucity of body hairs; (5) Primary amenorrhea; (6) Gonads (testis) may be intra-abdominal, inguinal, or palpable in labia.

Reifenstein Syndrome (Other Name: Lub Syndrome, Gilbert–Dreyfus Syndrome, or Rosewater Syndrome)

This is a hereditary male pseudohermaphroditism of X-linked recessive inheritance characterized by following features:
- Male baby with perineoscrotal hypoplasia at birth
- Normal axillary and pubic hair
- Scanty beard and body hair
- Pubertal gynecomastia (macromastia)
- Gonads (testes) are cryptocoid
- Wolffian derivatives develop in variable degrees
- Mullarian derivatives (uterus) absent

Pathology: Variable resistance to all actions of testosterone and dihydrotestosterone.

Postpubertal testosterone and FSH and LH levels vary. Usually testosterone is normal or high for adult male and estrogen high for adult male.

Karyotype: Normal male (46,XY).

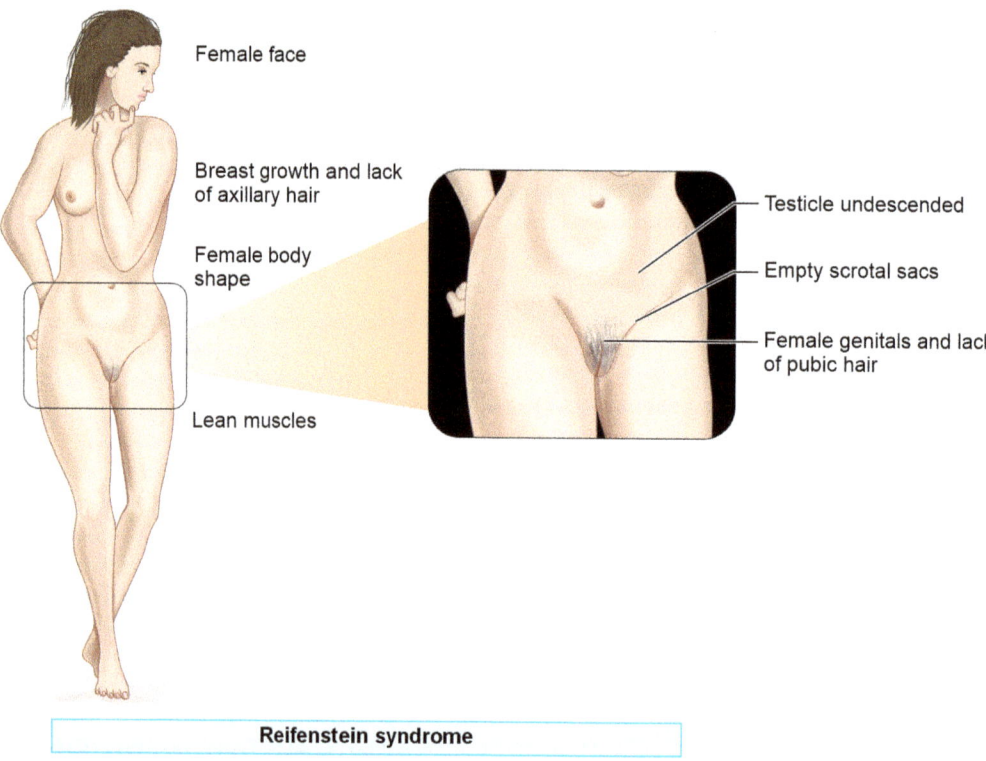

FIG. 37: Incomplete testicular feminization.

Treatment: Two options:
- For postpubertal boys, surgery is done to reduce breasts, repair undescended testicles, or/and reshape the penis to provide a more male appearance. They may also receive androgens to help facial hair grow and deepen the voice.
- For early cases and rearing sex is decided as female surgery is to remove the testicles and reshape the genitals to provide a more female appearance. The female hormone estrogen is then given during puberty **(Fig. 37)**.

FURTHER READINGS

1. Betts JG, Wise J, Young KA, Desaix P, Johnson E, Johnson JE, et al. Anatomy and Physiology. Acton, MA, Houston, Texas: XanEdu; OpenStax College, Rice University; 2017.
2. Standring S. Gray's Anatomy: The Anatomical Basis of Clinical Practice, 41st edition. Philadelphia: Elsevier; 2015.
3. Barrett KE, Barman SM, Yuan J, Brooks HL, Yuan JXJ. Ganong's Review of Medical Physiology, 26th edition. New York: McGraw-Hill Education; 2019.
4. Melmed S, Koenig R, Rosen CJ, Auchus RJ, Goldfine AB. Williams Textbook of Endocrinology, 14th edition. Philadelphia, PA: Elsevier; 2019.
5. Gardner D, Shoback D. Greenspan's Basic and Clinical Endocrinology, 10th edition. New York: McGraw-Hill Education; 2018.
6. Coleman WB, Tsongalis GJ. Molecular Pathology: The Molecular Basis of Human Disease, 2nd edition. San Diego, CA, USA: Academic Press. 2017.
7. Kliegman RM, St. Geme III JW. Nelson Textbook of Pediatrics, 21st edition. Philadelphia, PA: Elsevier; 2019.

CHAPTER 8

Reproductive Medicine

- ❏ Introduction to the reproductive medicine
  - ➢ Anatomy of the female reproductive system
  - ➢ Anatomy of the male reproductive system
  - ➢ Important anomalies of the reproductive organs
  - ➢ Amenorrhea
  - ➢ Classification of amenorrhea
  - ➢ Causes of amenorrhea
  - ➢ Evaluation of amenorrhea management
  - ➢ Cryptomenorrhea (other name hematocolpos)
  - ➢ Asherman syndrome
  - ➢ Müllerian dysgenesis [Mayer–Rokitansky–Küster–Hauser (MRKH) syndrome]
- ❏ Menopause
  - ➢ Problems (symptomatology) of menopause
  - ➢ Hormone replacement therapy for menopause
  - ➢ Osteoporosis
  - ➢ Premature ovarian failure
  - ➢ Hirsutism
- ❏ Gynecomastia
  - ➢ Causes of gynecomastia
  - ➢ Diagnostic evaluation of gynecomastia
- ❏ Microphallus
  - ➢ Common causes of microphallus
  - ➢ Treatment of microphallus
- ❏ Cryptorchidism
  - ➢ Classification of undescended testis or cryptorchidism
  - ➢ Evaluation of undescended testis or cryptorchidism
  - ➢ Treatment of cryptorchidism
- ❏ Ambiguous genitalia
  - ➢ Causes of ambiguous genitalia
  - ➢ Diagnosis of ambiguous genitalia
- ❏ Infertility
  - ➢ Causes of infertility
  - ➢ Infertility management
  - ➢ Management options for Infertility
- ❏ Contraceptives/birth control
  - ➢ Sterilization
  - ➢ Long-acting reversible contraceptives
  - ➢ Contraceptive injection
  - ➢ Short-acting contraceptive hormonal methods
  - ➢ The patch
  - ➢ Barrier methods
  - ➢ Emergency contraception
- ❏ Sexual problem
  - ➢ Sexual response cycle
  - ➢ Sexual dysfunction

This chapter is about Reproductive Medicine, which begins with an introduction to normal growth and development of reproductive organs. It covers 10 different important clinical issues, namely (1) amenorrhea, (2) menopause, (3) hirsutism, (4) gynecomastia, (5) microphallus, (6) cryptorchidism, (7) ambiguous genitalia, (8) infertility, (9) contraception, and (10) sexual problem. This chapter consists of 32 Figures, 19 Tables, and 7 Flowcharts to illustrate its text.

REPRODUCTIVE MEDICINE

The section "Reproductive Medicine" will cover applied anatomy and physiology of the female and male reproductive system in its introduction heading and thereafter will cover clinically important topics as separate sections of the chapter.

INTRODUCTION TO THE REPRODUCTIVE MEDICINE

■ Anatomy of the Female Reproductive System

The organs belong to female reproductive system are: (1) Two ovaries; (2) uterus, and (3) vagina.

Ovaries

The ovaries are located in the lateral wall of two sides of the pelvis and place is called the ovarian fossa. The fossa lies beneath the external iliac artery and in front of the ureter and internal iliac artery. The ovaries lie on either side of the uterus and are attached with uterus by a fibrous cord called the ovarian ligament. The ovaries are attached to the body wall by a ligament called suspensory of the ovary. A part of the broad ligament of the uterus covers the ovary and is called the mesovarium. The ovary is totally invaginated into the peritoneum, so it is an intraperitoneal organ. One end of an ovary which is attached with the fallopian tube via the infundibulopelvic ligament is called tubal extremity and the other extremity is pointed down to the uterus and is attached to that via the ovarian ligament. During reproductive life ovaries produce/ovulate one mature egg (ova) cyclically and hormones, i.e., estrogen and progesterone.

The ovaries are surrounded by a capsule, and have an outer cortex and an inner medulla. The capsule is of dense connective tissue and is known as the tunica albuginea. The surface of the ovaries is covered with membrane consisting of a lining of simple cuboidal-to-columnar shaped mesothelium, called the germinal epithelium. The outer layer is the ovarian cortex, consisting of ovarian follicles and stroma in between them. Included in the follicles are the cumulus oophorus, membrana granulosa (and the granulosa cells inside it), corona radiata, zona pellucida, and primary oocyte. Theca of follicle, antrum, and liquor folliculi are also contained in the follicle. Also in the cortex is the corpus luteum derived from the follicles. The innermost layer is the ovarian medulla. It can be hard to distinguish between the cortex and medulla, but follicles are usually not found in the medulla.

Follicular cells are flat epithelial cells that originate from surface epithelium covering the ovary. They are surrounded by granulosa cells that have changed from flat to cuboidal and proliferated to produce a stratified epithelium.

The ovarian artery arises from the abdominal aorta below the renal artery. It can be found in the suspensory ligament of the ovary, anterior to the ovarian vein and ureter.

The ovarian vein drains blood from ovary to inferior vena cava or one of its tributaries (**Figs. 1A to C**).

Lymphatics drainage: There are three pathways for lymphatic flow from the ovaries:
1. Superiorly, to the para-aortic lymph nodes adjacent to the ovarian artery
2. Inferiorly, to the medial group of superficial inguinal nodes through the inguinal canal alongside the round ligament
3. Horizontally, to the opposite ovary across the uterine fundus

Uterus

The uterus is located in the middle of the pelvis behind the urinary bladder and in front of the rectum. It is

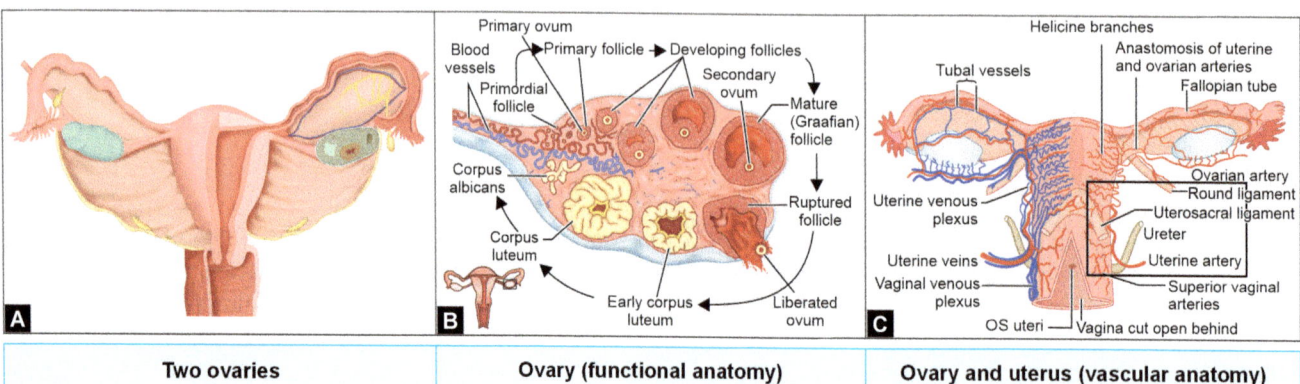

FIGS. 1A TO C: Anatomy of ovary.

pear-shaped and about 7.6 cm long. The uterus can be divided anatomically into four segments: (1) Fundus, (2) corpus or body, (3) cervix, and (4) the internal os. The fundus of the uterus is the top, rounded portion, opposite from the cervix. The vaginal part of the cervix does not extend below interspinal line. The uterus is mobile and moves under the pressure of the surrounding structures. Under normal circumstances, the uterus in anteflexion and anteversion (in 90% of women) and keeps it "floating" in the pelvis.

The uterus mostly consists of smooth muscle, known as myometrium. The innermost layer of myometrium is known as the junctional zone. The parametrium is the loose connective tissue around the uterus. The perimetrium is the peritoneum covering of the fundus and ventral and dorsal aspects of the uterus. The uterus is primarily supported by the pelvic diaphragm, perineal body, and the urogenital diaphragm. It is also supported by ligaments and the peritoneum called broad ligament of uterus. The lining of the uterine cavity is called the endometrium. It consists of the functional endometrium and the basal endometrium from which the former arises. The endometrium builds a lining periodically, which is shed or reabsorbed if no pregnancy occurs. Shedding of the functional endometrial lining is the menstrual bleeding. It occurs in cycle of approximately 28 days, ±7 days of flow and ±21 days of progression, throughout the fertile years of a female **(Figs. 2A to C)**.

Vagina

The vagina is a fibromuscular tubular tract, and it opens at valve behind the opening of urethra and ends at cervix of uterus. During childbearing age, length of the vagina in the front wall is approximately 7.5 cm long, and the back wall is approximately 9 cm long. Its functions include sexual intercourse, childbirth, and outflow tract for menses.

The vaginal wall from the lumen outward consists of three different layers—first (inner), second (middle), and third (inner).
- *First layer* is composed of nonkeratinized mucosa of stratified squamous epithelium and a lamina propria (a thin layer of connective tissue) underneath the epithelium.
- *Secondly layer* is a muscle layer—smooth muscle with bundles of circular fibers internal to longitudinal fibers run lengthwise.
- *Third one* is the outer layer of connective tissue, which is also called the adventitia **(Figs. 3A to C)**.

Blood, Lymphatic, and Nerve Supply
- Arterial blood is supplied to the vagina mainly via the vaginal artery. It emerges from a branch of the internal iliac artery or the uterine artery. The vaginal arteries anastomose along the side of the vagina with the cervical branch of the uterine artery. The middle rectal artery, the internal pudendal artery, and branches of the internal iliac artery also provide arterial supply to the vagina.
- Two main veins drain blood from the vagina, one on the left and one on the right. These form a network of smaller veins, the vaginal venous plexus, on the sides of the vagina, connecting with similar venous plexuses of the uterus, bladder, and rectum. They ultimately drain into the internal iliac veins.
- Lymphatic drainage of vagina occurs in three groups of lymph nodes. Lymphatic vessels accompany vaginal arteries; the upper group accompanies the vaginal branches of the uterine artery; a middle group accompanies the vaginal arteries; and the lower group, draining lymph from the area outside the hymen, drain to the inguinal lymph nodes.

Nerve supply: The upper vagina is provided by the sympathetic and parasympathetic areas of the pelvic

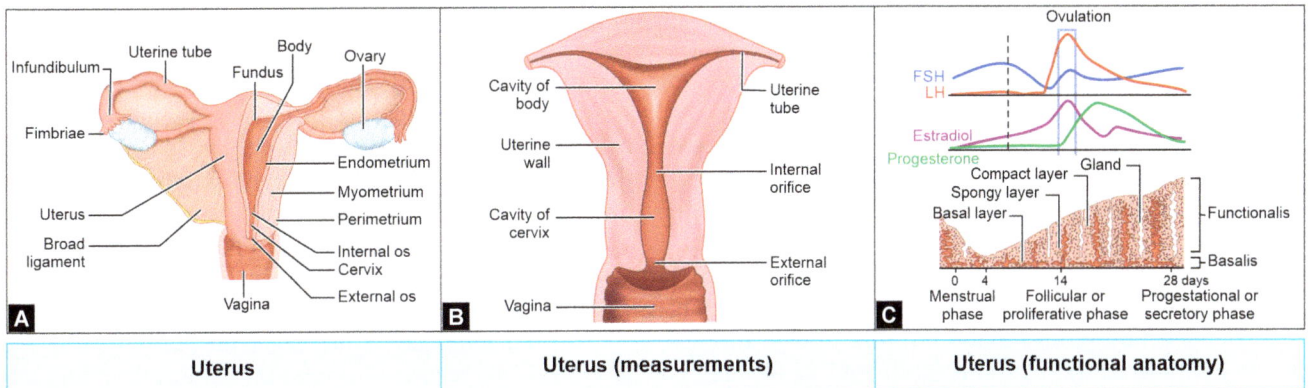

FIGS. 2A TO C: Anatomy of uterus.

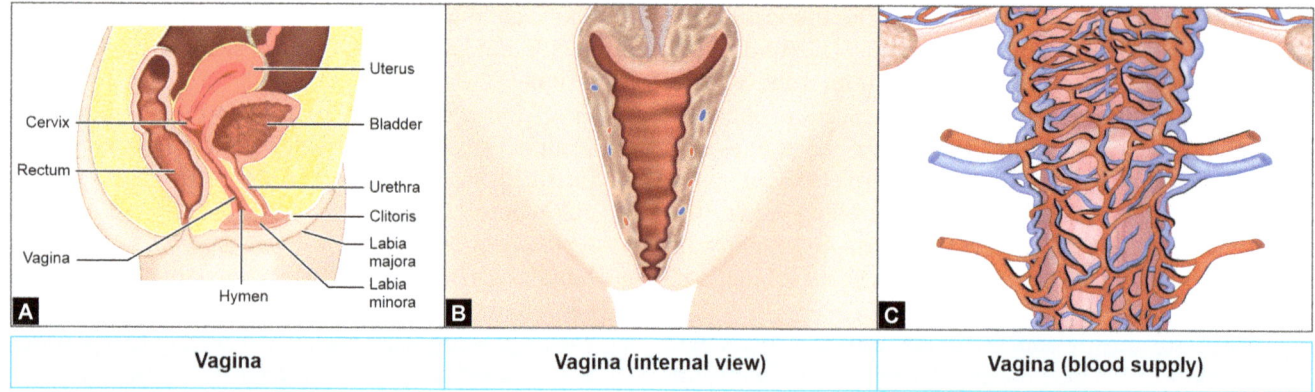

FIGS. 3A TO C: Anatomy vagina.

plexus. The lower part of vagina is supplied by the pudendal nerve.

Anatomy of the Male Reproductive System

The organs belong to male reproductive system are: (1) Two testes and (2) a penis.

Testes

The *testes* are the male reproductive organs—*gonads*. The testes are located in the scrotum in a muscular sack called scrotum behind the penis. This special location is to keep testes 2–4°C below core body temperature, which is required for efficient sperm production. They produce testosterone during the reproductive life of male.

Testes are ovals in shape with approximately 4–5 cm in length. Each one has two different layers of connective tissues:
1. The outer one is named the tunica vaginalis. It a serous membrane with parietal and visceral layers.
2. The inner one is named the tunica albuginea. It is a connective tissue covering tough, white and dense in nature. The tunica albuginea invigilates into the testis as septum and divides it into 300–400 structures called lobules. Sperm develops in structures called seminiferous tubules within the testicular lobules. During 7th month of gestation the testis migrates into the scrotal cavity through the inguinal canal from the abdomen. This phenomenon is known as the "descent of the testis."

The *seminiferous tubules* are tightly coiled and form the bulk of the testis.

Sperms are formed from the cells of tubules and released into the duct system of the testis. The lumens of the coiled seminiferous tubules become straight tubules (called tubuli recti). The fine meshwork of tubules is called the rete testes. Sperms leave the rete testes through 15–20 efferent ductules, which cross the tunica albuginea. There are six different types of cells in the seminiferous tubules. One is sustentacular cell, which works as the supporting structure of rest five types of cells. They are all developing sperm cells in different stages. Germ cell development progresses from the basement membrane toward the lumen.

Sertoli Cells

Sertoli cells are especial type of epithelial cells, having branching process, and found in seminiferous tubules of testis. They provide support to the growing sperm, so also called sustentacular cell or sustenocyte. Sertoli cells secrete signaling molecules that promote sperm production and can control spermatogenesis. Tight junctions between these Sertoli cells create the *blood–testis barrier*. This barrier prevents blood-borne substances from reaching the germ cells and surface antigens on developing germ cells from escaping into the bloodstream.

Spermatogenesis

Spermatogenesis means sperm production. It takes place in the seminiferous tubules of testes almost throughout the adult life. Spermatogonia are diploid cells. They differentiate into primary spermatocytes by mitosis. The primary spermatocytes undergo cell division twice by meiosis I and meiosis II to produce secondary spermatocytes(n) and spermatids(n), respectively. Mature sperms (spermatozoa) are produced by metamorphosis of spermatids. This spermatogenesis process occurs throughout adult life. Approximately 64 days are required for one production cycle. Spermatogenesis is not synchronous across the seminiferous tubules; each tubule starts a new cycle approximately in every 16 days. Sperm counts slowly decline after the age of 35 years **(Fig. 4)**.

The *testicular arteries* also called the *internal spermatic arteries* are the branch of the abdominal aorta that supplies blood to the testis **(Figs. 5A to C)**.

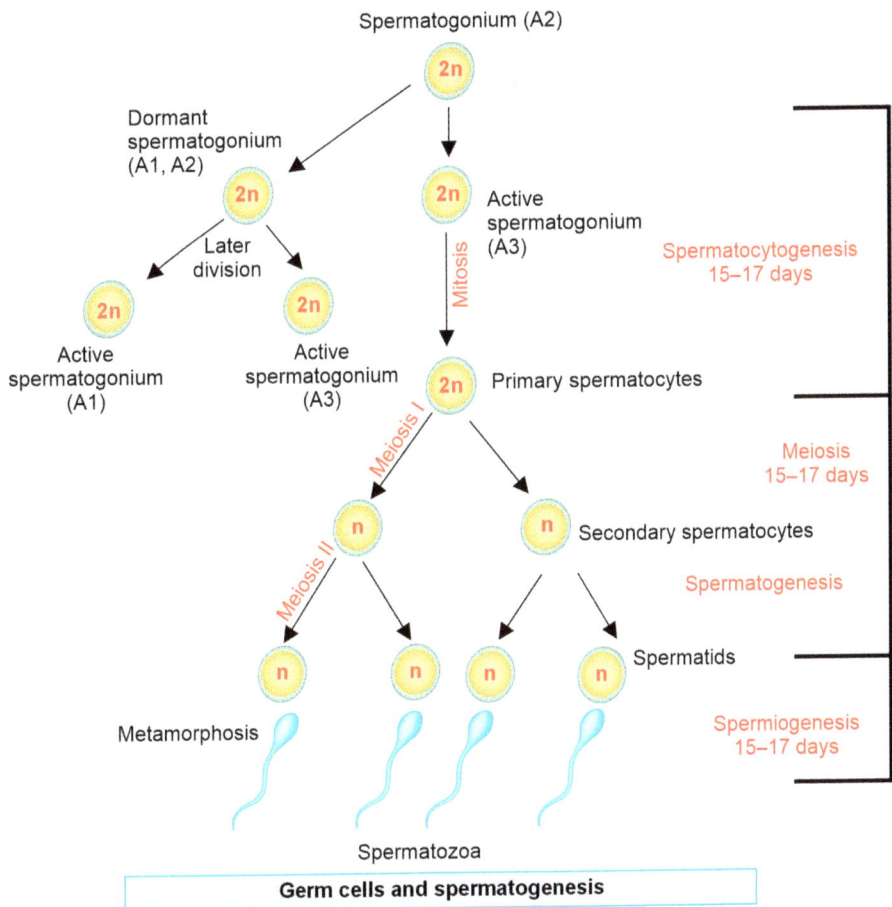

FIG. 4: Spermatogonia are the male germ cells. They differentiate into primary (2n) and then by meiosis to secondary (n) spermatocytes, then mature to spermatids, and finally become sperm. This spermatogenesis process occurs throughout adult life. Each production cycle takes approximately 64 days.

Venous drainage: Testicular veins of the right testis go to the right testicular vein, which joins the inferior vena cava and that of the left testis go to the left testicular vein, which joins the left renal vein.

Lymphatic drainage occurs via the testicular vessels, passes into the abdomen, and ends in the lateral aortic and preaortic nodes.

Nerve supply: The 10th and 11th thoracic spinal nerves supply the testes via the renal and aortic autonomic plexuses.

Important Anomalies of the Reproductive Organs

- Anomalies of the female reproductive organs may include:
  - Absence of one or both ovaries; an extra ovary; extra tissue attached to an ovary, and ovotestis, which contain both male and female tissue.
  - Fallopian tube agenesis—absence of one or both fallopian tubes.
  - Vaginal anomalies include vaginal agenesis, obstruction, duplication, and fusion.
  - MRKH (Mayer-Rokitansky-Küster-Hauser) syndrome is a congenital condition of the female reproductive system that affects approximately 1 in 5,000 women. Girls diagnosed with MRKH have vaginal agenesis, which refers to an absent or incomplete vagina. The uterus is also very small or absent **(Flowchart 1)**.
- Anomalies of the male reproductive organs may include:
  - Undescended testis (cryptorchidism of one or both testis) or agenesis/anorchia, etc.
  - Microphallus with or without hypospadias
  - Scrotal anomalies include scrotal agenesis, hypoplasia, ectopia, or hemangioma; penoscrotal transposition; and bifid scrotum **(Flowchart 2)**.

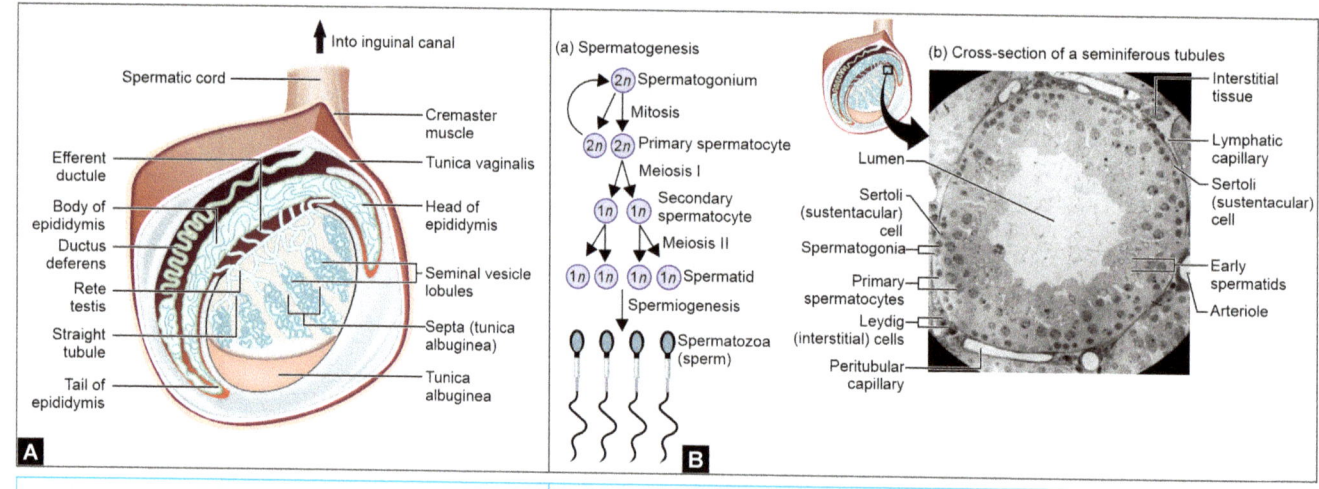

| Testis: Parts | Testis: Seminiferous tubules |

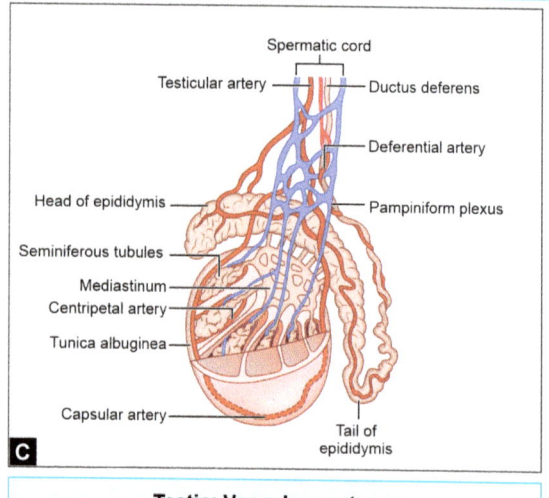

Testis: Vascular anatomy

FIGS. 5A TO C: Anatomy of testes.

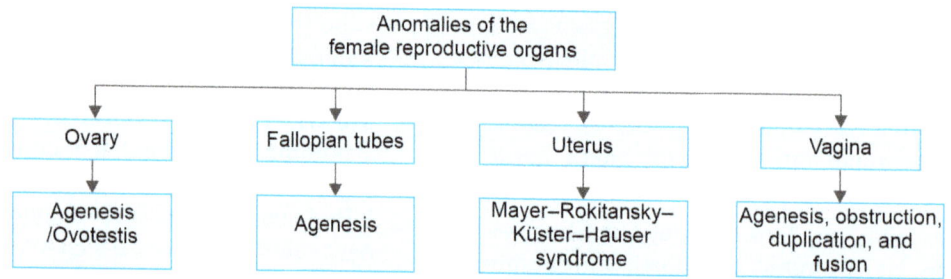

FLOWCHART 1: Anomalies of the female reproductive organs.

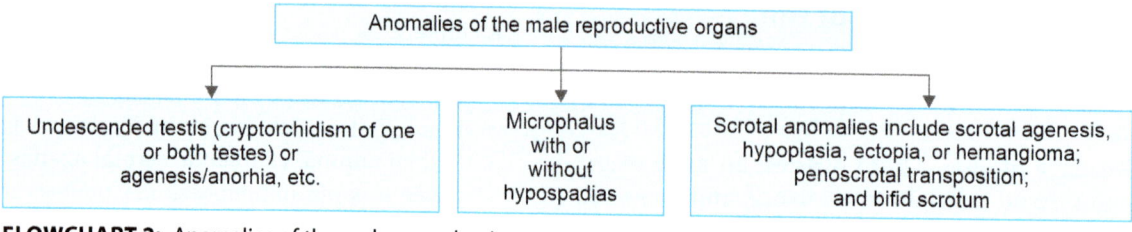

FLOWCHART 2: Anomalies of the male reproductive organs.

Amenorrhea

Amenorrhea means cessation of menstruation. Lay concept is missing one or more menstrual periods. It is stoppage of menstruation in an adult woman during reproductive age. But menstruation not started by 16 years of age and permanent stoppage of menstruation when reproductive age is over also fall in spectrum of amenorrhea, and they are termed as delayed puberty/pubertal failure, and menopause, respectively. Amenorrhea during reproductive age, termed as secondary amenorrhea, is common due to pregnancy or lactation and can also be due to other pathological reasons **(Table 1)**.

Classification of Amenorrhea

Amenorrhea can be classified as *primary* or *secondary*. In *primary amenorrhea*, menstrual periods have never begun (by the age of 16 year), whereas *secondary amenorrhea* is defined as the absence of menstrual periods for three consecutive cycles or a time period of more than 6 months in a woman who was previously menstruating. There is a big cause list of amenorrhea and that can be grouped into categories such as anatomical, gonadal (acquired/genetic), hormonal, etc. **(Flowchart 3)**.

Causes of Amenorrhea

Table 1 summarizes the causes of amenorrhea.

Evaluation of Amenorrhea Management

History and physical examination are to be used to categorize amenorrhea cases. Thereafter, a category-specific decision-making investigation steps (DMIS) make its management relatively simple.

Step 1: Clinical evaluation/history

Step 2: Physical evaluation

Step 3: Investigation according to category of amenorrhea, namely (i) Primary, (ii) Secondary, or (iii) Galactorrhea—amenorrhea syndrome.

Table 2 summarizes the components of evaluation of cases with amenorrhea.

For clinical category of amenorrhea cases for DMIS, see **Tables 3 to 5**.

Table 3 provides DMIS for primary amenorrhea (category I).

Table 4 provides DMIS for secondary amenorrhea (category II).

Table 5 provides DMIS for amenorrhea–galactorrhea Syndrome (category III).

TABLE 1: Causes of amenorrhea.

Group	Causes
Anatomical causes	Müllerian dysgenesis (Mayer–Rokitansky–Küster–Hauser syndrome) <ul><li>Cryptomenorrhea:<ul><li>Vaginal agenesis</li><li>Transvaginal septum</li><li>Imperforated hymen</li></ul></li><li>Asherman syndrome</li></ul>
Gonadal failure (steroidogenic enzymatic defects)	<ul><li>Cholesterol decleavage chain defects</li><li>3β-ol-dehydrogenase defects</li><li>17-hydroxylate defects</li><li>17-deslolase defects</li><li>17-ketoreductase defects</li></ul>
Gonadal dysgenesis	<ul><li>Turner syndromes and its variants</li><li>Pure gonadal dysgenesis</li></ul>
Postinfections (mumps)	
Postirradiation	
Postchemotherapy	
Postoophorectomy	
Autoimmune oophoritis	
Idiopathic premature ovarian failure	
Ovarian resistance syndrome	
Endocrine imbalance	<ul><li>Hypothalamic defects (functional amenorrhea):<ul><li>Anorexia nervosa</li><li>Bulimia</li><li>Weight loss</li><li>Obesity</li><li>Pseudocyesis</li><li>Systemic illness</li></ul></li><li>Pituitary defects:<ul><li>Isolated gonadotropin deficiency (Kallmann syndrome)</li><li>Panhypopituitarism (Sheehan's syndrome)</li><li>Somalomamalotropic hypersecretions (acromegaly, galactorrhea-amenorrhea syndrome)</li></ul></li><li>Other hormone defects<ul><li>Hypothyroidism</li><li>Hyperthyroidism</li><li>Hypercortisolemia (Cushing's syndrome)</li><li>Hyperandrogenism (CAH and PCOS)</li></ul></li></ul>
Amenorrhea in XY females	<ul><li>Testicular feminization</li><li>Pure gonadal dysgenesis</li><li>Anorchia</li><li>True hermaphrodism</li></ul>

(CAH: congenital adrenal hyperplasia; PCOS: polycystic ovarian syndrome)

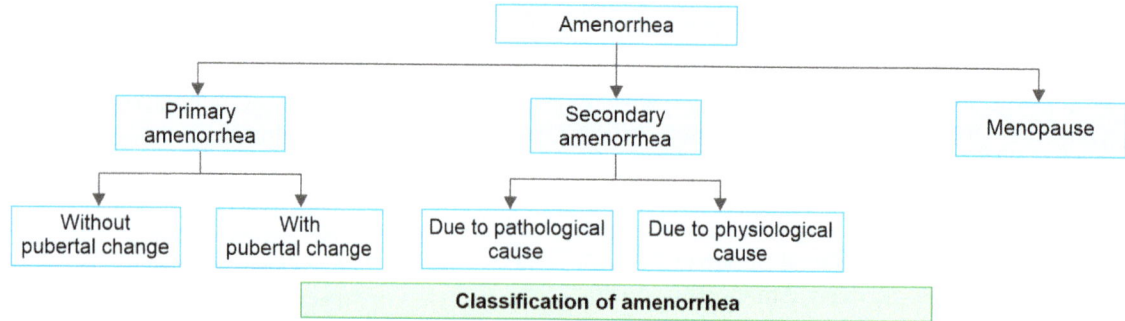

FLOWCHART 3: No menstruation after the age of 16 years in women may be: (1) Primary amenorrhea, (2) secondary amenorrhea, or (3) menopause.

TABLE 2: Components of evaluation of amenorrhea.		
Step 1	Clinical evaluation/ history	• Pubertal developments • Medication or drugs • Lifestyle, employment, dietary, and exercise habits • Environmental and psychological stress • Family history of amenorrhea or genetic disorders
Step 2	Physical evaluation	• Anthropometry (dimensions and habitus) • Pubertal development check (Tanner stage) • Physical signs of androgen excess (hirsutism, clitoromegaly) • Sigma of anatomical anomaly (uterus, cervix, vagina, and hymen)

TABLE 3: Decision-making investigation steps (DMIS) in a case of primary amenorrhea.			
Step	Investigations	Finding	Action
Initial step	Look for uterus*	Normal	Go to step 2
		Absent	Go to step 4
Step 2	Look for vagina	Normal	Go to step 3
		Absent	Go to step 4
Step 3	Look for breast and pubic hair stage	Stage 4 (normal)	Go to step 6
		Stage <4	Go to step 4
Step 4	Karyotype	Normal	Go to step 5
		Abnormal	Go to step 7
Step 5	Induction of menses by hormone therapy**	Positive	Follow-up
		Negative	Evaluate as normoestrogenic secondary amenorrhea case
Step 6	Look for cryptomenorrhea***	Present	Management by surgery
		Absent	Evaluate as normoestrogenic secondary amenorrhea case
Step 7	Look for stigma of genetic lesion/syndrome	Specific disease	Treat as per diagnosis
		Nonspecific disease	Supportive treatment

* By sonography/laparoscopy/digital rectal examination.
** By cyclical estrogen and progesterone.
*** By laparoscopy/sonography.

Cryptomenorrhea (Other Name Hematocolpos)

It is a condition where menstruation occurs but is not visible due to an obstruction of the outflow tract. Specifically, the endometrium is shed, but a congenital obstruction such as a vaginal septum or on part of the hymen retains the menstrual flow.

The affected girls have normal breast and pubic hair development (Tanner's B4 and PH4 stage). Cyclical (monthly) lower abdominal pain is the chief presenting complaint. They may be brought in emergency for urinary retention.

On examination, lower abdominal mass and vulva look tense and bulging; a large bulging mass is felt on digital rectal examination.

It can be easily diagnosed using ultrasound and/or magnetic resonance imaging (MRI). The vagina is commonly seen filled with blood and the uterus usually appears pushed upward. Other findings may include cervical stenosis and hematosalpinx (bilateral) **(Fig. 6)**.

The treatment of cryptomenorrhea is surgery.
- A cruciate incision followed by excision of tags of hymen allows the drainage of the retained menstrual blood.

TABLE 4: Decision-making investigation steps (DMIS) in a case of secondary amenorrhea.

Step	Investigations	Finding	Action
Initial step	Progesterone challenge test	Positive	Go to step 2
		Negative	Go to step 4
Step 2	Look for androgen excess*	Present	Go to step 3
		Absent	Go to step 4
Step 3	Look for endocrine disorders**	Present	Treat accordingly
		Absent	Go to step 4
Step 4	Look for hypothalamic disorders	Present	Treat accordingly
		Absent	Go to step 5
Step 5	Look for Asherman syndrome (hysteroscopy)	Positive	Treat accordingly
		Negative	Go to step 6
Step 6	Check FSH level	FSH level >40 IU/mL	Treat accordingly
		FSH level <40 IU/mL	Repeat Steps 3 and 4

* Serum testosterone.
** FT_4 and TSH; cortisol and ACTH.
(ACTH: adrenocorticotropic hormone; FSH: follicle-stimulating hormone; FT_4: free thyroxine; TSH: thyroid-stimulating hormone)

TABLE 5: Decision-making investigation steps (DMIS) in a case of amenorrhea–galactorrhea syndrome.

Step	Investigations	Finding	Action
Initial step	Check serum PRL and TSH level	Both elevated	Go to step 2
		Only PRL elevated	Go to step 3
Step 2	Treat hypothyroidism	Both normal	Continue treatment
		PRL elevated	Go to step 3
Step 3	Imaging of sellar region (MRI)	Normal/microadenoma	Go to step 4
		Macroadenoma	Go to step 4
Step 4	Treat with cabergoline	PRL normal	Continue treatment
		PRL elevated	Go to step 5
Step 5	Surgery/Gama knife	PRL normal/low	Cure
		PRL elevated	Go to step 4

(MRI: magnetic resonance imaging; PRL: prolactin; TSH: thyroid-stimulating hormone)

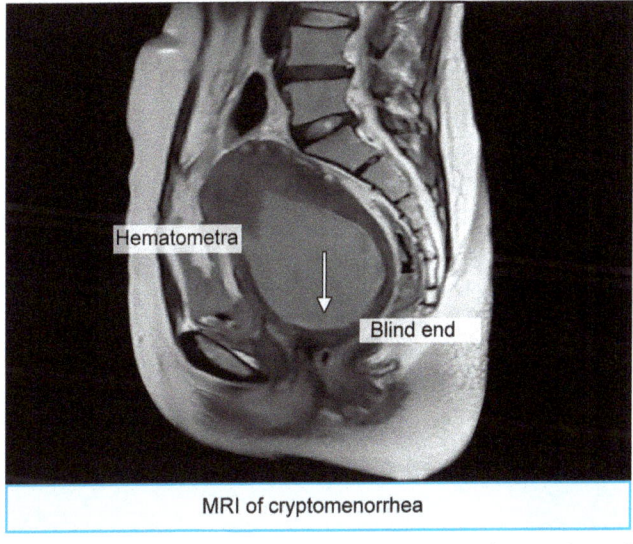

MRI of cryptomenorrhea

FIG. 6: MRI showing hematometra with cervical stenosis and hematosalpinx (bilateral). Hematometra was ending blindly with no communication with the vagina.

- A thicker transverse vaginal septum can be treated with Z-plasty.
  - A blind vagina will require a partial or complete vaginoplasty.
  - Hematosalpinx may require laparotomy or laparoscopy for removal and reconstruction of the affected tube.
  - Infertility may require assisted reproductive techniques (ARTs).

Asherman Syndrome

Asherman syndrome is in a fibrotization of endometrium due to an intrauterine trauma. Trauma occurs during uterine curettage, myomectomy, caesarean section, or by tuberculous endometriosis.

It is clinically characterized by secondary amenorrhea with normal secondary sex characters.

Diagnostic workup includes **(Table 4)**:
- No withdrawal bleeding on estrogen plus progesterone.
- Gonadotropins [follicle-stimulating hormone (FSH) and luteinizing hormone (LH)] are not elevated (exclude menopause).
- Serial serum progesterone level may show postovulatory level
- Hysterosalpingogram or hysteroscopy may document absent functional endometrial **(Fig. 7)**.

Treatment options:
- Treatment of the cause (if feasible) as in tuberculous endometriosis
- Trial with high dose estrogen plus progesterone [hormone replacement therapy (HRT)]
- For fertility, ART option like surrogacy with couple's embryo

■ Müllerian Dysgenesis [Mayer–Rokitansky–Küster–Hauser (MRKH) Syndrome]

Müllerian dysgenesis is an autosomal dominant congenital malformation characterized by a failure of the Müllerian duct to develop, resulting in a missing uterus and variable degrees of vaginal hypoplasia. It is clinically characterized by primary amenorrhea with normal secondary sex characters.

Diagnostic workup includes **(Tables 3 and 4)**:
- Ultrasonography/MRI documentation of missing uterus; absent or hypoplastic vagina **(Figs. 8A and B)**

- Karyotype—46,XX
- Gonadotropins (FSH and LH) are not elevated.

Treatment options include:
- Construction of vagina by surgery and dilatation
- For fertility, ART option like surrogacy with couple's embryo

MENOPAUSE

Menopause is permanent cessation of menstrual bleeding of a woman. It is the end point of declining ovarian function, and so it is transition of reproductive stage of life to postreproductive stage. Usually, it occurs between 45 to 55 years of age. It can occur prematurely because of bilateral oophorectomy (surgical menopause), irradiation, and abnormalities of ovaries.

Climacteric period denotes period of premenopause, menopause, and postmenopause during which most women experience a variety of disturbances, which is called climacteric syndrome. The disturbances include hot flash, night sweating, vaginal irritation, insomnia, and depression.

Investigation list includes:
- Serum gonadotropin and estradiol levels. FSH and LH are elevated (>40 µIU/mL); estradiol (E_2) low or low normal.
- For premature menopause (before 40 years), karyotype and examination of pelvis (ultrasound and/or endoscopy) should be included.

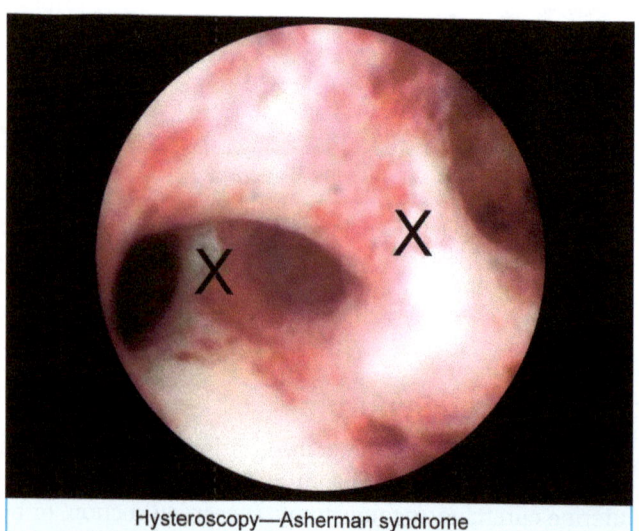

Hysteroscopy—Asherman syndrome

FIG. 7: Absent functional endometrial, intrauterine adhesions, and scar tissue in uterine cavity.

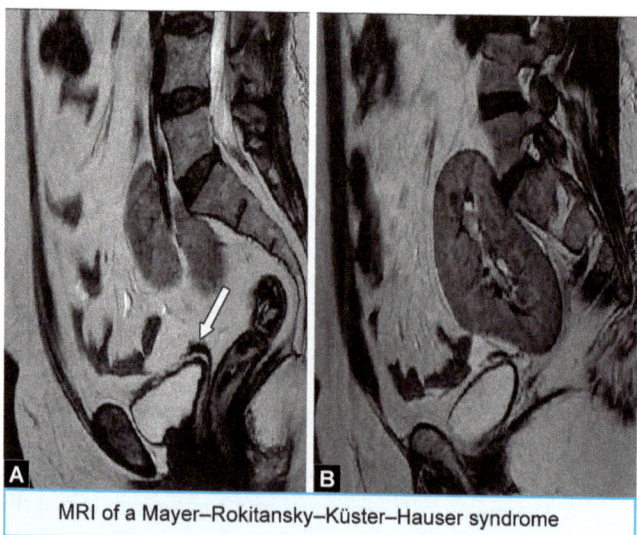

MRI of a Mayer–Rokitansky–Küster–Hauser syndrome

FIGS. 8A AND B: Missing uterus and hypoplastic vagina.

Problems (Symptomatology) of Menopause

Problems (symptomatology) of menopause are: (1) Vasomotor symptoms, (2) urogenital problems, (3) psychotogenic problems, (4) osteoporosis, (5) coronary heart diseases, and (6) other problems.

- *Vasomotor symptoms of menopause*: Most women seek medical attention for menopausal symptoms with complaints of vasomotor symptoms. This is described as hot flashes or flushes or night sweat. This is experienced by about 65-80% of women for about 1-2 years during her climacteric period. Constellation of symptoms is: (1) Preceded by an aura, (2) finger temperature raises by 6°C, and (3) pulse rate raises by 10 beats/min. It is usually transient, but may last up to 30 minutes. It is the major cause of insomnia.
- *Urogenital problems of menopause*: Vaginitis, sexual dysfunctions, and urinary dysfunctions are the major urogenital problems of menopause.
  - Vaginitis is due to the atrophy of the genital epithelium and its symptoms include: (1) irritation, (2) burning, (3) pruritus, and (4) leukorrhea.
  - Sexual dysfunctions are due to the vaginal mucosal changes and its symptoms include: (1) Dyspareunia, (2) vaginitis, (3) vaginismus, (4) physical discomforts, and (5) loss of sexual interest.
  - Urinary dysfunctions are due to atrophy of the lower urinary tract mucosa, and its symptoms include: (1) Dysuria, (2) cystitis, (3) urethral caruncles, and (4) urethritis.
- *Psychotogenic problems of menopause*: These problems include: (1) Anxiety, (2) depression, (3) insomnia, and (4) headache.
- *Osteoporosis due to menopause*: Exaggerated bone mass (particularly of trabecular bones) leads to disabilities, such as (1) back pain, (2) loss of height, (3) decreased mobility, and (4) increased risk of fractures (vertebral, hips, etc.)
- *Coronary heart diseases during menopause*: There is significant lower incidence of (1) coronary artery diseases (CAD), (2) congestive heart failure (CHF), and (3) atherosclerotic cardiovascular diseases (ACD) in women than man during before menopause but menopause those goes above than age-matched man.
- *Other problems during menopause*: The list includes: (1) Marked thinning and wrinkling of skin, (2) loss of axillary and pubic hairs, (3) hirsutism (mild), (4) atrophy of breast, (5) infra umbilical obesity, (6) low high-density lipoprotein (HDL) and high low-density lipoprotein (LDL) cholesterol (increases risk of cardiovascular events).

Hormone Replacement Therapy for Menopause

Menopause is a deficiency state, so its treatment is replacement of estrogen only or estrogen and progesterone combination. To combat the health problems of menopause, HRT is indicated for all menopausal women if there is no specific contraindication.

Regimens of HRT include:
- Standard regime
- Estrogen-only regime
- Tibolone regime

Standard regime of HRT: It is chosen if uterus is present and menopause is of recent onset. It consists of:
- Estrogen orally, once daily for 21 days
- Oral progesterone is added with estrogen from day 12th to 21st day
- No drugs for 7 days from 22nd to 28th day

Table 6 shows the oral estrogen and progesterone preparations used for HRT.

Estrogen-only Regime of Hormone Replacement Therapy (Also Called ERT)

It is used when uterus is absent. Classically, oral estrogen preparation (conjugate estrogen 0.625-1.25 mg) is given continuously. Surgical menopause requires initially higher dose to control climacteric features.

Nonoral ERT is also available. They are:
- Vaginal estrogen creams (conjugate estrogen 0.625 mg/g; 17β-estradiol 0.1 mg/g, and estropipate 1.5 ng/mg)

TABLE 6: Oral estrogen and progesterone preparations used for hormone replacement therapy (HRT).

Estrogen preparations	Dose
Conjugate estrogen	0.3, 0.625, 0.9, 1.25, and 2.5 mg
Estropipate	0.625, 1.25, 2.5, 5 mg
Micronized estradiol	1.0, 2.0 mg
Esterified estrogens	0.3, 0.625, 1.25, 2.5 mg
Ethinylestradiol	0.02, 0.05 mg
Quinestradiol	0.1 mg
Progesterone preparations	
Medroxyprogesterone	5 and 10 mg
Norethindrone	5 mg
Norgestrel	0.075 mg
Megestrol	20 and 40 mg

- Vaginal ring of estradiol (estring)
- Subcutaneous pellets (estradiol pellets 25 mg)
- Transdermal estradiol patches (estraderm 0.05 or 0.1 mg/day)

Tibolone Regime of Hormone Replacement Therapy

Tibolone is a synthetic steroid structurally related to norethynodrel and is used when women with uterus and do not want to have withdrawal bleeding. Dose is 2.5 mg daily and is to be started at least 1 year after spontaneous menopause.

Benefit and Risk of HRT/ERT

- Benefit of HRT/ERT:
    - Relieves vasomotor symptoms
    - Improves emotional wellbeing
    - Prevents bone loss
    - Promote new bone formation
    - Restore normal epithelium and skin
- Some points to be noted on risk of HRT/ERT:
    - ERT is cardioprotective; contraindicated during active thromboembolic disease
    - Risk of breast cancer is significantly lower than the untreated women.
    - Risk of endometrial cancer is increased in ERT but not with HRT.
    - Hypertension in postmenopause is due to increasing age, and there is no role of estrogen. BP should be monitored routinely and manage accordingly.
    - There is no valid data on increased risk for new occurrence of gallstone with ERT.

Contraindications of ERT

- Absolute estrogen-dependent/estrogen receptor positive neoplasm
- Relative:
    - Undiagnosed abnormal genital bleeding
    - Active thromboembolism

Osteoporosis

Osteoporosis in postmenopausal women is type 1 primary osteoporosis. It is caused by increased activity of osteoclasts, related to decreased levels of estrogen in the circulation. Lack of estrogen is associated with an increased release of cytokines, such as interleukin (IL)-1 and IL-6, which stimulate osteoclasts. For management of postmenopausal osteoporosis, bisphosphonates drugs play an important role in addition to HRT. For details, see Chapter 4.

Premature Ovarian Failure

It is defined by menopause before the age of 35 years. This is because of early exhaustion of ovarian follicle by (1) autoimmune disease, (2) chromosomal defects, (3) 17-hydroxylase deficiency, or (4) malignancy.

Diagnosis is confirmed by documenting high gonadotropins (>40 IU of FSH and LH). Other relevant tests for premature ovarian failure (POF) include ultrasonography (USG), karyotype, ovarian biopsy, etc.

Treatment is done by HRT and psychological support.

Hirsutism

Increased terminal hairs in androgen-sensitive areas such as face and body of women is called hirsutism.

Understanding of normal hair distribution and their types is prerequisite of understanding and evaluating hirsutism:

- Terminal hairs are normal hairs for male and female. They are course and pigmented hairs of scalp, eyelashes, eyebrows, and axilla.
- Vellus hairs are soft and nonpigmented hair that may even cover most of the body normally.
- Transitional hair represents an intermediate state between vellus and terminal hairs and may predominate in some hirsute women.
- Hypertrichosis is a state different from hirsutism, where diffuse excessive terminal hairs is seen in both androgen-sensitive and androgen-nonsensitive areas of the body.
- Hirsutism with virilization may be present where features of masculinization and defeminization are present. It represents severe form of hirsutism.

Table 7 summarizes the features of defeminization and virilization.

Hirsutism results from androgen-mediated conversion of vellus to terminal hair of androgen sensitive hair follicles of the body. Every woman has her fixed number of androgen-sensitive hair follicles; these are located in those regions in which adult men develop hairs, namely

TABLE 7: Features of defeminization and virilization.	
Defeminization	**Virilization**
• Amenorrhea	• Masculine habitus
• Diminished breast size	• Deepening of voice (Adam's apple)
• Temporal balding	
• Acne	• Clitoromegaly
Note: Size of clitoris is determined by formula height × widths. Normal is up to 35 mm and hirsute women with clitoris >100 mm constitutes virilization.	

pubis, axilla, face, chest, abdomen, and back (listed on decreasing sensitivity to androgen). About 10-15% women have terminal hairs in face and perioral region. 2% women have terminal hairs on sternum. Normal women rarely have hairs in upper abdomen or back.

Management of Hirsutism

It is done by (1) clinical confirmation of hirsutism, (2) severity assessment by using scoring system, (3) identification of cause, and (4) treatment—(i) specific to the cause (if found) and (ii) general treatment for hirsutism.

Clinical Confirmation of Hirsutism

It can be done by documentation of terminal hairs in androgen-sensitive.

Scoring of Hirsutism

The Ferriman-Gallwey scale is used for *hirsutism*. A *score* of 1-4 is given for 11 areas of the body. A total score <8 is considered normal, a score of 8-15 indicates mild *hirsutism*, and a score >15 indicates moderate or severe *hirsutism*. A score of 0 indicates absence of terminal hair **(Fig. 9 and Table 8)**.

Causes of Hirsutism

The causes of hirsutism are grouped into two: (1) Hirsutism without virilization and (2) hirsutism with virilization.

Cause list of hirsutism is shown in **Table 9**.

Diagnostic Evaluation of Hirsutism

Table 10 provides DMIS for cases with hirsutism.

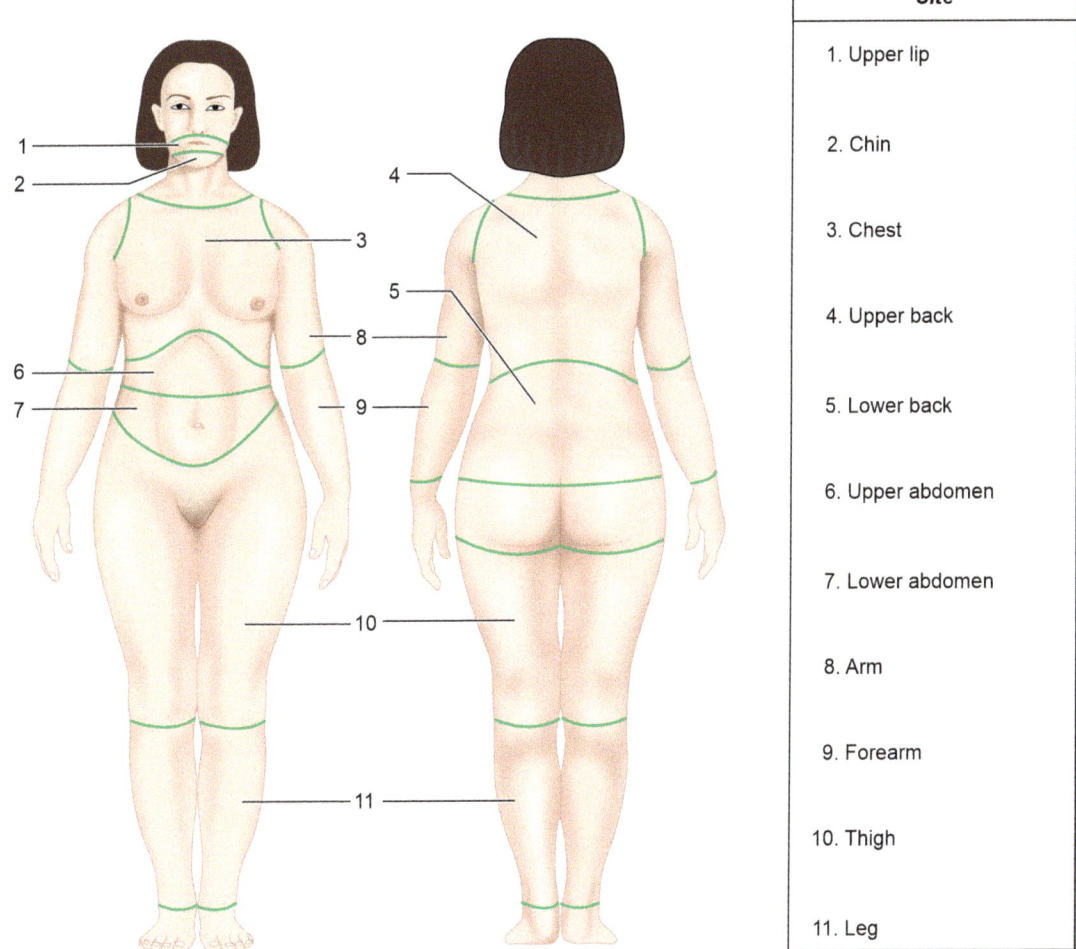

Eleven areas of Ferriman–Gallwey scale for hirsutism

FIG. 9: A score of 1–4 is given for eleven areas of the body. A total score <8 is considered normal, a score of 8–15 indicates mild hirsutism, and a score >15 indicates moderate or severe hirsutism. For score point, see **Table 8**.

TABLE 8: Ferriman–Gallwey scale for hirsutism.

Sl. no.	Site	Score	Definition
1	Upper lip	1	A few hairs at outer margin
		2	A few moustaches at outer margin
		3	Moustaches extending halfway from outer margin
		4	Moustaches extending to midline
2	Chin	1	A few scattered hairs
		2	Scattered hairs with small concentrations
		3 and 4	Complete cover, light, and heavy hairs
3	Chest	1	Circumareolar hairs
		2	Circumareolar plus midline hairs
		3	Fusion of above areas with three quarter cover
		4	Fusion of areas with full cover
4	Upper back	1	A few scattered hairs
		2	More but still scattered
		3 and 4	Complete cover, light, and heavy hairs
5	Lower back	1	A sacral tuft of hairs
		2	A sacral tuft of hairs with lateral extension
		3	Three quarter cover
		4	Complete cover
6	Upper abdomen	1	A few midline hairs
		2	More, still midline hairs
		3 and 4	Half and full cover
7	Lower abdomen	1	A few midline hairs
		2	Midline streak of hairs
		3	Midline band of hairs
		4	An inverted V-shaped growth
8	Arm	1	Sparse growth; affected < quarter of limb surface
		2	Affected > quarter of limb surface but incomplete
		3 and 4	Cover complete; light and heavy
9	Fore arm	1 and 2	Cover complete; light and heavy—dorsum
		3 and 4	Cover complete; light and heavy—ventrum
10	Thigh (as arm)	1	Sparse growth; affected < quarter of limb surface
		2	Affected > quarter of limb surface but incomplete
		3 and 4	Cover complete; light and heavy
11	Leg (as arm)	1	Sparse growth; affected < quarter of limb surface
		2	Affected > quarter of limb surface but incomplete
		3 and 4	Cover complete; light and heavy

Continued

TABLE 9: Causes list of hirsutism.

Hirsutism without virilization

Polycystic ovarian syndrome	
Idiopathic simple hirsutism	
Familial/genetic hirsutism	
Drug-induced hirsutism	• Androgens • Progesterogenal compounds • Anabolic steroids • Glucocorticoids • Phenytoin • Minoxidil, diazoxide, cyclosporine, etc.
Endocrine disorders	• Cushing syndrome • Hypothyroidism • Acromegaly
Postmenopausal state	
Pregnancy	Androgens of corpus luteum/placenta

Hirsutism with virilization

Virilizing ovarian tumors	Arrhenoblastoma
	Androblastoma
Virilizing adrenal tumors	
Hyperplasia of ovarian androgen-producing cells	
Congenital adrenal hyperplasia (CAH)	• 21-hydroxylase deficiency (classical CAH) • 11-hydroxylase deficiency • 3β-hydroxysteroid dehydrogenase deficiency

Treatment of Hirsutism

Treatment of hirsutism consists of (1) drug therapy of hirsutism, (2) cosmetic measures, and (3) treatment of cause.

Drug therapy of hirsutism

Cyproterone acetate (CPA), oral pills, and spironolactone are the drugs used in hirsutism treatment. CPA, sold alone under the brand name Androcur or with ethinylestradiol under the brand names Diane or Diane-35 among others.

TABLE 10: Decision-making investigation steps (DMIS) in a case of hirsutism.		
Step 1	Clinical confirmation/ history	• Documentation of terminal hairs in androgen sensitive area • Exclusion of hypertrichosis • Use of drugs causing hirsutism
Step 2	Severity assessment	Score (Ferriman–Gallwey scale for hirsutism)
Step 3	Examination of virilization	• Masculine habitus • Adam's apple • Clitoromegaly
Step 4	Serum androgen profile	Hyperandrogenemia
Step 5	Search of etiology	Endocrine function tests Imaging (if applicable)

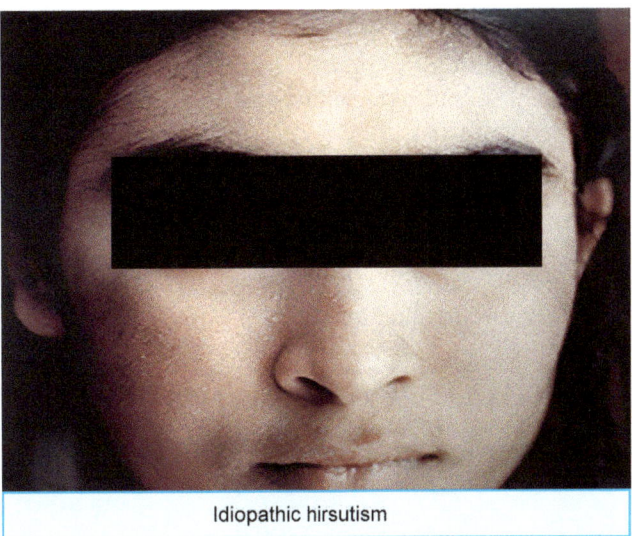

FIG. 10: Age of onset 15–25 years. Absence of menstrual disturbance and virilization. Exclusion of use of drugs that cause hirsutism. Exclusion of disease: (1) ovarian disorders; (2) congenital adrenal hyperplasia (CAH), and (3) polycystic ovarian syndrome (PCOS).

Idiopathic/Simple Hirsutism

Hirsutism affects between 5% and 10% of women without any obvious cause. It is seen commonly in young girls. Usually, age at onset is 15–25 years. There is no menstrual disturbance, and no sign of virilization is seen. Diagnosis is confirmed by exclusion of (1) use of drugs causing hirsutism, (2) ovarian disorders, (3) congenital adrenal hyperplasia (CAH), and (4) PCOS. Treatment consists of cosmetic measures and drug treatment **(Fig. 10)**.

Hirsutism of Polycystic Ovarian Syndrome

Hirsutism of polycystic ovarian syndrome (PCOS) is characterized by: (1) Age of onset of hirsutism along with acne is peripuberty and gradually progressive; (2) menstruation may be normal, irregular, or absent; (3) usually, there is weight gain; (4) there is no virilization; and (5) infertility may be a complaint. Diagnostic parameters include (1) enlarged polycystic ovaries by ultrasonogram or laparoscopic examination and (2) altered hormonal profile, such as absolutely raised LH, LH/FSH ratio >2.8, raised testosterone, 17-OH progesterone level is normal, usually raised DHAS, and raised prolactin in about 10% cases **(Flowchart 4)**.

Treatment of hirsutism consists of weight correction (if obese), cosmetic measures, and drug treatment and for fertility ovulation induction.

GYNECOMASTIA

Enlargement of male breast is called gynecomastia. Enlargement is measured by using Tanner scale of breast development for female (Stage: Tanner's BII or more). Fatty tissue deposition without glandular enlargement (particularly in in obese individual) is called lipomastia. During neonatal life, puberty, and in old age, gynecomastia (usually <Tanner's BIII) may appear without significant underlying pathology called "physiological gynecomastia."

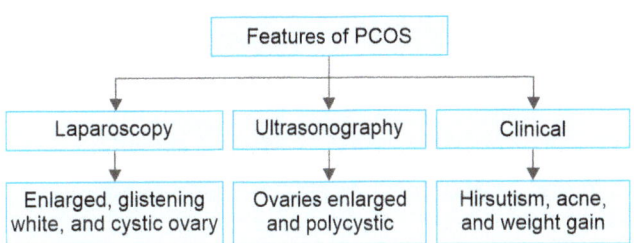

FLOWCHART 4: Features of polycystic ovarian syndrome (PCOS).

Almost all neonatal gynecomastia subsides spontaneously. Around 70% boys do have mild degree (up to Tanner's stage II) of gynecomastia during puberty majority of which regress within 2 years. A few of them may become more severe (more than Tanner's BII) called Pubertal Macromastia and do not restresses spontaneously.

Pathogenesis of gynecomastia is due to glandular enlargement, which is due to imbalance between estrogen and androgen. So causes of gynecomastia can be grouped into: (1) Gynecomastia of testosterone deficiency, (2) gynecomastia of estrogen excess, (3) drugs-related gynecomastia, and (4) idiopathic gynecomastia **(Fig. 11)**.

Causes of Gynecomastia

Gynecomastia develops by estrogenic excess over androgen. So, causes are either androgen lack or estrogen excess, or both.

Table 11 summarizes the causes of gynecomastia.

Diagnostic Evaluation of Gynecomastia

Step 1: Clinical evaluation/history

Step 2: Physical evaluation

Step 3: Investigations

Table 12 provides DMIS for case with gynecomastia.

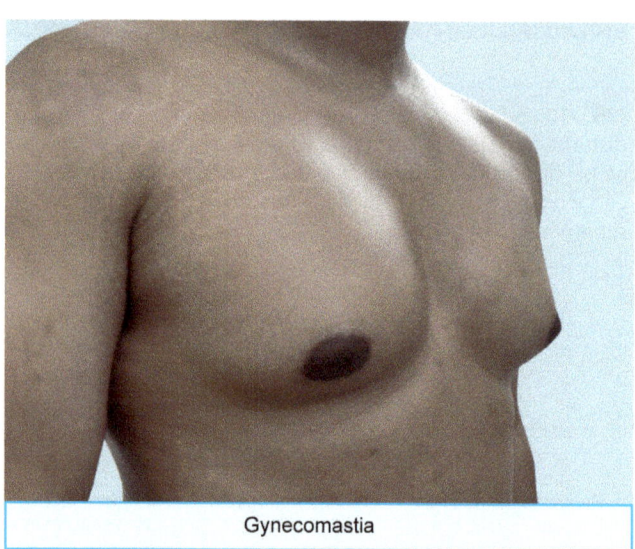

Gynecomastia

FIG. 11: Gynecomastia can be grouped into: (1) Gynecomastia of testosterone deficiency, (2) gynecomastia of estrogen excess, (3) drugs-related gynecomastia, and (4) idiopathic gynecomastia.

TABLE 11: Causes of gynecomastia.

Testosterone deficiency	• Anorchia • Klinefelter syndrome • Androgen resistance • Orchitis, castration, trauma, renal failure, spinal cord injury, etc.
Estrogen excess	• Increased production of estrogen • Estrogen-secreting testicular tumor, bronchogenic carcinoma, true hermaphroditism • Increased conversion of androgen to estrogen • Familial/genetic, starvation, liver disease, thyrotoxicosis
Drugs related	• Estrogen/drugs acting like it • Diethylstilbestrol, estrogen ointments, milk/meat of estrogen-injected cow, digitalis • Drugs acting with unknown mechanism • Antituberculosis—isoniazid, ethambutol; anticancer—busulfan; drug of Wilson's disease—penicillamine; antipsychotic tricyclic antidepressant; sedative diazepam; drug of addiction—marijuana and heroines • Drugs inhibit testosterone synthesis: Antifungal—ketoconazole • Drugs enhance estrogen production: Fertility—human chorionic gonadotropin (hCG) and clomiphene • Drug inhibits testosterone action: Spironolactone, cimetidine
Idiopathic	By exclusion of all causes listed above and physiological gynecomastia. It constitutes significant bulk gynecomastia

TABLE 12: Decision-making investigation steps (DMIS) in a case of gynecomastia.

Step 1	Clinical evaluation/history	Drug history	
Step 2	Physical evaluation	Examination of breast	• Grade (Tanner's stage) • Unilateral or bilateral • Galactorrhea present or absent • Tenderness present or absent • Exclude neurofibroma (unilateral) Carcinoma (tender), etc.
		Examination of testes	• Anorchia/cryptorchidism • Volume and consistency
		Anthropometry	Height, span, upper and lower segments
		Sigma of disorders	Klinefelter syndrome, hepatic/renal failure, thyrotoxicosis
Step 3	Investigations	Hormone	FSH, LH, testosterone, estrogen, prolactin
		Biochemistry	Creatinine, ALT, AST
		Imaging	Mammography, sonography

(ALT: alanine transaminase; AST: aspartate transaminase; FSH: follicle-stimulating hormone; LH: luteinizing hormone)

Treatment of Gynecomastia
- Treatment of underlying disorder(s) if treatable
- If breast size is up to Tanner's stage II then wait
- If breast size is more than Tanner's stage II, plastic surgery can be done.

MICROPHALLUS

Definition: A phallic length which is 2.5 or more standard deviations below the mean is microphallus.

An infant of 0–5 months of age, the lower limit of phallic length is 1.9 cm. The Stretched Penile Length (SPL) increases with age until the pubertal development is complete and the adult SPL varies with ethnicity. There is significant increase in SPL, especially from birth to the age of 5 years but mildly increased from 5 to 10 years, after that high growth rate occurred again and statistical differences remain from age 10 to 13 years. **Figures 12 and 13** show SPL measurement procedure and a nomogram for SPL, respectively.

Common Causes of Microphallus
- Congenital hypopituitarism
- Isolated gonadotropin deficiency
- Use of progesterone preparations for mother in early pregnancy
- Intrauterine testicular failure (late variants)

Treatment of Microphallus
After exclusion of definite causes, short-term testosterone therapy is given. Intramuscular testosterone 50–75 mg is given once every 21 days. Response is considered adequate if final SPL crosses the average SPL for the age. Usually, 2–4 shorts are required.

CRYPTORCHIDISM

Failure of descent of testis at its normal position, bottom of the scrotal sac, is called undescended testis or cryptorchidism. It may be unilateral or bilateral. Normally, descent of testis occurs during third trimester of intrauterine life. Rate of incidence of incomplete descent is high in premature babies. At full term, incident is about 3.4% but at the endo of 1 year the figure spontaneously drops to 0.8%. Consequences of cryptorchidism are:
- Intra-abdominal testis is likely to fail spermatogenesis in adult life
- Histological deterioration may occur by high temperature of abdomen
- Testicular malignancy is about 10% of cryptorchidism cases.

Classification of Undescended Testis or Cryptorchidism

Classification of cryptorchidism is done on the basis of: (1) Position of the undescended testes, (2) site/number of testes involved, or (3) it is due absence of testes.

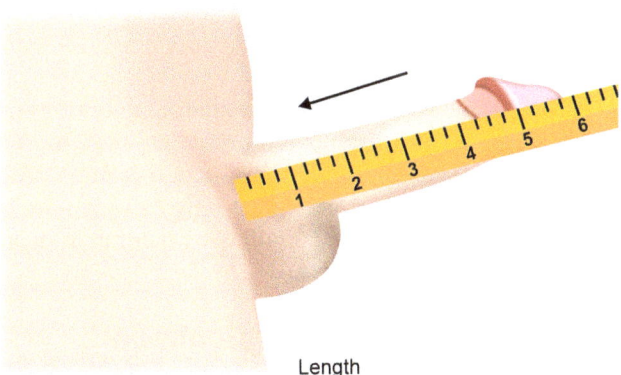

How to measure stretched penile length (SPL)?

FIG. 12: SPL is length stretched penis from the base at pubic bone up to tip of glans penis.

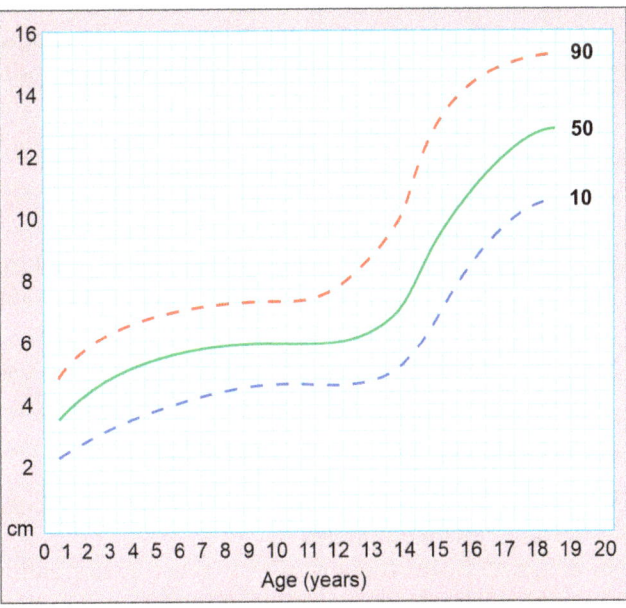

Stretched penile length (SPL)–nomogram

FIG. 13: Nomogram of SPL expressed as 10th, 50th, and 90th percentile.

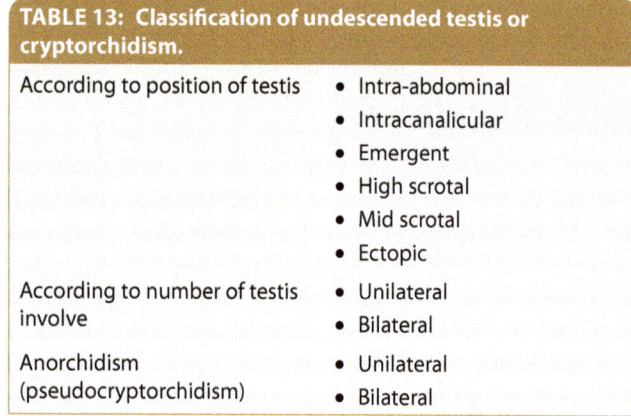

TABLE 13: Classification of undescended testis or cryptorchidism.

According to position of testis	• Intra-abdominal • Intracanalicular • Emergent • High scrotal • Mid scrotal • Ectopic
According to number of testis involve	• Unilateral • Bilateral
Anorchidism (pseudocryptorchidism)	• Unilateral • Bilateral

Table 13 describes the classification of undescended testis.

Evaluation of Undescended Testis or Cryptorchidism

- Gentle physical examination should be done by experienced physician. In the hands of an experienced provider, >70% of cryptorchid testes are palpable by physical examination and need no imaging. In the remaining 30% of cases with a nonpalpable testis, the challenge is to confirm absence or presence of the testis and to identify the location of the viable nonpalpable testis.
- Ultrasound has only 45% and 78% sensitivity and specificity, respectively to localize nonpalpable testes.
- MRI with or without angiography has been more widely used with greater sensitivity and specificity and has chances to provide misleading information (such as absence when actually present or vice versa).
- A karyotype can confirm or exclude dysgenetic primary hypogonadism.
- Hormone levels, such as gonadotropins and post hCG stimulated a rise in the testosterone level, can be useful in cases with bilateral cryptorchidism.
- In some cases, further testing is crucial and has a high likelihood of detecting intersex conditions **(Fig. 14)**.

Treatment of Cryptorchidism

- hCG stimulation test is done for bilateral nonpalpable testes to exclude anorchia.
- hCG and GnRH therapy has variable role in treating cryptorchidism.
    - For bilateral cryptorchidism, 3,000–5,000 units of hCG are given intramuscularly every alternate day for 5 days (total three injections)—called short course of hCG therapy.

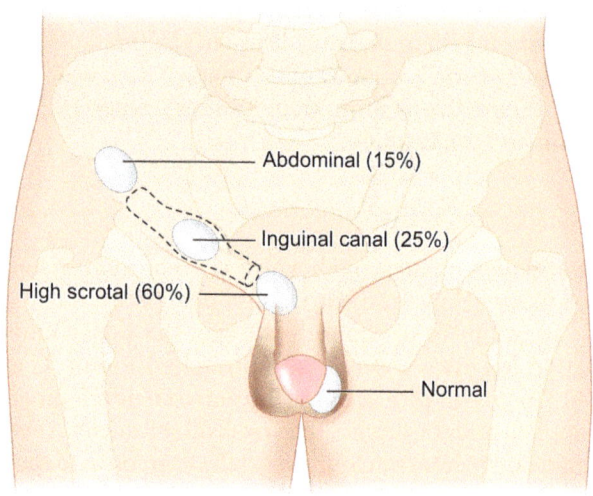

Undescended testis or cryptorchidism

FIG. 14: Evaluation of cryptorchidism. (1) Physical examination by expert, (2) USG, (3) CT/MRI with/without angiogram, and (4) Karyotype and hormonal study.

- For unilateral cryptorchidism, 500 units of hCG are given intramuscularly every third day for 45 days (total 20 injections)—called long course of hCG therapy.
- Surgery—*orchiopexy* (or *orchidopexy*) to move an undescended (cryptorchid) testicle into the scrotum and permanently fix it. This is considered when response hormone therapy is not satisfactory.

AMBIGUOUS GENITALIA

Ambiguous genitalia is a condition in which an infant's external genitals do not appear to be clearly either male or female. It is a disorder of sex development and is obvious at or shortly after birth.

It should be considered as neonatal emergency, because there may be immediate problems, like symptoms of diarrhea, vomiting, shock, etc., or salt-losing CAH. A rapid exploration of its cause not only can save life but also minimize anxiety of the family by helping in proper sex assignment of the neonate.

Causes of Ambiguous Genitalia

Causes can be grouped into: (1) Anatomical disruption giving rise to opposite sex outlook of external genitalia, (2) virilizing of female baby, (3) incomplete virilizing of male baby, and (4) gonadal intersex.

Table 14 shows the causes of ambiguous genitalia.

TABLE 14: Causes of ambiguous genitalia.

	Anatomical disruptions
Female with	• Clitoromegaly and prominent labia minora • Redundant prepuce • Hypertrophy of vaginal mucosa • Prolapse of vaginal tissue to uterus • Duplication of labia • Abnormal relation between rectum, vagina, and urethra
Male with	• Microphallus • Buried phallus • Absence or vestigial phallus • Absent scrotum and gonads
	Virilization of female
Congenital adrenal hyperplasia	• 21-hydroxylase deficiency • 11β-hydroxylase deficiency • 3β-hydroxylase deficiency
Maternal source androgen	• Taking of progesteronal agents • Luteoma of pregnancy • Adrenal tumor • Use of anabolic steroids (athletic/medical ground)
Idiopathic	
	Incomplete virilization of male

	• Androgen resistance syndromes (complete/incomplete)
	• 5α-reductase deficiency
	• Bilateral cryptorchidism/anorchia
	• Denys–Drash syndrome
	• Hypopituitarism
	• Male with microphallus syndrome:
	  ○ Robinow syndrome
	  ○ Septo-optic dysplasia
	  ○ Pallister–Hall syndrome

	Gonadal intersex
	• True hermaphroditism • Mixed gonadal dysgenesis (45,X/46,XY)

Diagnosis of Ambiguous Genitalia

Diagnostic studies of ambiguity of sex include:
- *Imaging study*: (1) Pelvic ultrasonogram, (2) contrast genitogram, and (3) renal ultrasonogram
- *Genetic study*: (1) Karyotype and (2) family study
- *Endocrine study*: (1) CAH, (2) gonadal stimulation with hCG, (3) adrenal stimulation with ACTH, and (4) adrenal suppression with dexamethasone.

Table 15 shows DMIS of a case genital ambiguity.

INFERTILITY

If a woman fails to conceive after 1 year of try without contraception than the couple is labeled as infertile.

Infertility may be primary—never conceived or secondary—previously conceived.

Causes of Infertility

Factors responsible for infertility are grouped into four categories plus one idiopathic:
1. Male factor infertility
2. Ovulatory and luteal factor
3. Tubal, uterine, and pelvic factors
4. Cervical factor
5. Idiopathic/unexplained (**Fig. 15**)

Male factor infertility is practically reflected as defect in the semen/sperm analysis report:
- Congenital factors (cryptorchidism and testicular dysgenesis, congenital absence of the vas deferens)
- Acquired urogenital abnormalities (obstructions, testicular torsion, testicular tumor, orchitis)
- Urogenital tract infections
- Increased scrotal temperature (e.g., due to varicocele)
- Endocrine disturbances
- Genetic abnormalities
- Immunological factors (autoimmune diseases)
- Systemic diseases (diabetes, renal and liver insufficiency, cancer, and hemochromatosis)
- Exogenous factors (medications, toxins, and irradiation)
- Lifestyle factors (obesity, smoking, drugs, and anabolic steroids)

According to semen analysis report, sperm abnormalities are of five types (**Fig. 16**):
1. Azoospermia—absent sperm
2. Oligozoospermia—diminished sperm count (<15 million/mL and severe <5 million/mL)
3. Asthenozoospermia—increased nonmotile sperm (motility <60%)
4. Necrozoospermia—increased dead sperm (alive <60%)
5. Teratozoospermia—increased sperm with abnormal morphology (normal <60%)

Ovulatory and luteal factor infertility: (1) Ovarian failure including POF, (2) unruptured luteum as in PCOS, (3) hypothyroidism, hyperprolactinemia, hypercortisolemia, etc., and (3) luteal insufficiency—short luteal phase.

Tubal, uterine and pelvic factors infertility: (1) Tubal blockage, (2) large myoma, (3) endometriosis, and (4) salpingitis (**Fig. 17**).

TABLE 15: Decision-making investigation steps in a case of genital ambiguity.

Steps	Investigations	Finding	Action/inference
Initial step	Look for palpable gonad(s)	Absent	Go to step 3
		Present	Go to step 2/(step 5 if enlarged breast during puberty)
Step 2	Check for microphallus	Present	Go to step 4
		Absent	Go to step 3/(step 5 if enlarged breast during puberty)
Step 3	Check for uterus (cryptorchidism) (sonogram/laparoscopy/PR examination)	Present	Go to step 4
		Absent	Go to step 7
		Cryptorchidism	Management accordingly
Step 4	Investigate for hypopituitarism	Present	Treat hypopituitarism and microphallus
		Absent	Go to step 7
Step 5	Investigate for androgen resistance and 5α-reductase deficiency	Present	Management accordingly
		Absent	Go to step 7
Step 6	Investigate for CAH and maternal source androgen	Positive	Management accordingly
		Absent	Go to step 7
Step 7	Karyotype	46, XY	Anatomical disruption of male—corrective surgery
		46, XX	Anatomical disruption of female—corrective surgery
		46, XY/46, XX	True hermaphroditism management accordingly
		45, XO/46, XX	Mixed gonadal dysgenesis management accordingly

(CAH: congenital adrenal hyperplasia; PR: per rectal)

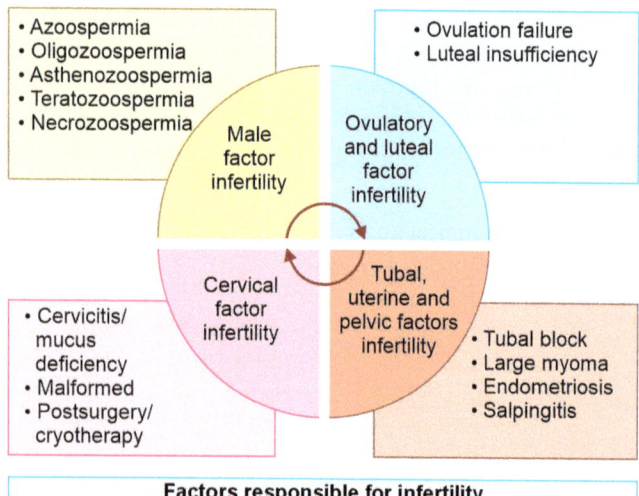

FIG. 15: Factors responsible for infertility are grouped into four categories plus one idiopathic.

Infertility Management

With the rapid advancement in ART such as intrauterine insemination (IUI) and in vitro fertilization (IVF), scope to have babies by infertile couples has becoming more feasible than ever before; some of them can provide full/partial biological parenthood while other are not.

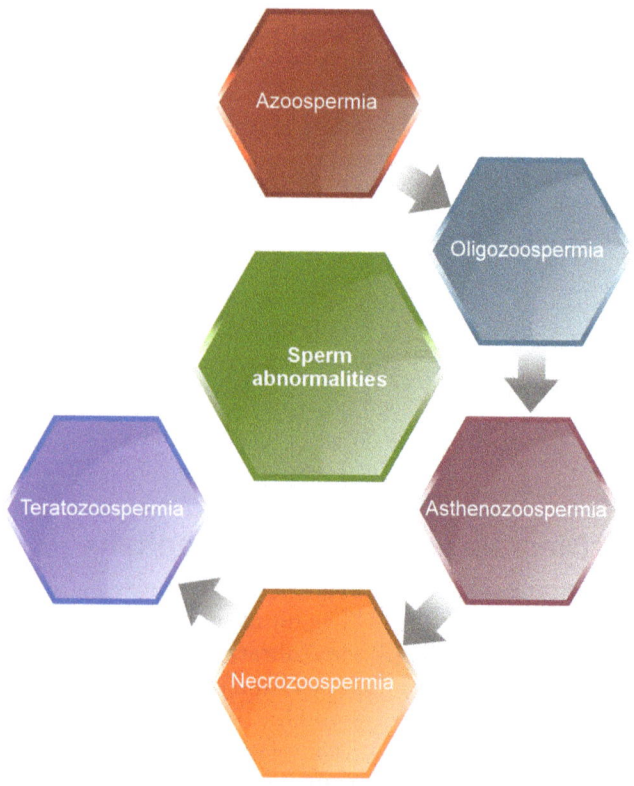

FIG. 16: Types of sperms in semen analysis.

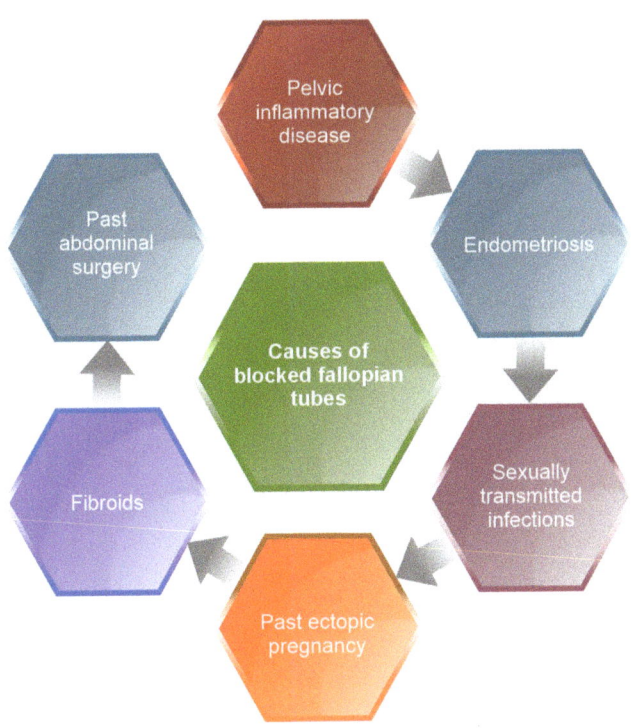

FIG. 17: Causes of blocked fallopian tubes.

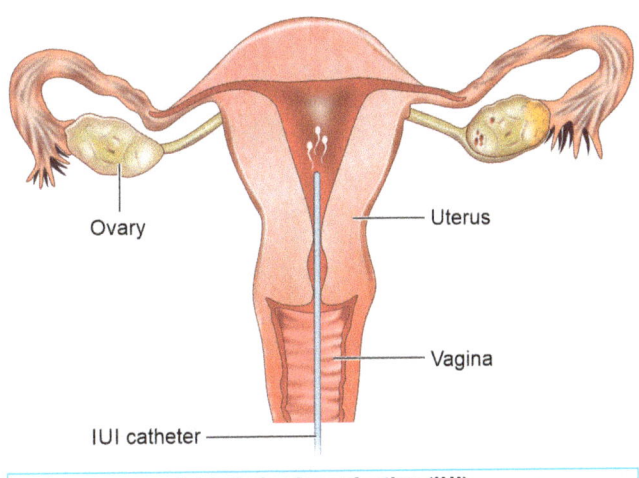

Intrauterine insemination (IUI)

FIG. 18: Insemination: 0.3–0.5 mL of semen (containing at least 10×10^6/mL actively motile sperm density) is pushed in the uterine cavity using IUI catheter. *Timing*: Ovulation period—on natural cycle/stimulated cycle. *Luteal phase support*: Micro dose of human chorionic gonadotropin (hCG) injection.

Intrauterine Insemination

Semen either freshly collected or stored previously with or without laboratory treatment (washed/concentrated) is introduced in the uterine cavity in and around the time of ovulation is called IUI.

Procedure of IUI
- The recipient is at ovulation time either on her natural cycle or after induction of ovulation by a specific protocol.
- Semen used is either freshly collected or after treatment (semen wash and centrifuged).
- Following a gentle speculum examination, 0.3–0.5 mL of semen (containing at least 10×10^6/mL actively motile sperm density) is injected into the uterine cavity via cervix using a fine atraumatic IUI catheter attached to a 1-mL syringe.
- Luteal support is given by hCG injection (daily micro dose of hCG 100 IU/day for 5 days from 1 or 2 days after ovulation) and pregnancy check is made after 16 days after ovulation **(Figs. 18 and 19)**.

Types of IUI with Indications
- IUI with husband's semen (full biological parenthood)—(1) idiopathic infertility, (2) sperm factor (Oligo-/astheno-/teratozoospermia) infertility, and (3) cervical factor infertility.
- IUI with donor's semen (only maternal biological parenthood)—(1) azoospermia and (2) major hereditary disease.

In Vitro Fertilization

In vitro fertilization process involves development of embryo of 8–16 cells size in specialized ART laboratory using egg and sperm either of a couple or one/both from donor(s). Fertilization is done by insemination in a Petri dish called Nunc or by other technique like intracytoplasmic sperm injection (ICSI). The source of sperm may be freshly collected or stored previously with or without laboratory treatment (washed/concentrated) or by special technique. The embryo is transferred to uterus of mother or surrogate mother and pregnancy check is done subsequently.

Procedure of IVF
1. The eggs are collected from female partner or donor who is on an ovarian stimulation protocol.
2. Egg retrieval/collection of eggs by transvaginal ultrasound aspiration—day 0
3. Sperm source may from male partner or donor from fresh or treated semen or microsurgery like testicular sperm aspiration (TESA).
4. Fertilization of egg by insemination of good sperms in a Petri dish called Nunc or other techniques such as ICSI where single sperm is injected into an egg by a microneedle under an inverted microscope vision—day 0

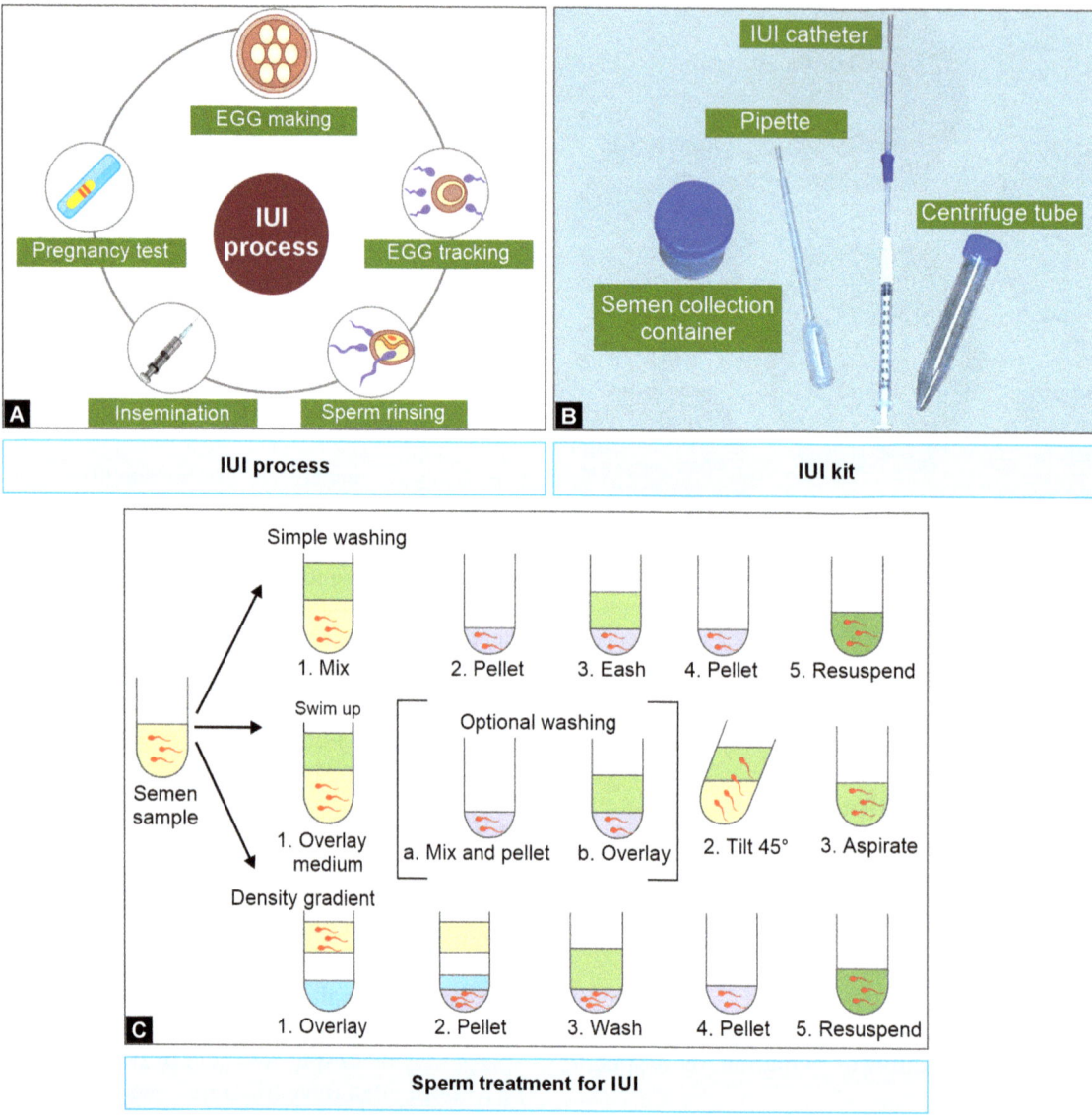

FIGS. 19A TO C: Intrauterine insemination (IUI) process.

5. Embryo culture is done in special media and serial check for 2 pronucleus (2pn) to 16 cells stage is done—day 0–5.
6. Embryo transfer (ET) is done to uterine cavity of mother or surrogate mother. Good quality embryo (1–3) is inserted to the recipient uterus by using transferred to day 3–5.
7. Pregnancy test 14 days after ET **(Figs. 20 to 22)**

Type of IVF with Indications

- IVF with couple's egg and sperm (full biological parenthood): (1) Idiopathic infertility; (2) sperm factor (such as severe oligo-/astheno-/terato-/necrozoospermia) infertility; (3) tubal, uterus, and pelvic factor infertility; and (4) cervical factor infertility with failed IUI.
- IVF with couple's egg and sperm with surrogate mother (full biological parenthood): (1) Asherman syndrome; (2) hysterectomy; (3) uterine a developmental defect including agenesis (Mayer-Rokitansky-Küster-Hauser syndrome); and (4) choice of the couple.
- IVF with donor's semen (only maternal biological parenthood): (1) Azoospermia and (2) major hereditary disease.
- IVF with donor's egg (only paternal biological parenthood): (1) Ovarian failure—Turner syndrome and (2) bilateral oophorectomy.

Management Options for Infertility

Table 16 summarizes the management options for infertility.

Table 17 describes DMIS of an infertile couple.

CONTRACEPTIVES/BIRTH CONTROL

Contraception means *prevention of pregnancy*. It is done by (1) keeping the ovum and sperm apart, (2) prevention of egg production, or (3) stopping the fertilized egg implantation in the uterus.

There are six types of medicines and devices for birth control **(Flowchart 5)**.

■ Sterilization

Sterilization is a permanent form of birth control that is extremely effective at preventing pregnancy. But it is difficult to reverse if you change your mind, and it does not protect against STDs. Both men and women can be sterilized. For women, a tubal ligation is performed; for men, a vasectomy is performed **(Figs. 23A and B)**.

■ Long-acting Reversible Contraceptives

There are two types of long-acting reversible contraceptive (LARC): (1) The intrauterine device (IUD) and (2) the birth control implant. Both are highly effective in preventing pregnancy. They last for several years and are easy to use. Both methods are reversible—if couple wants to get pregnant or if you want to stop using them, these can be removed at any time **(Fig. 24)**.

■ Contraceptive Injection

The contraceptive injection (medroxyprogesterone acetate or norethisterone enanthate) releases the hormone progestogen in blood to prevent pregnancy. Medroxyprogesterone acetate (Depo-Provera or Sayana Press) is most commonly used, and its contraceptive action lasts for 13 weeks. Norethisterone enanthate (Noristerat) is effective for 8 weeks.

■ Short-acting Contraceptive Hormonal Methods

In these methods, hormones are dispensed as *pill, patch, or ring* such as NuvaRing. These contain hormones,

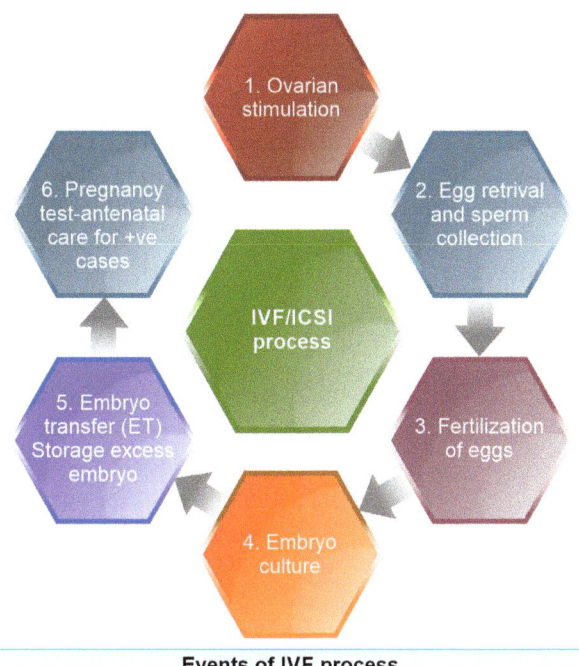

FIG. 20: Steps of in vitro fertilization (IVF) process. (1) Ovarian stimulation for eggs; (2) Egg retrieval—day 0; (3) Fertilization of egg with good sperm(s) by insemination/intracytoplasmic sperm injection (ICSI)—day 0; (4) Embryo culture—day 0–5; (5) Embryo transfer (ET)—day 3–5; (6) Pregnancy test 14 days after ET.

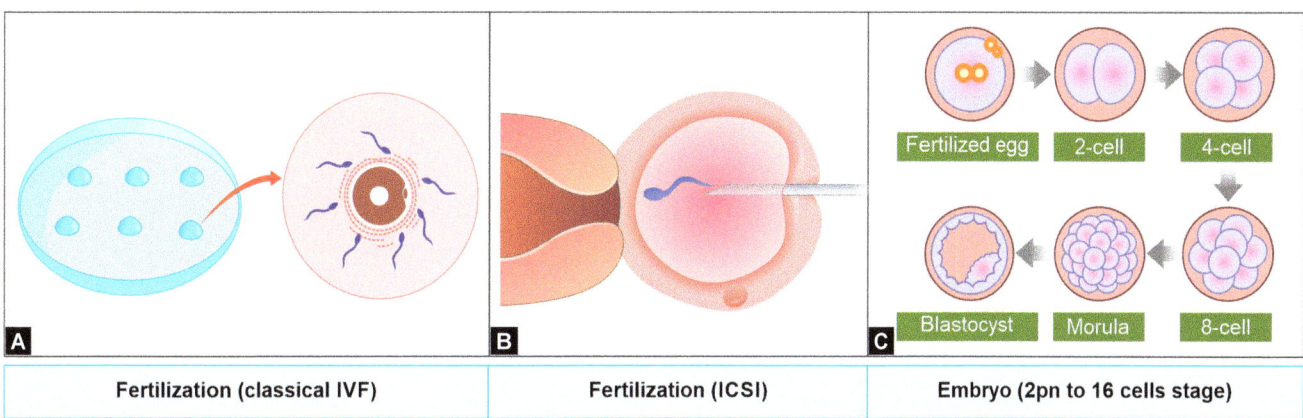

FIGS. 21A TO C: IVF process.
(IVF: in vitro fertilization; ICSI: intracytoplasmic sperm injection)

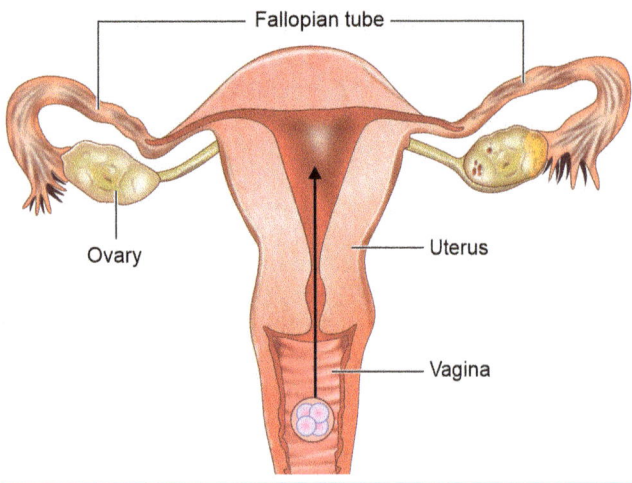

FIG. 22: After fertilization by IVF/ICSI the embryo development is done in the laboratory. On day 2–5 healthy *embryo(s) are transferred* in uterine cavity.
(ICSI: intracytoplasmic sperm injection)

either both estrogen and progestin or only progestin. The combined preparations act by interfering with ovulation and thicken the cervical mucosa but progestin-only preparations predominantly thicken the cervical mucosa.

Progestin-only preparations are used in woman who should not take estrogen due to certain medical conditions, examples blood clots, pulmonary embolism, deep vein thrombosis, high blood pressure, smokers, age over 35 years, and migraine. Breastfeeding mothers also should not take estrogen, because it can decrease milk production.

The types of birth control pills include:
- Combined oral contraceptives (also called COCs or "the pill") contain a combination of the female hormones estrogen and progestin and are taken orally once daily, usually at the same time each day.
- Progestin-only pills (POPs, also called "the mini pill") are taken orally once daily, usually at the same time of day.

TABLE 16: Management options for infertility.

Infertility factor	Investigation	Disorder	Management options
Male	Semen analysis	Azoospermia	• Counseling • IUI/ART (donor's sperm) • Treatment of obstruction (in obstructive azo)
		Oligozoospermia	• IUI/IVF/ICSI • Treatment trail in vivo
		Asthenozoospermia	
		Necrozoospermia	
		Teratozoospermia	
Ovulatory and Luteal	Hormone study	Ovarian failure	• Counseling • ART (superovulation) • ART with donor's egg
		Unruptured luteum	Treatment of cause + ovulation induction
		Luteal insufficiency	Luteal support
Tubal, uterine and pelvic	HSG/hysteroscopy/laparoscopy	Tubal blockage	IVF
		Large myoma	Myomectomy
		Endometriosis	Medical therapy + IVF
		Salpingitis	Medical therapy + IVF
Cervical	Cervical mucosa study/HSG	Inadequate cervical mucosa in mid cycle	IUI
		Cervicitis	IUI
		Congenital malformation of cervix	IUI/IVF
		Postsurgery/cryotherapy of cervix	IUI
Idiopathic	Exclusion of above factors		IUI/IVF/ICSI

(ART: assisted reproductive technique; HSG: hysterosalpingography; ICSI: intracytoplasmic sperm injection; IUI: intrauterine insemination; IVF: in vitro fertilization)

TABLE 17: Decision-making investigation steps (DMIS) in case of an infertile couple.

Steps	Investigations	Finding	Action/inference
Initial step	Check for menses and coital practice	Normal	Go to step 2
		Abnormal	Educate and go to step 2
Step 2	Male factor evaluation—complete semen analysis	Normal	Go to step 3
		Abnormal	Management accordingly*
Step 3	Investigate for ovulatory and luteal factors	Normal	Go to step 4
		Abnormal	Management accordingly*
Step 4	Investigate for tubal, uterine, and pelvic factors	Normal	Go to step 5
		Abnormal	Management accordingly*
Step 5	Investigate for cervical factors	Normal	Go to step 6
		Abnormal	Management accordingly*
Step 6	Manage the couple as idiopathic infertility	IUI/IVF/ICSI	

Note: Management accordingly* see in the Table 16.
(ICSI: intracytoplasmic sperm injection; IUI: intrauterine insemination; IVF: in vitro fertilization)

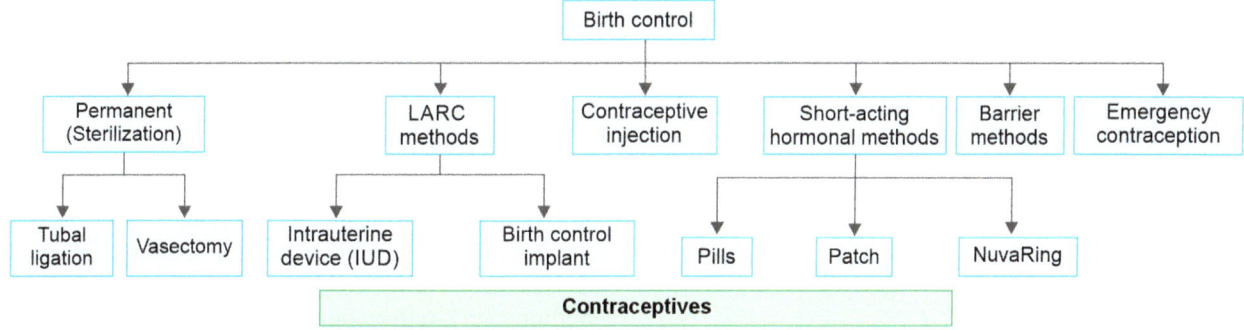

FLOWCHART 5: Six types of medicines and devices for birth control.
(LARC: long-acting reversible contraceptives)

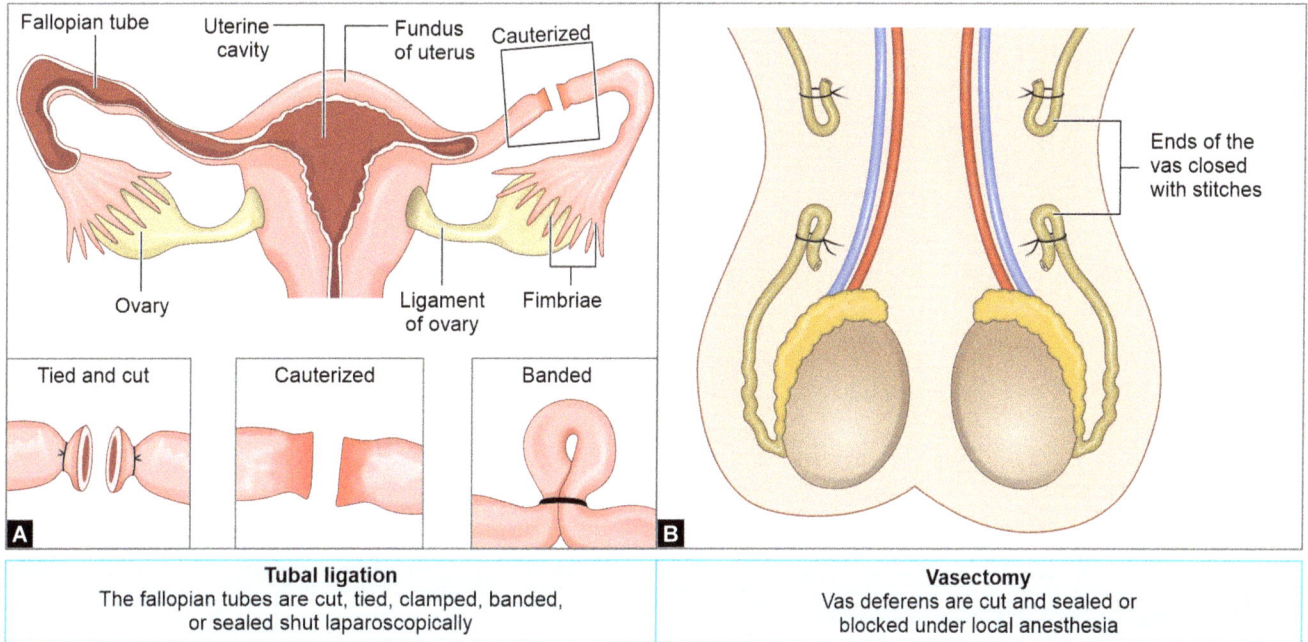

FIGS. 23A AND B: Sterilization for male and female.

Monophasic oral contraceptive pills contain the same amount of estrogen and progestin in each active pill:
- Ethinylestradiol and norethindrone
- Drospirenone and ethinylestradiol
- Drospirenone, ethinylestradiol, and levomefolate
- Ethinylestradiol and norgestrel
- Ethinylestradiol and desogestrel
- Ethinylestradiol and levonorgestrel
- Ethinylestradiol and levonorgestrel extended-cycle
- Estetrol and drospirenone

Biphasic oral contraceptive pills contain the same amount of estrogen each day and the dose of progestin is increased halfway through cycle:
- Ethinylestradiol and levonorgestrel extended-cycle
- Ethinylestradiol and desogestrel.
- Ethinylestradiol and levonorgestrel

Triphasic oral contraceptive pills have three different doses of progestin and estrogen that change about every 7 days:
- Ethinylestradiol and norethindrone
- Ethinylestradiol and levonorgestrel
- Ethinylestradiol and desogestrel

Four-phasic oral contraceptive pills deliver four different doses of progestin and estrogen during a 28-day cycle:
- Dienogest and estradiol
- Ethinylestradiol and levonorgestrel extended-cycle (Quartette)

Ninety-one-day oral contraceptive pills contain a constant dose of estrogen and progestin for 84 days:
- Ethinylestradiol and levonorgestrel
- Ethinylestradiol and levonorgestrel extended-cycle

Progesterone-only oral contraceptive pills provide a constant dose of progestin:
- Norethindrone **(Flowchart 6)**.

■ The Patch

They are dermal patches that contain both estrogen and progestin. Hormones are released transdermally and prevent pregnancy in similar mechanism as oral-combined pills. The patch is worn for consecutive 3 weeks followed by 1 week that is patch free. The patch needs to be replaced weekly.

Ring (NuvaRing): It is a soft ring that contains both estrogen and progestin. It is placed in vagina for 21 days and then removed for a 7-day break. Regularly checking that NuvaRing is in vagina (for example, before and after intercourse) is required to ensure its efficacy **(Fig. 25)**.

■ Barrier Methods

Barrier methods of birth control prevent pregnancy by blocking sperm from reaching egg. Types of barrier methods include condoms (male or female), diaphragms, cervical caps, and the contraceptive sponge. Barrier methods work better when you use them with a spermicide.

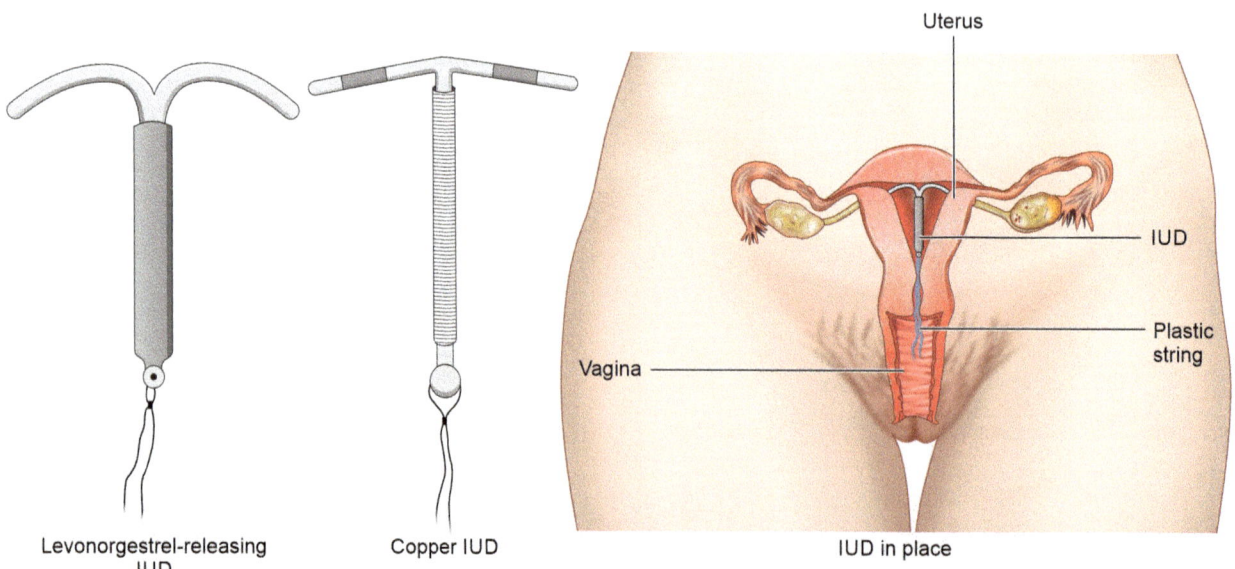

FIG. 24: Long-acting reversible contraceptives (LARC).

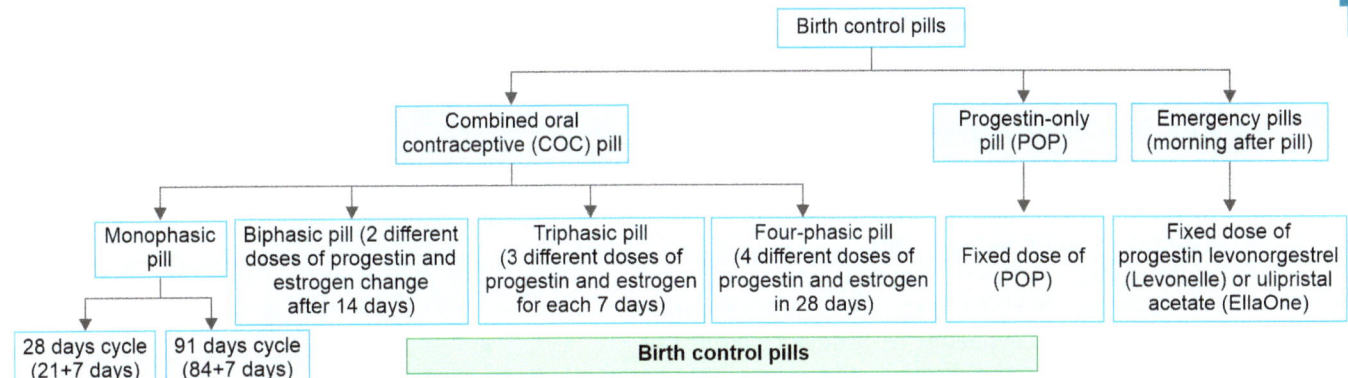

FLOWCHART 6: Types of birth control pills.

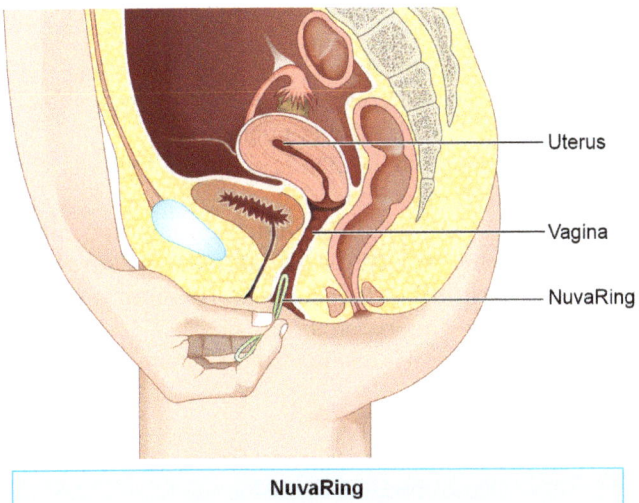

FIG. 25: It is placed in vagina. It releases a continuous low dose of estrogen and progestin to prevent pregnancy. It is kept for 3 weeks continuously than 1 week off.

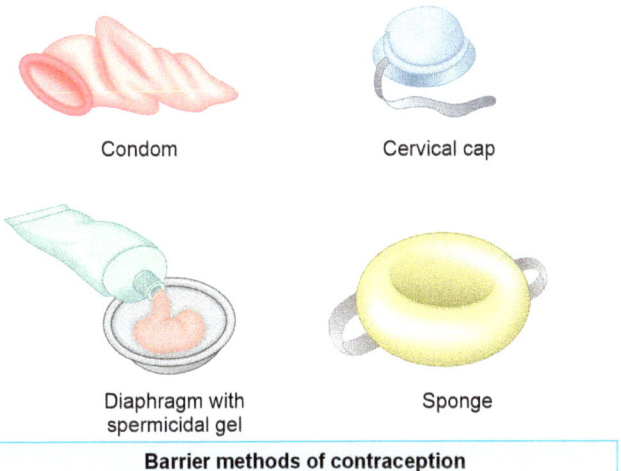

FIG. 26: Male condoms and female diaphragms, cervical caps, and the contraceptive sponge are used as barrier methods of contraception.

Some barrier methods of birth control are described here:
- *Male condom*: This is a thin tube, which is made of rubber (latex), plastic, or lambskin. It is fitted over the penis to prevent sperm from getting into the vagina. Rubber and plastic condoms can protect against sexually transmitted infections (STIs). A new condom must be used each time of sex.
- *Female condom*: It is a thin plastic pouch with open on one end. It is placed inside the vagina, keeping the closed end up. So, this condom lines the walls of the vagina and thus prevents sperm from getting into the vagina. It also protects against STIs. A new condom is to be used each time of sex.
- *Diaphragm*: This is a dome with firm, flexible rim, which is made of rubber or silicone. It is fitted inside a woman's vagina to cover the cervix of uterus. A diaphragm is used with spermicide. A woman should put in the diaphragm no more than 6 hours before she had sex.
- *Cervical cap*: This is a rubber device, fits inside the vagina, right up against the cervix. It should always be used with a spermicide. A cervical cap can last for up to 2 years.
- *Contraceptive sponge*: This is a disk made of thick plastic foam. It is fitted inside the vagina and covers the cervix. It also contains spermicide. A woman wets the sponge and then inserts it into her vagina. It can provide protection against pregnancy for the next 24 hours, even if she has sex more than once.
- *Spermicide*: It kills sperm. It is available as jelly, foam, cream, suppository, and film. The most commonly used spermicide is nonoxynol-9. It is put into the vagina about 15 minutes before sex by usually an applicator **(Fig. 26)**.

Emergency Contraception

Emergency contraception can prevent pregnancy after unprotected sex or if the contraception you have used has failed; e.g., a condom has split or you have missed a pill.

There are two types of emergency contraception:
1. The emergency contraceptive pill—Levonelle or Ellaone (the "morning after" pill)
2. The intrauterine device (IUD or coil)

You need to take the emergency contraceptive pill within 3 days (Levonelle) or 5 days (Ellaone) of unprotected sex for it to be effective—the sooner it can be taken, the more effective it will be.

The IUD can be fitted up to 5 days after unprotected sex, or up to 5 days after the earliest time you could have ovulated, for it to be effective.

SEXUAL PROBLEM

Failure of achieving target(s) of sexual performance by either one or both the partner is termed as sexual problems. Most often it is due to unrealistic target settings but it may due to dysfunctions like premature ejaculation (PE), erectile dysfunction, dyspareunia vaginismus, etc. These may result in personal, interpersonal even social damage. Most problems are successfully managed by education, correction of organic problem(s), and reassurance. Knowledge on human sexual response cycle (SRC) is essential to develop skill on the subject. Physicians in general and endocrinologist in particular should enable themselves to identify to solve the common sexual disorders. Intense psychological problems should be managed by specifically trained persons called sex therapist.

Sexual Response Cycle

For descriptive purpose, SRC is divided into four phases:
1. Excitement phase
2. Plateau phase
3. Orgasmic phase
4. Resolution phase **(Fig. 27)**

Description of SRC is given below:
1. *Excitement phase*: During this phase sexual arousal is initiated by stimuli such as psychic, visual, or tactile. These result in:
    i. In male:
        a. Enlargement and erection of penis
        b. Increase of penile angle of protrusion from the body
        c. Retraction of testis
    ii. In female:
        a. Vaginal lubrication (sweating reaction)
        b. Clitoral engorgement

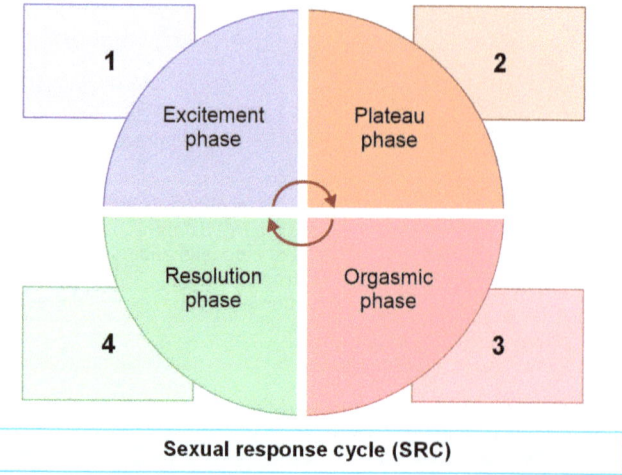

Sexual response cycle (SRC)

FIG. 27: Four phases of sexual response cycle of man and woman.

   c. Nipple erection
   d. Increased breast size
   e. Vaginal vessel engorgement
   f. Vaginal wall expands in inner two-thirds
  iii. In both male and female:
     a. Erotic tension leading to increased muscle tone, tachycardia, and raised blood pressure
     b. Sex flushes spread as morbilliform rash from upper abdomen toward chest.
2. *Plateau phase*: It is distinct from excitement phase and is imprecise.
    i. In male:
        a. Diameter of penis increases
        b. Glands become reddish purple
        c. Progressive excitement
        d. Volume of testis increase
        e. A few drops of fluid may appear from bulbourethral (Cowper's) gland. It contains active sperm, so pregnancy is possible before ejaculation.
        f. Respiratory rate, pulse rate, muscle tone, and blood pressure changes intensify
        g. Muscle tension increases in buttocks and sphincter.
    ii. In female (also called orgasmic platform):
        a. Engorgement and swelling of outer third of vagina
        b. Elevation and ballooning of inner two-third of vagina
        c. Erection of clitoris
        d. Engorgement of labia
3. *Orgasmic phase*:
    i. In male:
        a. Increased tension in seminal vesicles causes semen empty in bulbous urethra
        b. Rhythmic contraction of bulbocavernosus muscle

c. Prostatic contraction expelling fluid into bulbous urethra
d. A series of rhythmic contraction of bulb eject semen with great pressure
e. A series of minor contractions in the urethra for several seconds continues even after complete expulsion of semen.
  ii. In female:
   a. Rhythmic contraction of vaginal muscle begins at a rate of 3–10 per minutes
   b. Contractions are intense at first, but subsides quickly.
   c. A series of uterine contractions quickly follows, begin in the upper portion, and move down toward the cervix.
   d. Occasionally, rhythmic contraction of anal sphincter occurs.
  iii. In both male and female:
   a. Pulse rate, blood pressure, and respiratory rate reach a peak and quickly dissipates.
   b. There is marked generalized muscle tension.
   c. Facial muscles tighten; muscles of neck, extremities, abdomen, and buttocks are strongly contracted.
   d. There may be grasp movement by both followed by clutching and even carpopedal spasm.
   e. A fleeting period occurs in which each individual withdrawal physiologically, but not physically, concentrating almost solely on genital sensation, unaware perhaps of cries and uncomfortable behavior.
4. *Resolution phase*:
  i. In both male and female:
   a. Muscle tension released
   b. Engorgement of genitalia subsides
   c. As sex flash fades, there appears sight sweating.
  ii. In female:
   a. Clitoris returns to unstimulated state.
   b. Relaxation of orgasmic platform occurs, diameter of outer third of vagina increases.
   c. Vaginal ballooning diminishes, uterus shrinks, and cervix descent to its normal position.
   d. Time for total resolution varies, as much as 30 minutes may elapse before an woman is in true unstimulated state.
  iii. In male:
   a. Loss of erection occurs in two stages:
    – First stage, most of the erection volume is lost
    – Second or refractory stage during which period he is unable to arose again and remaining shrinkage occurs.
   b. In a young man the refractory period may be very short but lengthen with age; it may last for seral minutes to hours or even days.

Sexual Dysfunction

Failure of normal sexual performance is a common problem that occurs during lifetime of all individuals. Sexual dysfunctions are defined mostly on the basis of the component(s) of the SRC involved. Definitions of sexual dysfunctions are given here:
- *Problems in excitement phase*:
  o Inhibited sexual desire (ISD): Decreased interest in sex by male or female. Another name is loss of libido.
  o Excessive sexual desire (ESD): Increased interest in sex by male or female. Another name is nymphomania.
- *Problems in plateau phase*:
  o Excitement phase dysfunction (EPD): Decreased lubrication
  o Erectile dysfunction (ED)/impotence—difficulties/nonerection
- *Problems in orgasmic phase*:
  o Anorgasm—no orgasm
  o Premature ejaculation—too early ejaculation (male only)
  o Anejaculation—no ejaculation (male only)
  o Dry drive—no emission (male only)
- *Problems in satisfaction*:
  o Sexual failure—no satisfaction
  o Dyspareunia—pain during intercourse (female)
  o Vaginismus—spasm of circumvaginal muscle (female)
  o Sex phobia—fear of sex (female)

Inhibited Sexual Desire

Decreased interest in sex may be lifelong (primary) or occurs after normal period (secondary). Its presence does not necessarily imply to lack of ability to response psychosociologically.
- Primary ISD is caused by (1) poor partner relationship or (2) women are mostly from sexually repressive background—sexually traumatized in childhood or adolescence. But secondary ISD is due to (1) problem with partner, (2) physical or emotional trauma (rapid onset), or (3) drugs or alcohol.
- Diagnostic evaluation includes: (1) Careful history to revel recent life change, loss, (2) medical and drug history, (3) concern of pregnancy, (4) partner with very different sex appetite, and (5) change in body image (for sex).

- Treatment consists of (1) behavior and psychological methods and (2) hormone therapy for hypogonadism or hyperprolactinemia.

Premature Ejaculation

Premature ejaculation is a condition when sexual desire is normal, erection is either normal or partial, and emission and fleeting take place before or immediately after penetration. So, female partner fails to experience orgasm.
- Premature ejaculation is caused by (1) over excitement and inexperience (as in early days of marriage) or (2) attempt at coitus before adequate erection.
- Treatment consist of: (1) Treatment of the cause, (2) supportive treatment, (3) for overexcitement advice frequent coitus, (4) use of condom to reduce phallic stimulation, (5) pelvic floor exercise (deliberate contraction of muscles to interrupt micturition may allow to gain control over ejaculation, and (6) use of monoamine oxidase inhibitor, e.g., isocarboxazid 20-40 mg daily to delay ejaculation by inhibiting sympathetic nerves.

Orgasmic Dysfunction

No orgasm during coitus is called orgasmic dysfunction. It may be lifelong (primary) or occurs after normal period (secondary). It is characterized by: (1) Women may lubricate easily; (2) enjoy love making; and (3) feel satisfaction but they get stuck in the plateau phase of SRC.
- It is caused by: (1) Inadequate sensory input from brain and periphery (clitoris, nipple, and other place), (2) fear about sexuality and relationship, and (3) fear of losing control, urination, getting pregnant, etc.
- Treatment consists of: (1) Improvement of sensory stimuli by educating on SRC, (2) teaching technic of stimuli, and (3) To extinguishing involuntary control of women due to fear of sex and its consequences.

Dyspareunia

Dyspareunia is pain during intercourse. It is very distressing and may be lifelong (primary) or occurs after normal period (secondary).
- It is characterized by: (1) Women may lubricate easily; (2) enjoy love making; and (3) Feel satisfaction but they get stuck in the plateau phase of SRC. So, women may have strong preoccupied idea that sex will be pain full, they associate menstruation and childbirth with pain.
- It is caused by: (1) Hymen, tender episiotomy scar, and Bartholin's gland abscess, (2) infected clitoris, (3) vaginal—infection, dry vagina, atrophic vagina, and (4) pelvic disorders like endometriosis, ectopic pregnancy, and pelvic inflammatory disease.
- Treatment is the treatment of its cause(s).

Vaginismus

Painful reflex spasm of the perivaginal and thigh adductor muscle that occurs in anticipation of any vaginal penetration is called vaginismus.
- It is caused (1) most often in young, newly married inexperienced women from strict home. Some of them may have been subjected to rape or incest as children. (2) Severe pain due to trauma or medical procedures in vaginal area may sometimes cause this problem, or (3) insufficient lubrication from lack of arousal or sex phobias, etc.
- Treatment is the treatment of its cause(s).

Sexual Failure

Decreased or no satisfaction of sex may loosely have termed as sexual failure.
- Its causes include: (1) From ignorance, cultural taboos and myths, poor communication between partners; (2) once there is sexual failure it brings fear of failure, and it may establish a vicious cycle; and (3) unrealistic goal-focused concept of success and (d) undue performance pressure may lead one to be trapped into a vicious cycle of sexual failure.
- Management includes (1) sex education, (2) permission giving (care full lessening of their problem in their language), (3) teaching communication skills, (4) redefinition of for themselves a broader and more realistic concept of normal successful sex life, and (5) removal of performance pressures may even be all that needed for a distressed couple **(Fig. 28)**.

Impotence

Impotency is the inability to initiate and sustain a penile erection to allow vaginal penetration long enough to

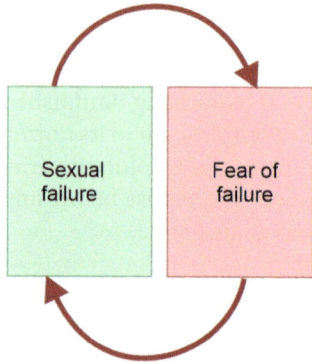

FIG. 28: Management includes: (1) Sex education, (2) teaching communication skills, (3) redefinition of for realistic goals, and (4) removal of performance.

complete sexual intercourse. Potency is one of the basic characters of a man. Impotence is a fairly common problem and caused by wide variety of reasons. **Table 18** summarizes the cause of impotence.

TABLE 18: Cause list of impotence.	
Disorders	**Due to**
Psychogenic disorders	Sex phobia, poor understanding with partner, religious orthodoxy, depressive disorders, lack of sex education
Nervous system disorders	
Central nervous system disorder	• Brain—Parkinsonism, epilepsy, cerebrovascular accident (CVA), tumors, etc. • Spinal cord—multiple sclerosis, syringomyelia, injury, tumor, lumbar intervertebral disc protrusion (LIDP), etc.
Peripheral nervous system disorder	Diabetic neuropathy, vitamin B12 deficiency, chronic alcoholism, and surgical injury of nerves
Vascular disease	
Arterial	Atherosclerosis, aortoiliac disease, diabetic microangiopathy
Venous sinusoidal disease	• Excessive draining veins • Poor neurotransmitters release • Fibrosis, e.g., Peyronie's disease, penile contusion/fracture, and priapism
Endocrine disease	Testicular failure, hyperprolactinemia, hyperthyroidism, Cushing syndrome, and Addison's disease
Systemic disorders	Cirrhosis of liver, renal failure, congestive heart failure, angina pectoris, and chronic disabling disease
Drug	
Antihypertensive	Methyldopa, reserpine, guanethidine, phenylbenzamine, thiazide, spironolactone, and clonidine
Antipsychotic	Phenothiazine, butyrophenones, thioxanthene, thioridazine
Antidepressant	Tricyclic antidepressant, monoamine oxidase inhibitor
Sedatives and drugs of abuse	Alcohol, barbiturate, cannabis, chlordiazepam, diazepam, methadone, and heroin
Anticholinergic	Atropine, benztropine, trihexyphenidyl, and scopolamine
Antihistamine	Cimetidine, diphenhydramine, and hydroxyzine
Others	Fenfluramine, levodopa, clofibrate, aminocaproic acid, baclofen, and ethionamide

Assessment of Patient with Impotence
- History
- *Physical assessment*:
    o Pubertal developments
    o Stigmata of cardiovascular and endocrine disorders
    o Neurological examination:
        – Qauda equine lesion—loss of bulbocavernosus reflex, lax anal sphincter, and saddle anesthesia
        – Evidence of lumbar intervertebral disc prolapse (LIDP) and spinal tumor
    o Examination of genitalia:
        – Testicle—volume, consistency, position, and reflex
        – Microphallus
        – Epispadias
        – Hypospadia with chordee externa
- *Investigation*:
    o To differentiate between psychogenic and organic impotence:
        – Nocturnal penile erection or real-time monitoring of penile tumescence
            ▪ Result:
                ♦ Normal response—rule out organic cause.
                ♦ Abnormal response does not have any specific diagnostic value **(Figs. 29A to C)**.
    o To differentiate between vasculogenic and neurogenic organic impotence
        – Papaverine test:
            ▪ Procedure: Penile arterial blood flow and penile diameter are measured after intracavernosal injection of papaverine by color Doppler and duplex ultrasonography recorder.
            ▪ Result:
                ♦ Normal response—(diameter increases by >75% and very fast blood flow) rule out vasculogenic cause.
                ♦ Abnormal response—atherosclerotic cavernosal problems **(Fig. 30)**
    o To establish neurogenic impotence:
        – Neurogenic test:
            ▪ Procedure: Cavernous electromyography (EMG) or single potential analysis of cavernous electrical activity (SPACE) is measured for indignity of cavernous autonomic innervation and smooth muscle actions.
            ▪ Result:
                ♦ Normal response—rule out neurogenic cause.
                ♦ Abnormal response confirms neurogenic cause.

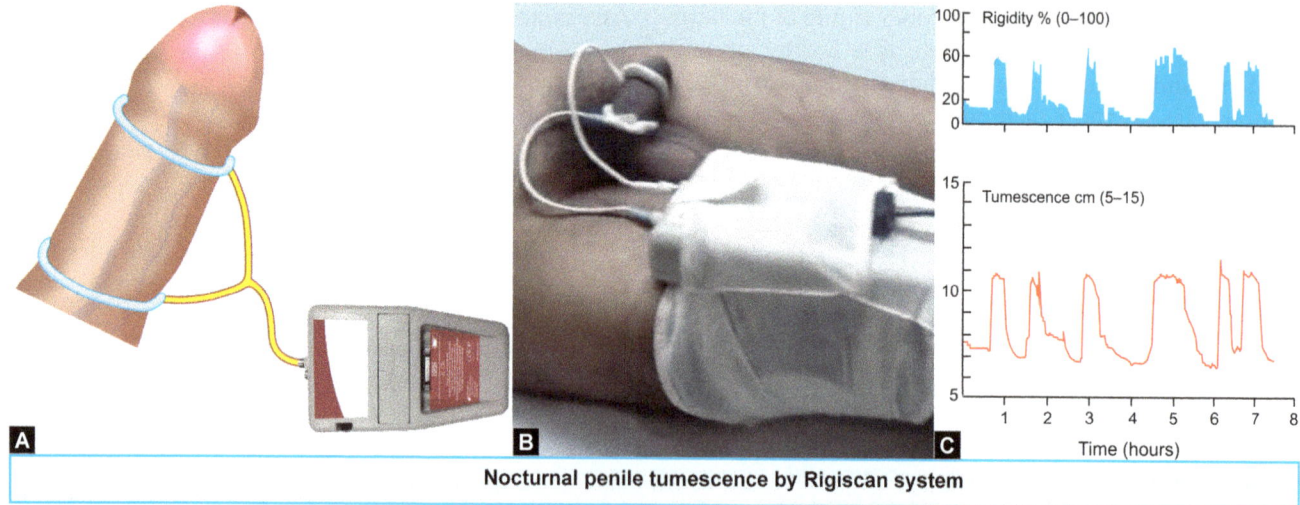

Nocturnal penile tumescence by Rigiscan system

FIGS. 29A TO C: A normal response to rule out organic cause; abnormal response does not have diagnostic value.

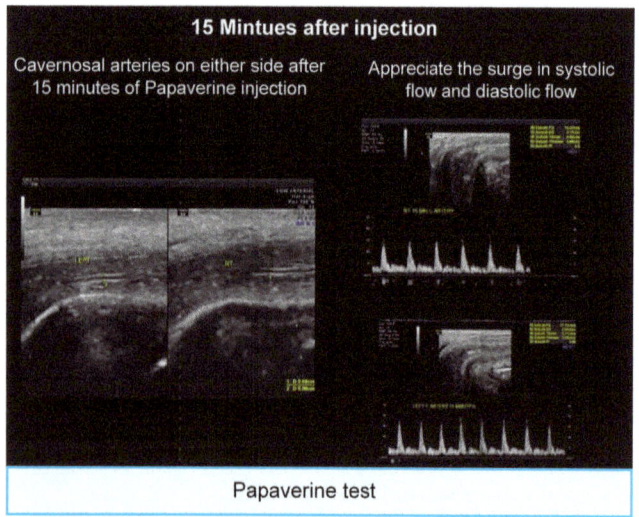

FIG. 30: Penile arterial blood flow and penile diameter are measured after intracavernosal injection of papaverine by color Doppler and duplex ultrasonography recorder. Normal response—(diameter increases by >75% and very fast blood flow) rule out vasculogenic cause. Abnormal response—atherosclerotic cavernosal problems.

- To establish endocrine impotence:
  - Endocrine test:
    - Procedure: After clinical evaluation for hypothalamic-pituitary-gonadal axis, thyroid and adrenal dysfunctions at least testosterone, and prolactin levels are determined.
    - Result:
      - Normal response—rule out endocrine cause.
      - Abnormal response confirms endocrine cause.

Treatment of Impotence

- Treatment of cause (when identified and treatable)
- *For psychogenic impotence:*
  - Individual and couple counseling on performance pressure
  - Behavioral therapy
  - Hypnotherapy

  All these need to be done by professional psychotherapist.
- *For neurogenic impotence:*
  - Method of choice—vacuum and constriction device
  - Other options—vasoactive agents and penile implants
- *For endocrine impotence:*
  - Treatment should be preserved for proven abnormal cases only.

External Vacuum Constriction Device

- Noninvasive simple method
- Device consists of: (1) A cline plastic cylinder; (2) a pump (hand/battery operated), and (3) a special tension ring.
  - A tension ring is stretched around the opening end of cylinder.
  - Penis is inserted into the opening end of cylinder.
  - The device is hold firmly against the body to create an air seal.
  - The pump is activated to create vacuum around the penis causing entry of blood to enter into it and make engorgement.
  - The stretched ring is slipped on the base of penis.
  - The erection can be maintained for about half an hour **(Fig. 31)**.

Intracavernosal Vasoactive Drug Therapy

Drugs
Papaverine Hcl, papaverine, phentolamine, prostaglandin E1.

Usual dose of drugs
- Papaverine Hcl 15–30 mg
- Papaverine 30 mg
- Phentolamine 1 mg
- Prostaglandin E1 (PGE1) 10 µg

Procedure
Intracorporeal self-injection by automatic injector or syringe (insulin syringe).

Benefit
Repeated injections improve the hemodynamics of the penis. Some persons may achieve good erection without injection afterward.

Side effect
Failure to ejaculate, infection, priapism (painful persistent erection), and fibrosis.

Penile Implants

Types of penile prosthesis
There are two *types of penile prosthesis implants*: Inflatable and noninflatable types, and the inflatable *penile implants* can be subdivided into single-, two-, and three-piece devices. Noninflatable *penile prosthesis* (non-IPP) may be referred to as semirigid rod or malleable *prosthesis* **(Flowchart 7 and Figs. 32A and B)**.

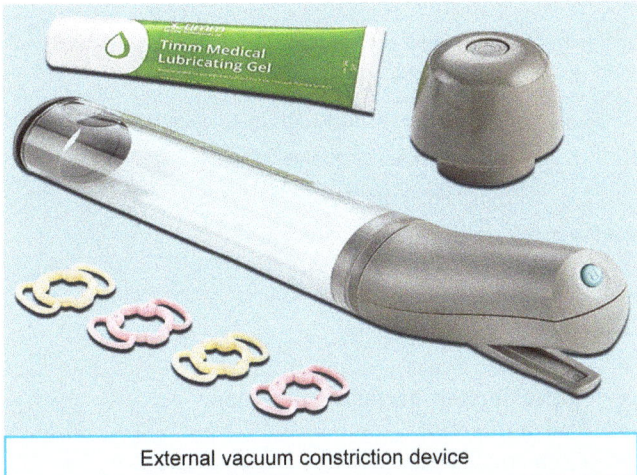

External vacuum constriction device

FIG. 31: A tension ring is stretched around the opening end of cylinder. Penis is inserted into the opening end of cylinder and hold firmly against the body to create an air seal. The pump is activated to create vacuum around the penis, causing entry of blood to enter into it and make engorgement. The stretched ring is slipped on the base of penis.

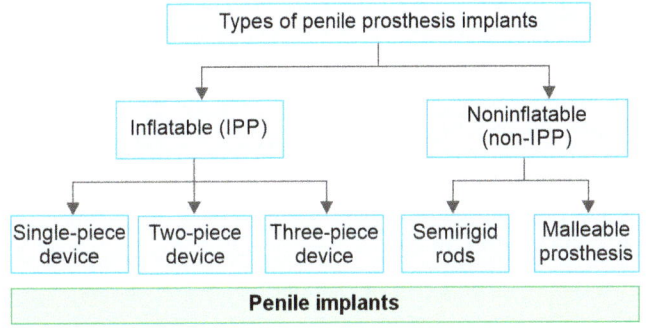

FLOWCHART 7: Two types of penile prosthesis.
(IPP: inflatable penile prosthesis)

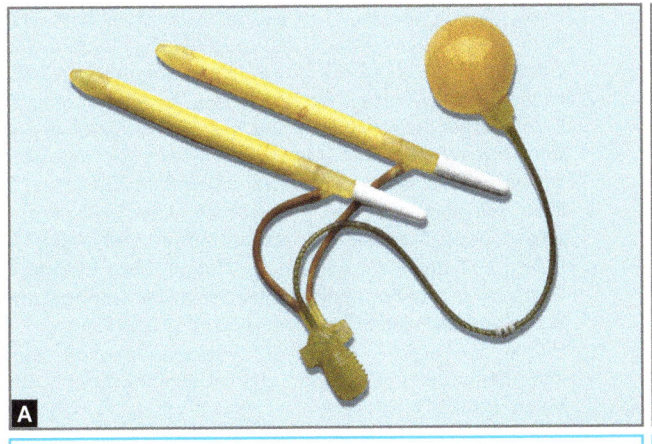

A — Three-piece CX AMS 700 penile prosthesis

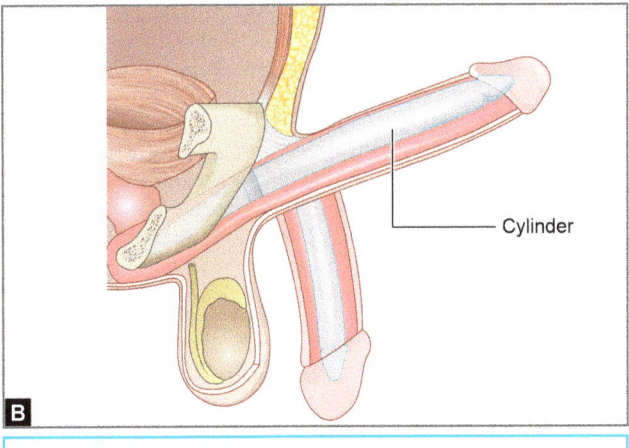

B — One-piece, positionable prosthesis (malleable)

FIGS. 32A AND B: Prosthesis.

TABLE 19: Decision-making investigation steps (DMIS) in a case suspected for impotence.

Step	Investigation	Result	Action/inference
1	Nocturnal penile erection or real-time monitoring of penile tumescence test	Normal	• Organic cause excluded • Got step 2
		Abnormal	Got step 5
2	Papaverine test	Normal	• Vascular cause excluded • Got step 3
		Abnormal	Got step 4
3	Cavernous EMG or SPACE	Normal	Got step 4
		Abnormal	• Vascular cause established • Got step 6
4	Hormone study	Normal	Got step 6/7/8
		Abnormal	Treat accordingly
5			Refer to psychotherapist
6			Offer vacuum and constriction device
7			Vasoactive agents
8			Penile implants

(EMG: electromyography; SPACE: single potential analysis of cavernous electrical activity)

Use
Implants are placed into the corpora by surgical procedure to provide as means of erection.

Advantage
- Natural appearance in erector face
- Full control on use

Disadvantage
- High cost
- Approximately 5% failure in 5 years
- Risk of infection

Table 19 describes DMIS of impotence.

FURTHER READINGS

1. Anatomy & Physiology by ©2017 Rice University. Textbook content produced by OpenStax. [online] Available from https://openstax.org/ [Last accessed September, 2023].
2. Standring S (Ed). Gray's Anatomy: The Anatomical Basis of Clinical Practice, 41st edition. [online] Available from https://www.amazon.com/Garys-Anatomy-Henry-Gray/dp/B00DXO9JRA) [Last accessed September, 2023].
3. Barrett K, Barman S, Yuan J, Brooks H (Eds). Ganong's Review of Medical Physiology, 26th edition. [online] Available from https://www.amazon.com/Ganongs-Review-Medical-Physiology-Twenty/dp/1260122409 [Last accessed September, 2023].
4. Melmed S, Koenig R, Rosen C, Auchus R, Goldfine A. Williams Textbook of Endocrinology, 14th edition. [online] Available from (https://www.elsevier.com/books/williams-textbook-of-endocrinology/bresnahan/978-0-323-55596-8 [Last accessed September, 2023].
5. Gardner D, Shoback D (Eds). Greenspan's Basic and Clinical Endocrinology, 10th edition. [online] Available from https://www.amazon.com/Greenspans-Basic-Clinical-Endocrinology-Tenth/dp/1259589285 [Last accessed September, 2023].
6. Coleman W, Tsongalis G (Eds). Molecular Pathology: The Molecular Basis of Human Disease, 2nd edition. [online] Available from https://www.elsevier.com/books/molecular-pathology/coleman/978-0-12-802761-5 [Last accessed September, 2023].
7. Kliegman RM, St. Geme III JW (Eds). Nelson Textbook of Pediatrics, 2-Volume Set (NelsonPediatrics), 21st edition. [online] Available from https://www.amazon.com/Nelson-Textbook-Pediatrics-2-Set/dp/032352950X [Last accessed September, 2023].
8. Khan MR, Ahmed T (Eds). The Essence of Endocrinology, 1st edition. Dhaka, Bangladesh: Asiatic Civil Military Press Dhaka; 1997.
9. Islam S, Pathan F, Ahmed T. Clinical and Biochemical Characteristics of Polycystic Ovarian Syndrome among Women in Bangladesh. Mymensingh Med J. 2015;24(2):310-8.
10. Huque M, Tofail T, Ahmed T. Response to short course androgenisation in late reported cases with micropenis. IMC J Med Sci. 2020;14(1):1.

Index

Page numbers followed by *b* refer to box *f* refer to figure, *fc* refer to flowchart, and *t* refer to table.

A

Acarbose 115, 116
Acidophils 12
Acquired growth hormone deficiency 134
Acromegaly 14, 16
   diagnosis of 17*f*
   physical features of 15*f*
   treatment for 17
Addison's disease 183
Adenocarcinoma 49
Adenoma-secreting aldosterone, large 78*f*
Adenosine
   monophosphate 6
   triphosphate 5
Adiposogenital dystrophy 144
Adrenal adenoma 77*f*
Adrenal arteries 69*f*
Adrenal cortex 69*f*, 70*f*, 71, 71*f*
   diseases of 73, 73*fc*
   physiology of 70
Adrenal crisis 83
   treatment of 84*t*
Adrenal disorders 72
Adrenal gland 68
   anatomy of 68
   diseases of 68, 72
   parts of 69*f*
   physiology of 70
Adrenal hyperplasia, congenital 73, 84, 84*fc*, 88, 88*f*, 89, 159, 167*f*, 172
   treatment of 85, 89*t*
Adrenal incidentaloma 90
Adrenal insufficiency 25, 73, 73*fc*, 81
   acute 83
   chronic 80*f*, 82*t*
   syndrome 81
Adrenal medulla 69*f*
   develop 70
   disease of 73, 73*fc*
Adrenal medullary glands 72
Adrenal steroids, deficiency of 89*f*
Adrenocortical insufficiency 83*t*
   primary 81*b*, 82
   secondary 82, 82*t*, 83*t*
   treatment of primary 82
Adrenocorticotropic hormone 2, 3*f*, 9, 13*f*, 14, 21, 71*f*, 77, 77*fc*, 83, 103, 161
   deficiency 22
   secretion 71, 75*t*
Adrenolytic test 89
Adrenomedullary hyperplasia 90
Aerobic exercise 109
Agranulocytosis 42
Alanine transaminase 168
Alcohol 106, 183
Aldosterone 71*f*
   lack, state of 70
   site of action of 70
Alendronate 65
Alpha-glucosidase inhibitors 115, 116*t*
Alström–Hallgren syndrome 144, 144*f*
Ambiguous genitalia 153, 170
   causes of 170, 171*t*
   diagnosis of 171
Amenorrhea 153, 159, 160*t*
   causes of 159, 159*t*
   classification of 159
   functional 159
   management 159
   primary 151*f*, 160*fc*, 160*t*
   secondary 160*fc*, 161*t*
Amenorrhea-galactorrhea syndrome 161*t*
Aminocaproic acid 183
Aminoglutethimide 36
Anaplastic carcinoma 46
Anatomic anomalies 53, 70, 93
Android obesity 143*f*
Angina pectoris 183
Anorchia 159
Anthropometry 109*f*, 168
Antibody
   antimicrosomal 44
   antithyroglobulin 44
Antidiuretic hormone 9, 12, 12*fc*, 14
Anti-inflammatory effects 72
Antithyroid
   antibody test 45
   drug, large dose of 43
   drugs 41, 42
Aorta
   abdominal 69*f*
   coarctation of 149
Aortic dissection 149
Aortic valve, bicuspid 149
Appetite, oncreased 39
Arial natriuretic factor 6
Arsenic 36
Asherman syndrome 161
Aspartate transaminase 168
Assisted reproductive technique 176
Atherosclerosis 100*f*
Atropine 183
Autoimmune 55
   disease 164
   thyroid
      disease 36, 45
      disorders 149
Autosomal recessive disorder 135*f*
Azoospermia 171

B

Baclofen 183
Balanced diet 105
Barbiturate 183
Bartter syndrome 81
Basal insulin secretion 98
Basal-bolus regimen 113*f*
Basophils 12
Beckwith–Wiedemann syndrome 139, 140*f*
Benztropine 183
Beta cells 93
Beta-blocker drugs 41, 44
Beta-cell
   failure, causes of 99
   function 97*f*
Biochemical euthyroidism, continued 35
Birth anomalies 70
Birth control 175
   pills, types of 179*fc*
   prevent pregnancy 178
Bisphosphonates 60, 65
Blocked fallopian tubes, causes of 173*f*
Blood
   pressure 57
   sugar, random 102
Blood glucose
   level, random 101
   molecules 95*f*
   targets of 104
Blood-testis barrier 156
Body hairs
   loss of 21
   paucity of 151*f*
Body mass index 107, 109, 142*t*
Body weight 105
Bone
   age 134
   maturity 134
Bonnevie-Ullrich-Turner's syndrome 148
Brain cell 96*f*

Breast
    development, Tanner's grades of 146c, 147f
    examination of 168
    fully developed 151f
    tanner's stage 150f
Butyrophenones 183

C

Cabergoline 20
Calcifediol 57
Calcitonin 60, 65
Calcitriol 57
Calcium 6, 53, 65, 66
    carbonate 57
    chloride 57
    entry from
        bone, reduction of 60
        gut, reduction of 60
    from blood, removal of 60
    gluconate 57
    lactate 57
    regulation, role in 53
Candidiasis 61
Cannabis 183
Carbamazepine 25
Carbimazole 41, 43
Carbohydrate 105, 106
Catecholamine, excess productions of 73
Cavernous sinuses 12f
Cell
    adenosine triphosphate 93
    chief 52
    membrane 6fc, 93, 95f
Central hypothyroidism 36
Central nervous system 21
    disorder 25, 148, 183
    tumors, primary 14
Cerebral gigantism 139, 139f
Cerebral thrombosis 25
Cerebrovascular disease 122f
Cervical cap 179
Chlodronate 60
Chlordiazepam 183
Chlorpropamide 25
Cholesterol desmolase deficiency syndrome 85, 89f, 89t
Chromophobes 12
Chromosomal defects 164
Chromosomal disorder 150
Cimetidine 183
Clofibrate 25, 183
Clonidine 183
Cobalt 36
Colloid 28
Communication skills 182f
Condom
    female 179
    male 179, 179f
Congenital adrenal hyperplasia, classification of 84t
Conjugate estrogen 163
Connective tissues, different layers of 156
Constipation 38
Constitutional delayed puberty 148
Constitutional precocious puberty 147
Contraception 153
Contraceptive
    hormonal methods, short-acting 175
    injection 175
    long-acting reversible 175, 178f
    sponge 179
Coronary artery bypass 23
Coronary heart disease 109
    during menopause 163
Corticotropes 12fc
Corticotropic hormone 1
Corticotropin-releasing
    factor 9, 14
    hormone 77f
Cortisol 3f, 72
Coupled hormone test 40
Cranial diabetes insipidus 14, 22fc, 23
Creatinine clearance 116
Cretinism 33
Cryptomenorrhea 160
Cryptorchidism 153, 169, 170
    classification of 170t
    evaluation of 170f
    treatment of 170
Cushing's disease 14
    stage of 7f
    treatment of 76
Cushing's syndrome 73, 73fc, 74, 74f, 74fc, 75, 76f, 103, 183
    causes of 73t
    diagnosis of 75
    drug therapies for 76
    surgeries for 76
    treatment of 76
Cyclic adenosine monophosphate 5, 6
Cyclophosphamide 25
Cyproterone acetate 166
Cytotoxic antibiotic 60

D

de Quervain's thyroiditis 40, 44
    phases of 44t
Defeminization 164, 164t
Deficient hormones, replacement therapy for 27
Dehydroepiandrosterone 87f
    sulfate 72
Delayed puberty 148
Denosumab 65
Deoxyribonucleic acid analysis 140
Desogestrel 178
Device delivers insulin 113f
Dexamethasone 76f
    suppression tests 9
    therapy 44
Dextrose normal saline 84
Diabetes insipidus 22
    symptoms of 22t
Diabetes management 117
    transplantation for 117fc
Diabetes mellitus 92, 101, 101fc, 102, 103, 105, 108, 111, 119
    chronic complications of 122
    classes of 103f
    classification of 101, 102
    clinical presentation of 101
    development of 97
    drugs for 110, 110f
    lifestyle modification in 105
    management of 103, 104
    pathogenesis of
        type 1 97
        type 2 98
    pathophysiology of 96, 97t
    prescription for 117, 119
    risk factors of 96, 97fc
    treatment of 104, 110, 114
        type 2 115t
    type 1 123fc
    type 2 98, 99, 99f, 100, 100f, 103, 114, 115, 123fc, 143, 143f
    type of 103
Diabetic ketoacidosis 119
    causes of 119
    complications of 120
    diagnosis of 119
    management 119
Diabetogenesis 100
Diaphragm 179
    female 179f
Diazepam 183
Diazoxide 103
Diet plan 105
Dietitian 105
Diffuse nontoxic goiter 45
Digeorge's syndrome 55
Dihydrotachysterol 57
Dipeptidyl peptidase-4 111, 116
    inhibitors 115
Diphenhydramine 183
Disabling disease, chronic 183
Dopamine 27, 72f
    agonists 19
Double collecting system 149
Drospirenone 178
Dyslipidemia 100f, 143f
Dyspareunia 181, 182

E

Early-onset genetic syndrome 55
Ectopic kidney 149
Edema 43
Ejaculation, premature 182
Electrocardiogram 57
Embryo
    culture 174
    transfer 174
Emergency contraception 180
    types of 180
Emergency therapy 57

Empty Sella syndrome 14
Encephalitis 25
Endemic goiter 45, 46
Endocrine
　disease 183
　function tests 6
　glands 2
　imbalance 159
　impotence 184
　neoplasia, multiple 50, 137
　test 16, 184
Enzymatic disorders 45
Epinephrine 72f
Epithelial cells, types of 28
Ergocalciferol 57
Ergosterol 57
Erythrocyte sedimentation rate 44
Esterified estrogens 163
Estetrol 178
Estraderm 164
Estradiol
　pellets 164
　vaginal ring of 164
Estrogen 145, 145f
　excess 168
　preparations 163
Estropipate 163
Ethinylestradiol 163, 178
Ethionamide 183
Eunuchoid 16
Euthyroid population 33f
Euthyroidism, continued clinical 35
Euvolemia 24
Excitement phase 180
　dysfunction 181
Exercise 108
　intensity of 109
Exocytosis 93, 114f
Exogenous obesity 143
External vacuum constriction device 184
Extracellular fluid volume, normal 24
Extrathyroidal soft tissue 49f
Extra-Y syndrome 141, 141f

F

Fallopian tube agenesis 157
Familial hypocalciuric hypercalcemia 61, 62, 62f
Familial medullary carcinoma 50
Fasting glucose, impaired 99, 100, 102
Fat 106
Fatty food 106
Female reproductive
　organs, anomalies of 157, 158fc
　system, anatomy of 154
Fenfluramine 183
Ferriman-Gallwey scale 165
　for hirsutism 166t
Fibrocalculous pancreatic diabetes 103
Fine needle aspiration cytology 45, 47t
Follicles 49

Follicle-stimulating hormone 2, 3f, 6, 9, 14, 36, 88, 146f, 161, 162, 168
Follicular carcinoma 46
Follicular cell 28, 154
Free fatty acid 100
Free thyroxine 32, 35, 44, 62, 161
Froehlich's syndrome 144, 145f

G

Gallium nitrate binds 60
Genetic short stature 135
Genetic syndrome 135, 136
Genetic tall stature 138, 139f
Genital ambiguity 172t
Genitalia development, Tanner's grades of 146fc
Genitalia, Tanner's grades of 146f
Gentle physical examination 170
Germ cells, male 157f
Gestational diabetes mellitus, prescription for 118
Giant cell 49f
Gigantism 14, 15, 15fc, 16, 17
　treatment for 17
Gilbert-Dreyfus syndrome 151
Gitelman syndrome 81
Glans penis, tip of 169f
Gliflozin 115, 116
Glinides 114
　mechanism of action of 113
Glitazones 115
Glucocorticoid 71, 71f, 103
　therapy 84
Glucose
　homeostasis 94
　tolerance, impaired 99, 100, 102, 143, 143f
　transporter-2 93
Goiter 44, 46
　causes of 45, 45t
　grade of 45f
　management of 45, 46t
　physiological 45
　simple 46
Goitrogen exposure 36
Gonadal dysgenesis 149, 159
Gonadal intersex 171
Gonadotropes 12fc
Gonadotropin 162
　deficiency 22
　dependent 147
Gonadotropin-releasing hormone 6, 9, 14
Gonads 151f
Granulomatous diseases 23
Granulomatous disorders 61
Graves' disease 39, 40, 41, 42f, 43
　management of 42
Graves' ophthalmopathy 39, 42, 43, 43f
　classification of 42t
　management of 42
　treatment of 43t

Growth and development, disorders of 125, 126
Growth hormone 1, 2, 3f, 9, 14
　antagonists 19
　deficiency 14, 126, 134
　inhibitory factor 14
　releasing factor 14
Guanethidine 183
Guanosine triphosphate 5
Guillain-Barré syndrome 25
Gut epithelial cell 96f
Gynecomastia 150f, 153, 167, 168f, 168t
　causes of 168, 168t
　diagnostic evaluation of 168
　treatment of 169

H

Hand and leg films 16
Hand's grip system 108f
Harrison's sulcus 63
Hashimoto's disease 38
　treatment of 39
Hashitoxicosis 40
Head injury 25
Heart failure, congestive 183
Hemangiomatosis 149
Hematometra 161f
Hemochromatosis 103
Hepatic glucose
　output 94
　production 100
Hepatosplenomegaly 140f
Hermaphrodism, true 159
Heroin 183
Herring bodies 12, 12fc
Hip circumference 108
Hirsutism 153, 164, 167t
　causes of 165, 166t
　clinical confirmation of 165
　diagnostic evaluation of 165
　management of 165
　scoring of 165
　simple 167
　treatment of 166, 167
Histochemical staining 12
Hodgkin's disease 61
Homocystinuria 140, 140f
　treatment of 140
Honeymoon phase 97
Hormonal deficiency, screening tests for 26
Hormonal disorders 1f
Hormonal excess, screening tests for 27
Hormonal regulation, metabolic areas of 4
Hormonal source 14t
Hormone 2, 4fc, 5f
　action of 1f
　chemical features of 2
　classification of 2
　different 126
　estrogen, female 152

regulates cell function 2
replacement therapy 65, 163, 163t
   tibolone regime of 164
structure 2
types of 6fc
Hormone-producing glands 1
Horseshoe kidney 149
Human chorionic gonadotropin 2, 3f, 9, 40
  injection 173f
Human insulin 93
  synthesis 93
Human leukocyte antigen 96, 97, 98f
Human monoclonal antibody 65
Hungry bone syndrome 61, 62
Hydroxylase deficiency 85f
Hydroxysteroid dehydrogenase deficiency 87f
Hydroxyzine 183
Hyoid bone 30f
Hyperaldosteronism 73, 78, 78t
  causes of 78
  diagnosis of primary 79
  primary 78, 79t, 80, 80t
  secondary 78, 80, 80t
Hypercalcemia 61, 61f
  acute 60
  causes of 61
  nonparathyroidal causes of 61b
  onset of 62
  severe 60
  treatment of 60
Hypercortisolemia 73, 73fc
Hyperglycemia 97f
Hyperinsulinemia 145
Hyperosmolar non-ketotic Coma 119, 120
  causes of 120
  clinical features of 120
  diagnosis of 120
  management 120
Hyperostosis frontalis interna 144
Hyperparathyroidism 58
  primary 59, 59t, 60b, 61
    management of 59, 60t
Hyperphosphatemia 57b
Hyperpituitarism 15
Hyperprolactinemia 19, 20f, 183
  cause of 19t
  diagnosis of 20f
Hypertension 100f, 143f
  essential 90
  secondary hyperaldosteronism 78, 80
Hyperthermia 43
Hyperthyroid
  disorders 40f
  phase 44
  states, treatment for 41
Hyperthyroidism 31, 39, 61, 183
  causes of 40t
  diagnosis of 40
  signs of 39, 39t
  subclinical 40
  symptoms of 39, 39t
  types of 41fc

Hypertriglyceridemia 145
Hyperuricemia 145
Hypocalcemia 23, 57b, 120, 140f
  prolonged 62
Hypoglycemia
  clinical features of 121t
  mild-to-moderate 121
  severe 121, 121t
  treatment of
    severe 121
    unaware 122
  unawareness 109
Hypogonadotropic hypogonadism 148
Hypomagnesemia 55, 62
Hypoparathyroidism 54-56, 56t, 57b, 57f, 57t, 58t
  causes of 55, 55t
  diagnosis of 56
  grading of severity of 56t
  severity of 55
  treatment of 57, 57b
Hypophosphatemia 62
Hypophosphatemic rickets 64
Hypopituitarism 20
  causes of 21, 37
Hypoplastic vagina 162f
Hypothalamic defects 159
Hypothalamic-pituitary thyroid 31f
Hypothalamus 145f
Hypothyroidism 25, 33, 35, 36, 38t, 135
  cause of 36t, 37t, 38
  congenital 33, 34, 34t
    stomata of 35t
  description of 33
  diagnosis of 38
  phase 44
  primary 37
  severe 148
  treatment of 36, 38
  types of 38fc
Hysterosalpingogram 162
Hysterosalpingography 176
Hysteroscopy 162

I

Ibandronate 65
Ibuprofen 44
Idiopathic hirsutism 167
Idiopathic infantile hypercalcemia 61
Idiopathic precocious puberty 147
Immunostaining 66
Impotence 182, 183
  cause of 183t
  treatment of 184
In vitro fertilization 173, 175-177
  procedure of 173
  steps of 175f
  type of 174
Infertile couple 177t
Infertility 153, 171
  causes of 171
  luteal factor 171
  management 172, 175, 176t

Inflammatory bowel disease 149
Inflatable penile prosthesis 185
Inguinal canal 156
Inhibits osteoclast 60
Insemination 175f
Insomnia 39
Insulin 3f, 93, 94f, 110, 111fc
  absolute lack of 98f
  action 96, 96t
  deficiency 97, 97f
  independent cells 96f
  preparations 110
  pump 112
    use, indications of 113
  regimen 111
  release 98
  resistance 97f, 100, 100t
    evidences of 100
  secretagogue 111fc, 113
  secretion 93
    increase 95
  sensitizers 115
  synthesis 93
  types of 111f, 112t
  use, indications of 111
Insulinoma 92, 123
Intestinal telangiectasia 149
Intracellular mobile receptors 5
Intracytoplasmic sperm injection 175, 175f, 176, 177
Intrauterine
  adhesions 162f
  growth retardation 135, 136f
Intrauterine insemination 173, 174f, 176, 177
  procedure of 173
  types of 173
Iodine 30
  deficiency 36, 46
  therapy 43
Iodothyroglobulin 28

K

Karyotype 151
Kidney 122f, 149
  disease, chronic 59
  inability of 80
Klinefelter's syndrome 125, 150
Kocher-Debre-Semelaigne syndrome 36

L

Labia, development of 151f
Lactic acidosis 120
  treatment of 120
Laparoscopic resection 123
Laron short stature 134, 135f
Laurence-Moon-Biedl syndrome 144, 144f
Lesion, management of 91
Lethargy 38
Levodopa 183
Levomefolate 178

Levonorgestrel 178
    extended-cycle 178
Leydig cells 145
Libido, loss of 21
Lingual thyroid 30*f*
Lipomatosis, multiple 144
Lipoprotein, high-density 100
Lisuride 20
Lithium 23, 36
Liver
    tissue insulin 96
    cirrhosis of 183
Lower abdominal mass 160
L-triiodothyronine 31
Luteinizing hormone 1, 2, 3*f*, 7*f*, 9, 12, 14,
    18, 36, 146, 162, 168
Lymph drainage 29
Lymphatic drainage 92
Lymphoproliferative disorders 61

M

Macroangiopathy, organ affected by 122
Macrocephaly 140*f*
Macroglossia 140*f*
Macroincidentaloma 27
Macronutrient
    composition of 105
    distribution of 105*t*
Male reproductive
    organs, anomalies of 157, 158*fc*
    system, anatomy of 156
Malignancy 61
Marfan's syndrome 140, 140*f*
Mayer–Rokitansky–Küster–Hauser
    syndrome 157, 162
McCune-Albright syndrome 137
Medical nutrition therapy 104*f*, 105
Medicines, types of 177*fc*
Medroxyprogesterone 163
Medullary carcinoma 46, 50
Megestrol 163
Meningitis 25
Menopause 153, 160*fc*, 162, 163
    psychotogenic problems of 163
    urogenital problems of 163
Menstrual disturbance, absence of 167*f*
Mental defect 61, 61*f*
Metabolic alkalosis, mild 70
Metabolic complications, acute 119
Metabolic syndrome 100, 100*t*, 143
Metastatic thyroid carcinoma 40
Metformin 115
Methadone 183
Methyldopa 183
Microangiopathy 122*f*
    organ affected by 122
Micronized estradiol 163
Microphallus 134, 153, 169
    causes of 169
    treatment of 169
Mineralocorticoids 70, 71*f*

Monoamine oxidase inhibitor 25, 183
Monophasic oral contraceptive pills 178
Monozygotic twins 98, 99*fc*
Müllerian dysgenesis 162
Multinodular goiter 46
    toxic 41, 43
Multiple mucosa neuroma 50
Myxedema coma 38

N

Nasal spray, desmopressin 24
Necrozoospermia 171
Neoplastic disorders 25
Nephrogenic diabetes insipidus 23, 23*fc*
Nervous system disorders 183
Neural crest cells 70
Neurogenic impotence 184
Neurohypophysis 11
Neuromuscular hyperactivity, features of
    56
Neuropathy renal failure 109
Nicotine 25
Nocturnal hypoglycemia 121
    treatment of 122
Nonosmotic polyuria
    cause of 23*t*
    pathophysiology of 23
Nonresectable malignant insulinomas 123
Norepinephrine 70*f*, 72*f*
Norethindrone 163, 178
Norgestrel 163, 178
Normal sexual performance, failure of 181

O

Obesity 141
    cause for 142*t*
    types of 142, 142*f*
Octreotide, injection of 123
Ocular hypertelorism 141*f*
Oligozoospermia 171
Omphalocele 140*f*
Oral administration 64
Oral antidiabetic
    class 116*t*
    drug 115-117
Oral contraceptive pills 178
    biphasic 178
    four-phasic 178
    triphasic 178
Oral estrogen 163*t*
Oral glucose tolerance test 9, 101, 102, 102*t*
Orgasmic dysfunction 182
Orgasmic phase 180
    problems in 181
Osmolality 23
Osteitis fibrosa 64
Osteomalacia 63, 63*fc*, 63*t*
    causes of 63*t*
Osteoporosis 63, 64, 163, 164
    female 65
    male 66

    monitoring of 65
    prevention of 63
    risk of 66
    therapeutic of 64
    treatment of 63
Ovarian disorders 167*f*
Ovarian failure, premature 164
Ovarian follicles 145*f*
Ovarian resistance syndrome 159
Ovary 154
    anatomy of 154*f*
Ovine-corticotropin-releasing hormone 83
Oxyphil cells 52
Oxytocin 25

P

Pain management 44
Pamidronate 60
Pancreas 93*f*, 123
    insulinoma of 123
    transplantation 117
Pancreatic disease 103
Pancreatic insulinomas, treatment for 123
Pancreatitis
    chronic 103
    recurrent 103
Papaverine 185
Papillary carcinoma 46, 48
Papillary nuclear features 49*f*
Para-aminosalicylic acid 36
Parafollicular cells 28
Parathormone 8*t*
Parathyroid
    adenomas 60*f*
    development 53
    disorders 54, 55*fc*
    superior 54*f*
    surgery 61
    vascular anatomy 53
Parathyroid gland 52, 53, 53*f*
    anatomy of 52, 54*f*
    disorders of 52
    function 8*t*
    physiology of 53
Parathyroid hormone 58-60, 62
    related protein 65
Parathyroidectomy, extent of 61*t*
Pelvic factors infertility 171
Penile
    arterial blood flow 184*f*
    contusion 183
    implants 185
    prosthesis, types of 185*fc*
Peptide hormone 60
Perchlorate 36
Peripheral nervous system disorder 183
Peyronie's disease 183
Phenobarbitone 41
Phenothiazine 183
Phentolamine 185
Phenylbenzamine 183
Phenylbutazone 36

Pheochromocytoma 50, 73, 73fc, 85
   diagnosis of 88
   missed 90
   treatment of 90
Phlebectasia 149
Phosphate
   homeostasis 53
   low 63
Phosphatidylinositides 6
Phrenic artery, inferior 69f
Physical activity, increase in 106
Pioglitazone 115
Pituitary cells, types of 12
Pituitary defects 159
Pituitary disorders 13
   posterior 22
Pituitary gigantism 137
Pituitary gland 11, 14fc, 145f
   disorders of 11
   microscopic structure 12
   tissue, histology of 12fc
   weighs, adult 11
Pituitary hormone deficiency 21t
   manifestations of 35
Pituitary incidentaloma 26
Pituitary incidentaloma 27
Pituitary lesion 26
Pituitary oxytocin, posterior 12fc
Pituitary surgery cases 17
Plasma
   potassium concentration 71
   renin activity 79, 79f
Plateau phase 180
Plicamycin 60
Polycystic ovarian syndrome 100, 159, 167, 167f, 167fc
Polydipsia, primary 24fc
Polygenic disorder 99fc
Polyglandular autoimmunity 149
Porphyria, acute intermittent 25
Postmeal insulin secretion 98
Post-thyroidectomy 36, 46
Potassium
   concentration of 71
   iodide, solution of 43
Prader-Willi-Lambert syndrome 143, 144f
Precocious puberty 147
   causes of 147t
   treatment of 148
Precursor hormone pro-opiomelanocortin 12
Predominantly cortisols 71f
Pregnancy test 174
Premenopause 162
Primary hyperparathyroidism, clinical features of 59, 59b
Progesterone 7f, 145, 163t, 178
   preparations 163
Prolactin 14, 161
   inhibitory factor 14
Prolactinoma 15fc, 19
   surgery for 20
   treatment of 19, 20

Proliferative retinopathy 109
Propranolol 44
Propylthiouracil 41
Prostaglandin E1 185
Prosthesis 185f
Protein 106
   intake 106
Provocative test 89
Psammoma bodies 48
Pseudo-Cushing's syndrome 73fc
Pseudohypoparathyroidism 57, 58, 58f, 58t
   treatment of 58
Pseudopseudohypoparathyroidism 57, 58, 58t
   treatment of 58
Psychogenic disorders 183
Pubertal goiter 46
Pubertal growth spurt 147
Puberty, causes of delayed 148t
Pubic hair development 146f
   Tanner's grades of 146f, 146fc
Pyelonephritis 23

Q

Quinagolide 20
Quinestradiol 163

R

Radioablation 41, 42
Radionuclear scan 45
Rathke's pouch 13f
Red blood cell 96f
Regulate cell function 5f
Rehydration 60
Reifenstein syndrome 151
Renal artery 69f
   ligation 90
Renal failure 183
   advance 109
Renal osteodystrophy 63, 64fc
   development of 64
   prevention of 64
Renal tubular acidosis 80
Renin-angiotensin system 71
Reproductive medicine 153, 154
Reproductive organs 157
Reserpine 183
Respiratory disorders 25
Retrosternal goiter 30f
Rickets 63, 63fc, 63t
   causes of 63t
   prevention of 63
   treatment of 63
Risedronate 65
Rosewater syndrome 151
Saline, normal 84

S

Sarcoidosis 23
Satellite nodule 48

Scar tissue 162f
Sclerosis, multiple 23
Scopolamine 183
Scrotal cavity 156
Secrete epinephrine 70
Sedatives 183
Semen analysis 171
Seminiferous tubules 156
Sertoli cells 156
Serum
   alkaline phosphate high 63
   calcium 56, 63
      normal 54f
   parathyroid hormone 62f
   sodium 24
   testosterone 161
   thyroid hormone levels 31
Sex education 182f
Sex hormones, male 72
Sex phobia 181
Sexual desire, inhibited 181
Sexual dysfunction 181
Sexual failure 181, 182
Sexual problem 153, 180
Sexual response
   cycle 180
   phases of 180f
Sheehan's syndrome 21, 23
   cause of 21t
   symptoms of 21t
   treatment of 22
Short stature 61, 61f, 126, 135, 136
   causes of 126, 133t
   constitutional 135
   endocrine causes of 126
   nonendocrine causes of 135
   psychological 135, 136
Silicosis 61
Skeletal developmental defects 149
Skeletal disorders 135
Sleep disturbance 39
Small cell carcinoma 49f
Smooth muscle 155
Sodium, concentration of 71
Sodium-glucose cotransporter 111, 115, 117
Somatostatin analogs 18, 27
Somatotropinomas 137
Sotos syndrome 139
Sperm 156
   develops 156
   in semen analysis, types of 172f
Spermatic arteries, internal 156
Spermatogenesis 156
Spermatogonia 157f
Spermicide 179
Spindle carcinoma 49f
Spironolactone 183
Spontaneous hypercortisolemia 77f
Stereotactic radiosurgery 77
Sterilization 175
Steroid hormones 5
   types of 71f

Steroid production, types of 84*fc*
Stigmata 16
Stimulation test 8, 9*t*, 21, 26
Subarachnoid hemorrhage 25
Subcutaneous insulin infusion, continuous 112
Sulfonylurea 113, 114
Superinvolution 21
Suppression test 9, 9*t*
Supravalvular aortic stenosis 61, 61*f*
Sweetening agents 106
Syndrome of inappropriate antidiuresis 24, 25*t*
  cause of 25*t*
  hormone secretion 22
  management of 24
Systemic disorders 183

T

Tall stature 137
  causes of 137*t*
  constitutional 138*f*
  nonendocrine causes of 138
Target gland hormone deficiencies, replacement of 22
Tension ring 185*f*
Teratozoospermia 171
Teriparatide 65
Testicular arteries 156
Testicular failure 183
Testicular feminization syndrome 151, 152*f*, 159
Testis 151*f*, 156
  anatomy of 158*f*
  descent of 156
  examination of 168
  failure of descent of 169
Testosterone 3*f*, 146*f*
  deficiency 168
  resistance syndrome 125
Thiazide 61, 183
  diuretics 25
Thiazolidinediones 115, 116*t*
Thiocyanate 36
Thioridazine 183
Thioxanthene 183
Thyrocytes, single layer of 48
Thyroglossal cyst 30*f*
Thyroglossal duct 30*f*
Thyroid 40*f*, 49*f*
  aberrant 30*f*
  anaplastic carcinoma of 49
  arteries 28, 53
  deficiency 35
  disorders 31
  dysfunction, management of 44
  follicular carcinoma of 48, 49
  function test 31
  incidentaloma 50
  malignancy 46
  medullary carcinoma of 50
  nodule 46, 47*fc*
  papillary carcinoma of 47, 47*b*, 48, 48*b*
  physiology of 30
Thyroid gland 28, 29, 30*f*
  anatomy 29*f*
  anomalies of 30*f*
  arteries 29*f*
  developmental anomalies of 30
  disorders of 28
  embryology of 30
Thyroid hormone
  fraction of 44
  resulting, excess of 39
Thyroidectomy 41
Thyroiditis 45
  chronic 38
  subacute 41, 44
Thyroid-stimulating hormone 2, 3*f*, 8, 8*t*, 9, 14, 21, 31*f*, 32, 33, 35-38, 41, 44, 46, 62, 161
  deficiency 22
  suppression test 9
Thyromegaly 44
Thyrotoxic crisis 43, 43*t*
  management of 43
Thyrotoxicosis 39*t*
  control of 43
  signs of 39
  symptoms of 39
Thyrotropes 12*fc*
Thyrotropin-releasing hormone 30, 36, 37
Thyroxine 1, 2, 8*t*, 9, 31*f*
  therapy 48
Tissue, loss of functional 37
Toxic adenoma 41
Toxic multinodular goiters 39
Transdermal estradiol patches 164
Tricyclic antidepressant 183
Triglyceride 100
Trihexyphenidyl 183
Tri-iodothyronine 2, 9, 31*f*
Tuberculosis 61
Tuberculous endometriosis 162
Tuberculous meningitis 23
Tuner's syndrome, growth in 150*f*
Tunica albuginea 154, 156
Turner's syndrome 125, 148, 149*fc*, 150*f*
  baby, management of 149
Tyrosine kinase inhibitors 50

U

Ullrich–Turner's syndrome 148
Undescended testis 170
  classification of 169, 170*t*
Ureter, double 149
Urine
  osmolality 24
  specific gravity 23
  volume 23
Uterine 171
  cavity 162*f*, 176*f*
Uterus 154, 155
  anatomy of 155*f*
  missing 162*f*

V

Vagina 155, 161*f*, 179*f*
  anatomy 156*f*
  blind-ending 151*f*
  upper 155
Vaginal anomalies 157
Vaginal estrogen creams 163
Vaginal muscle, rhythmic contraction of 181
Vaginal wall 155
Vaginismus 181, 182
Vaginitis 163
Van Wyk–Grumbach syndrome 36, 148
Vascular disease 183
Vasopressin 25
  deficiency of 22*fc*
Venous drain 29
Venous sinusoidal disease 183
Vinblastine 25
Virilization 164, 164*t*, 171
  incomplete 171
Visual symptoms 35
Vitamin 106
  A intoxication 61
  D_2 57
Vitamin D 57*t*, 65, 66
  dependent rickets 64
  intoxication 61
  large doses of 64
  level 63
  resistant rickets 64, 64*fc*
  supplement 63
  therapy 57
Voltage-gated calcium channels get opened 93
Vulva 160

W

Waist-Hip ratio 108
Warning symptoms 121
Water deprivation test 24
Whipple triad of insulinoma 123*f*
Widen epiphyseal bone 63
Williams syndrome 61
Williams–Beuren syndrome 61, 61*f*

Z

Zoledronic acid 65
Zona
  fasciculata 69*f*, 71, 71*f*
  glomerulosa 69*f*, 71*f*
  reticularis 69*f*

EU GSPR Authorised Reprsentative
Logos Europe, 9 rue Nicolas Poussin
1700, La Rochelle, France
Phone: +33 (0) 6 67 93 73 78
E-mail: contact@logoseurope.eu

www.ingramcontent.com/pod-product-compliance
Ingram Content Group UK Ltd.
Pitfield, Milton Keynes, MK11 3LW, UK
UKHW050942270226
468476UK00005B/57